Herbal
Drug Technology

Herbal
Drug Technology

Neelesh Malviya PhD

Professor and Principal
Smriti College of Pharmaceutical Education
Indore, Madhya Pradesh

Sapna Malviya PhD

Professor and Head
Department of Pharmacy
Modern Institute of Pharmaceutical Sciences
Indore, Madhya Pradesh

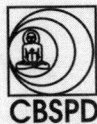

CBSPD

CBS Publishers & Distributors Pvt Ltd

New Delhi • Bengaluru • Chennai • Kochi • Kolkata • Lucknow • Mumbai
Hyderabad • Jharkhand • Nagpur • Patna • Pune • Uttarakhand

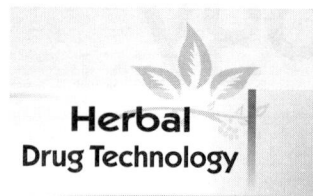

Herbal Drug Technology

ISBN: 978-93-87964-33-4

Copyright © Authors and Publisher

First Edition: 2019
   Reprint 2021, 2024

Published by Satish Kumar Jain and produced by Varun Jain for
CBS Publishers & Distributors Pvt Ltd
4819/XI Prahlad Street, 24 Ansari Road, Daryaganj, New Delhi 110 002, India
Ph: 011-23289259, 23266861, 23266867   Fax: 011-23243014
Website: www.cbspd.com   e-mail: delhi@cbspd.com; cbspubs@airtelmail.in

Corporate Office: 204 FIE, Industrial Area, Patparganj, Delhi 110 092, India
Ph: 011-49344934   Fax: 011-49344935   e-mail: publishing@cbspd.com; publicity@cbspd.com

Branches

- **Bengaluru:** Seema House 2975, 17th Cross, K.R. Road, Banasankari 2nd Stage, Bengaluru 560 070, Karnataka, India
  Ph: +91-80-26771678/79   Fax: +91-80-26771680   e-mail: bangalore@cbspd.com
- **Chennai:** 7, Subbaraya Street, Shenoy Nagar, Chennai 600 030, Tamil Nadu, India
  Ph: +91-44-26680620, 26681266   Fax: +91-44-42032115   e-mail: chennai@cbspd.com
- **Kochi:** 42/1325, 1326, Power House Road, Opposite KSEB, Power House, Ernakulum 682018, Kochi, Kerala, India
  Ph: +91-484-4059061–65, 67   Fax: +91-484-4059065   e-mail: kochi@cbspd.com
- **Kolkata:** 147, Hind Ceramics Compound, 1st Floor, Nilgunj Road, Belghoria, Kolkata 700056, West Bengal, India
  Ph: +91-33-25330055/56   e-mail: kolkata@cbspd.com
- **Lucknow:** Basement, Khushuma Complex, 7 Meerabai Marg (behind Jawahar Bhawan), Lucknow 226001, UP, India
  Ph: +91-522-4000032   e-mail: tiwari.lucknow@cbspd.com
- **Mumbai:** PWD Shed, Gala No. 25/26, Ramchandra Bhatt Marg, Next JJ Hospital Gate No. 2, Opp. Union Bank of India,
  Noorbaug, Mumbai 400009, Maharashtra, India
  Ph: +91-22-66661880/89   e-mail: mumbai@cbspd.com

Representatives

• **Hyderabad**	0-9885175004	• **Jharkhand**	0-9811541605	• **Nagpur**	0-9421945513
• **Patna**	0-9334159340	• **Pune**	0-9623451994	• **Uttarakhand**	0-9716462459

Printed at Glorious Printers, Delhi, India

This book is gratefully
dedicated to my
loving and caring
mother

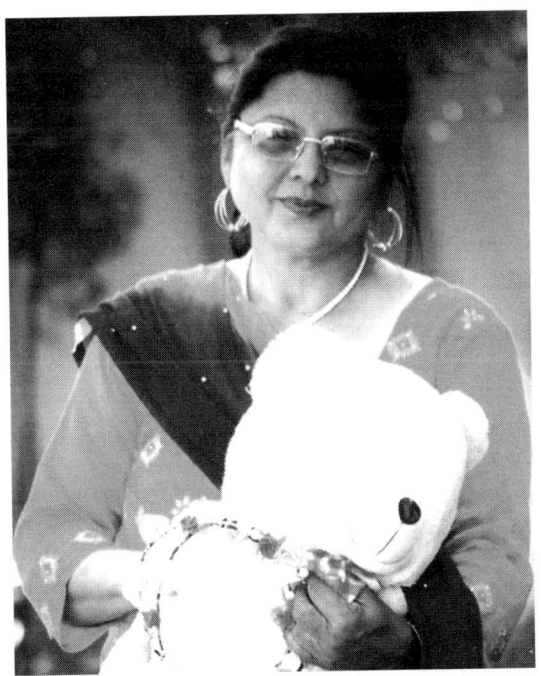

Mrs Nirmala Ashok Motwani

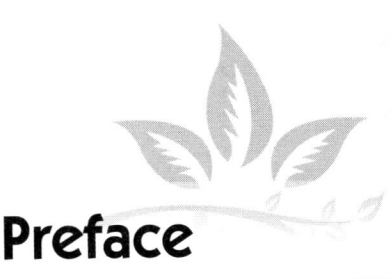

Preface

Herbal Drug Technology is the outcome of numerous efforts of the authors. We have given entire details, right from its impetus, the technology involved for applying herbs and its various benefits. The book accentuated on the technology and knowledge of traditional and modern pharmacognosy which can stand as a pilaster for all postgraduate and undergraduate students. This book furnished entire details on various evolving topics of herbal drug technology and highlighted its gravity.

Considering all comprehensive information of the subject, a textbook is enthralled to contribute indefatigable pronounce of pharmacognosy. This modern version of herbal drug technology emphasizes on herbs as raw materials, WHO guidelines for good agricultural practices in cultivation of medicinal plants, Indian systems of medicine, nutraceuticals, general introduction to herbaldrug and herb-food interactions and classification of herbal cosmetics, herbal excipients and various formulations containing herbs. The evolving topics included are evaluation of drugs, patenting and regulatory requirements of natural products and regulations in India (ASU DTAB, ASU DCC), regulation of manufacture of ASU drugs—Schedule Z of Drugs and Cosmetics Act for ASU drugs. The highlighted portion of the text focuses on general introduction to herbal industry and its present scope and future prospects. In addition, it includes Schedule T—good manufacturing practices of Indian systems of medicine.

The objective of the authors is fully achieved by systematic assemblage of the well-written chapters with neat and clean well-labelled diagram wherever necessary.

The authors convey deep sense of gratitude to their grandparents, parents and son to deeply motivating them to provide a kind of book required for undergraduate, postgraduate and researchers.

Doubtless authors are indebted to all who have supported in giving the present shape to the book.

Last but not the least authors express heartfelt gratitude towards Mr YN Arjuna for his support, guidance and cooperation to publish this book.

Suggestions and criticism will always be solicited by the authors to further improve the quality of book in real sense.

Neelesh Malviya
Sapna Malviya

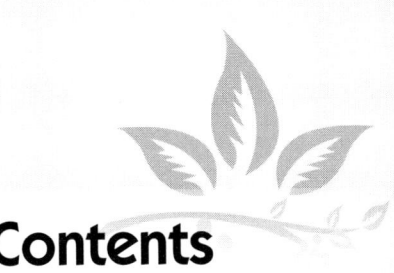

Contents

Fundamental Concepts of Herbs and its Production Ayurveda, Siddha, Unani and Homeopathy Systems of Medicine

☞ Herbs as Raw Materials

☞ Biodynamic Agriculture

☞ Indian Systems of Medicine

1 Herbs as Raw Materials

- Introduction
- Extraction and its quality assurance
- Identification and authentication of herbal materials
- Processing of herbal raw material
- Plant Metabolites
- Techniques for detection of phytochemical groups in extracts

INTRODUCTION

Nature always stands as a golden mark to symbolize the significant phenomenon of symbiosis. Natural products derived from various sources of plant, animal and minerals have been the basis of treatment of human disease.

The term **medicinal plant** includes various types of plants which contain substances that can be used for therapeutic purposes, or which are precursors for chemo-pharmaceutical semi-synthesis. These medicinal plants consider as a rich resources of ingredients which can be used in drug development and synthesis.

A plant is designated as 'medicinal' due to its use as a drug or therapeutic agent or an active ingredient of a medicinal preparation. Medicinal plants may be defined as a group of plants that possess some special properties or virtues that qualify them as articles of drugs and therapeutic agents and are used for medicinal purposes.

The term **herbal drugs** denotes plants or plant parts that have been converted into phytopharmaceuticals by means of simple processes involving harvesting, drying, and storage. Hence they are capable of variation. This variability is also caused by differences in growth, geographical location, and time of harvesting. Medical herbs and its application are shown in Fig. 1.1.

Several problems not applicable to synthetic drugs often influence the quality of herbal drugs. For instance:

- Herbal drugs are usually mixtures of many constituents.
- The active principle(s) is (are) in most cases unknown.
- Selective analytical methods or reference compounds may not be available commercially.

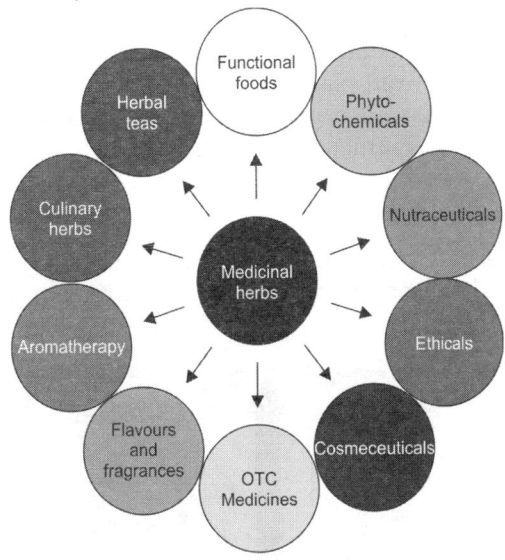

Fig. 1.1: Medicinal herbs and its application

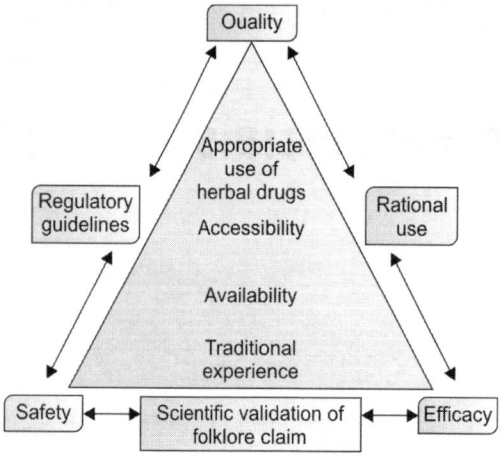

Fig. 1.2: Three pillars of herbal drugs and their rational use

- Plant materials are chemically and naturally variable.
- Chemo-varieties and chemo-cultivars exist.
- The source and quality of the raw material are variable.

Herbs

The term Herb is derived from the Latin word *herba* and old French word *herbe*. It refers to any part of plant like fruit, seed, stem, bark, leaf, flower and root as well as nonwoody plant. Otherwise stated, herbs are crude material derived from plant, fungi, algae and lichen roots, rhizomes or other plant parts, which may be entire fragmented or powdered.

Herbal Medicines

Herbal medicines, also called botanical medicine or phytomedicine, are the remedies and made from plants to prevent and treat an illness or to achieve good health. It includes herbs, herbal materials, herbal preparations and finished herbal products. Herbal medicines are accessible, affordable and safe. The global market of herbal medicines is increasing due to its assured benefits as shown in Fig. 1.3.

Herbal Materials

Herbal materials are either whole plants or parts of medicinal plants in the crude state which include herbs, fresh juices, gums, fixed oils, essential oils, resins and dry powders of herbs. These materials may be processed by various local procedures, such as steaming, roasting, or stir baking with honey, alcoholic beverages or other materials.

Herbal Preparations

Herbal preparations are the basis for finished herbal products and may include comminuted or powdered herbal materials, or extracts, tinctures and fatty oils, expressed juices and processed exudates of herbal materials. They are produced with the aid of extraction, distillation, expression, fractionation, purification, concentration, fermentation or other physical or biological processes. They also include preparations made by steeping or heating herbal materials in alcoholic beverages and/or honey, or in other materials. The classification and categorization of herbal medicine is illustrated in Figs 1.4 and 1.5.

EXTRACTION AND ITS QUALITY ASSURANCE

Extraction is the separation of medicinally active portions of plant (and animal) tissues using selective solvents through standard procedures. The extraction method separates the soluble plant metabolites (chemical constituents) and leave behind the insoluble cellular marc. The products obtained from plants are relatively complex mixtures of metabolites, in liquid or semisolid state or (after removing the solvent) in dry powder form, and are intended for oral or external use.

Galenicals (named after second century Greek physician Galen) include classes of preparations known as decoctions, infusions,

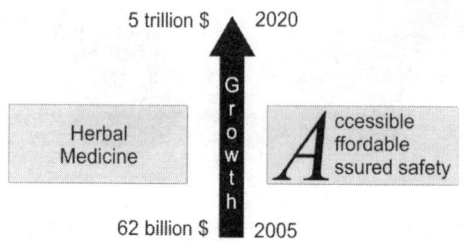

Fig. 1.3: Global market of herbal medicines

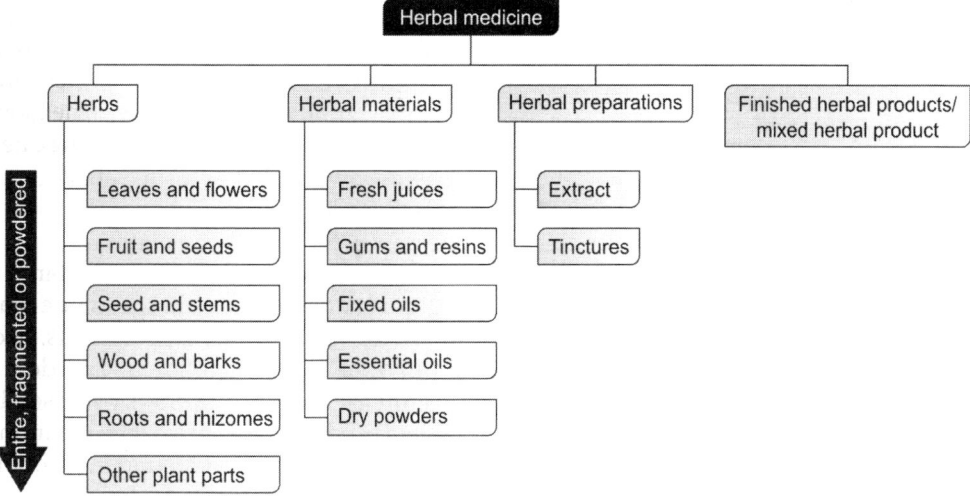

Fig. 1.4: Classification of herbal medicine

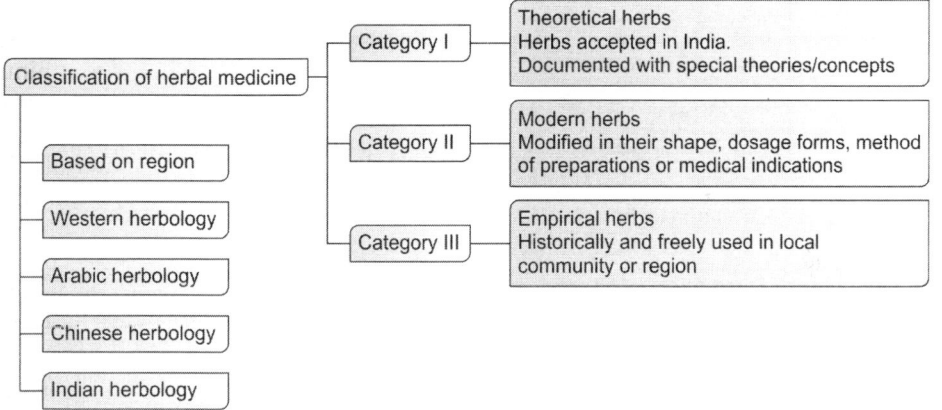

Fig. 1.5: Categorization of herbal medicine

fluid extracts, tinctures, semisolid extracts or powdered extracts.

The purpose of standardized extraction procedures for crude drugs (medicinal plant parts) is to attain the therapeutically desired portions and to eliminate unwanted material by treatment with a selective solvent known as menstruum. The extract thus obtained, after standardization, may be used as medicinal agent as such in the form of tinctures or fluid extracts or further processed to be incorporated in any dosage form such as tablets and capsules. These products all contain complex mixture of many medicinal plant metabolites, such as alkaloids, glycosides, terpenoids, flavonoids and lignans.

In order to be used as a modern drug, an extract may be further processed through various techniques of fractionation to isolate individual chemical entities such as vincristine, vinblastine, hyoscyamine, hyoscine, pilocarpine, forskolin and codeine.

The basic parameters influencing the quality of an extract are the plant parts used as starting material, the solvent used for extraction, the manufacturing process (extraction technology) used with the type of equipment employed, and the crude drug:extract ratio. From laboratory scale to pilot scale, all the conditions and parameters can be modelled using process simulation for successful industrial-scale production.

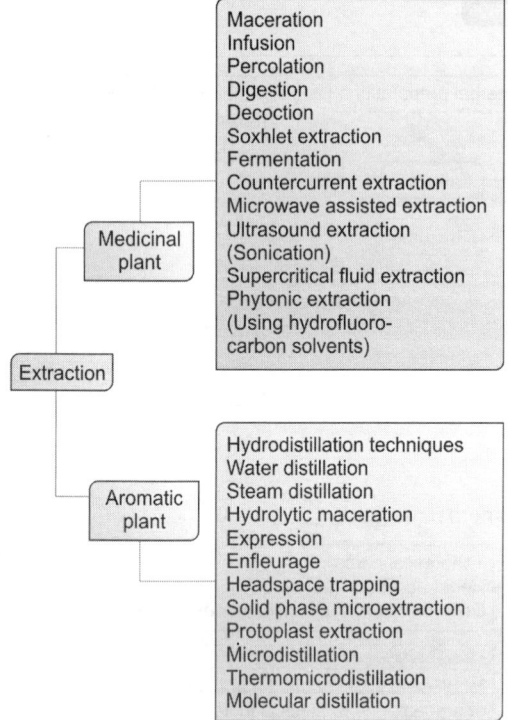

Fig. 1.6: Types of extraction techniques

General Methods of Extraction of Medicinal Plants

The methods of extraction of herbal medicinal plants are enlisted in Fig. 1.6.

Maceration

Maceration is a process in which powdered crude drug (whole or coarsely powdered) is placed with the solvent in a stoppered container and allowed to stand at room temperature for a period of at least 3 days with frequent agitation until the soluble matter has dissolved. The mixture then is strained, the marc (the damp solid material) is pressed, and the combined liquids are clarified by filtration or decantation after standing.

Percolation

It is the procedure used most frequently to extract active ingredients in the preparation of tinctures and fluid extracts.

A percolator is a narrow, cone-shaped vessel open at both ends. The powdered crude drug is moistened with an appropriate amount of the specified menstruum and allowed to stand for approximately 4 hours in a well-closed container, after which the mass is packed and the top of the percolator is closed. Additional menstruum is added to form a shallow layer above the mass, and the mixture is allowed to macerate in the closed percolator for 24 hours. The outlet of the percolator then is opened and the liquid contained therein is allowed to drip slowly. Additional menstruum is added as required, until the percolate measures about three-quarters of the required volume of the finished product. The marc is then pressed and the expressed liquid is added to the percolate. Sufficient menstruum is added to produce the required volume, and the mixed liquid is clarified by filtration or by standing followed by decanting.

Infusion

Fresh infusions are prepared by macerating the crude drug for a short period of time with cold or boiling water. These are dilute solutions of the readily soluble constituents of crude drugs.

The general principles and mechanisms involved in maceration, percolation and infusion for the extraction of the crude drugs are generally referred to as leaching. The processes of leaching may involve simple physical solution or dissolution.

The extraction procedures are affected by various factors, namely

1. Rate of transport of solvent into the mass
2. Rate of solubilization of the soluble constituents by the solvent and
3. Rate of transport of solution out of the insoluble material.

The extraction of crude drugs is mostly favoured by increasing the surface area of the material to be extracted and decreasing the radial distances traversed between the solids (crude drug particle). Mass transfer theory states that the maximum surface area is obtained by size reductions which entail reduction of material into individual cells. However, this is not possible or desirable in many cases of vegetable material.

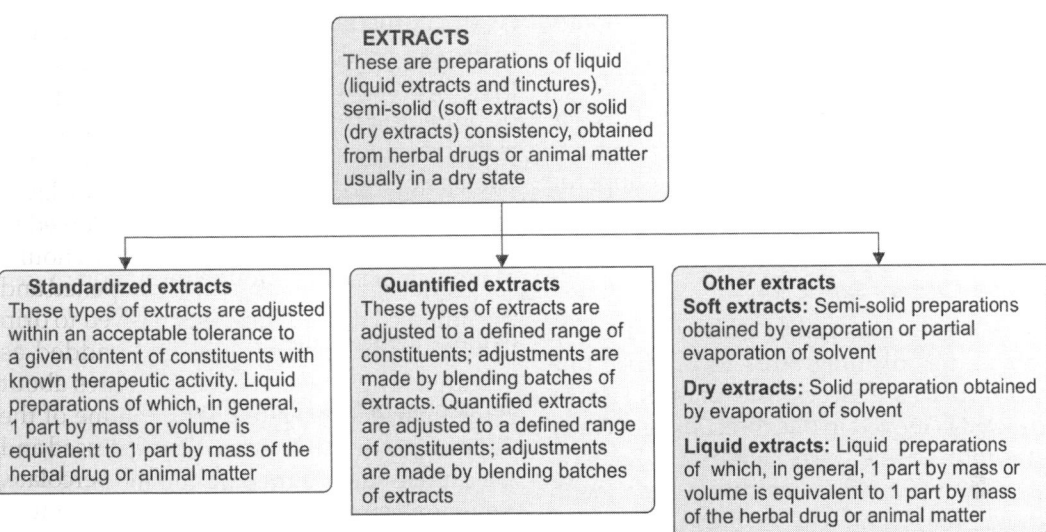

Fig. 1.7: Extracts and its types

Digestion

Digestion is a form of maceration used when moderately elevated temperature is not objectionable. It is done with gentle heating during the process of extraction. The solvent efficiency of the menstruum is thereby increased.

Decoction

Decoction is suitable for extracting water-soluble, heat-stable constituents. The crude drug is boiled in a specified volume of water for a defined time; it is then cooled and strained or filtered. This process is used for preparation of Ayurvedic extracts called 'quath' or 'kawath'.

The procedure for preparation includes starting ratio of crude drug to water is fixed, e.g. 1:4 or 1:16; the volume is then brought down to one-fourth its original volume by boiling during the extraction procedure. Then, the concentrated extract is filtered and used as such or processed further.

Hot Continuous Extraction (Soxhlet)

In this method, the finely ground crude drug is placed in a porous bag or 'thimble' made of strong filter paper, which is placed in chamber of the Soxhlet apparatus. The extracting solvent in flask is heated, and its vapors condense in condenser. The condensed extract drips into the thimble containing the crude drug, and extracts it by contact. When the level of liquid in chamber rises to the top of siphon tube, the liquid contents of chamber siphon into flask.

This process is continuous and is carried out until a drop of solvent from the siphon tube does not leave residue when evaporated.

The advantage is that large amounts of drug can be extracted with a much smaller quantity of solvent. This effects tremendous economy in terms of time, energy and consequently financial inputs. At small scale, it is employed as a batch process only, but it becomes much more economical and viable when converted into a continuous extraction procedure on medium or large scale.

Aqueous Alcoholic Extraction By Fermentation

The extraction procedure involves soaking the crude drug, in the form of either a powder or a decoction (kasaya), for a specified period of time, during which it undergoes fermentation and generates alcohol *in situ*; this facilitates the extraction of the active constituents contained in the plant material. The alcohol thus generated also serves as a preservative. If the fermentation is to be carried out in an earthen vessel, it should not be new: Water should first be boiled in the vessel. In large-scale manufacture, wooden vats, porcelain jars or metal vessels are used in place of earthen vessels. Some examples of such preparations are karpurasava, kanakasava, dasmularista. Some medicinal preparations of Ayurveda (like asava and arista) adopt the technique of fermentation for extracting the active principles.

Counter-Current Extraction

The wet raw material is pulverized using toothed disc disintegrators to produce fine slurry. In this process, the material to be extracted is moved in one direction (generally in the form of fine slurry) within a cylindrical extractor where it comes in contact with extraction solvent. The further the starting material moves, the more concentrated the extract becomes. Complete extraction is thus possible when the quantities of solvent and material and their flow rates are optimized. The process is highly efficient, requiring little time and posing no risk from high temperature. Finally, sufficiently concentrated extract comes out at one end of the extractor while the marc (practically free of visible solvent) falls out from the other end.

This extraction process has significant advantages:

  i. A unit quantity of the plant material can be extracted with much smaller volume of solvent as compared to other methods like maceration, decoction, percolation.
 ii. CCE is commonly done at room temperature, which spares the thermolabile constituents from exposure to heat which is employed in most other techniques.
iii. As the pulverization of the drug is done under wet conditions, the heat generated during comminution is neutralized by water. This again spares the thermolabile constituents from exposure to heat.
 iv. The extraction procedure has been rated to be more efficient and effective than continuous hot extraction.

Ultrasound Extraction (Sonication)

The procedure involves the use of ultrasound with frequencies ranging from 20 kHz to 2000 kHz; this increases the permeability of cell walls and produces cavitation. Although the process is useful in some cases, like extraction of rauwolfia root, its large-scale application is limited due to the higher costs. One disadvantage of the procedure is the occasional but known deleterious effect of ultrasound energy (more than 20 kHz) on the active constituents of medicinal plants through formation of free radicals and consequently undesirable changes in the drug molecules.

Supercritical Fluid Extraction

Supercritical fluid extraction (SFE) is an alternative sample preparation method with general goals of reduced use of organic solvents and increased sample throughput. The factors to consider include temperature, pressure, sample volume, analyte collection, modifier (cosolvent) addition, flow and pressure control, and restrictors. Generally, cylindrical extraction vessels are used for SFE and their performance is good beyond any doubt. The collection of the extracted analyte following SFE is another important step: significant analyte loss can occur during this step, leading the analyst to believe that the actual efficiency was poor. There are many advantages to the use of CO_2 as the extracting fluid. In addition to its favourable physical properties, carbon dioxide is inexpensive, safe and abundant. But while carbon dioxide is the preferred fluid for SFE, it possesses several polarity limitations. Solvent polarity is important when extracting polar solutes and when strong analyte-matrix interactions are present. Organic solvents are frequently added to the carbon dioxide extracting fluid to alleviate the polarity limitations. Of late, instead of carbon dioxide, argon is being used because it is inexpensive and more inert. The component recovery rates generally increase with increasing pressure or temperature: The highest recovery rates in case of argon are obtained at 500 atm and 150°C. The extraction procedure possesses distinct advantages:

  i. The extraction of constituents at low temperature, which strictly avoids damage from heat and some organic solvents.

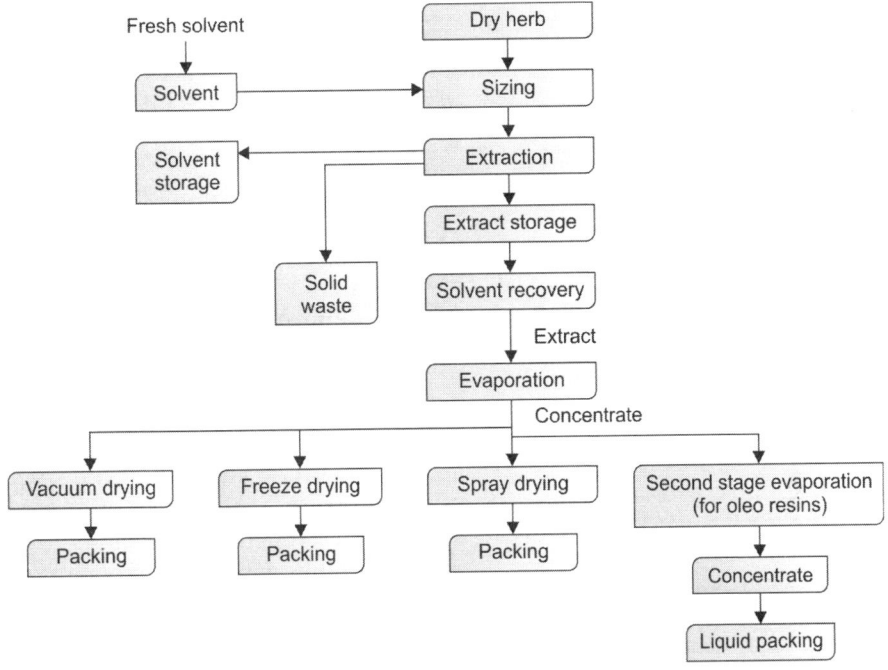

Fig. 1.8: Extraction of herbal drugs

ii. No solvent residues.

iii. Environmentally friendly extraction procedure.

The largest area of growth in the development of SFE has been the rapid expansion of its applications. SFE finds extensive application in the extraction of pesticides, environmental samples, foods and fragrances, essential oils, polymers and natural products. The major disadvantage in the commercial application of the extraction process is its prohibitive capital investment.

Phytonics Process

A new technology to optimize its remarkable properties in the extraction of plant materials offer significant environmental advantages and health and safety benefits over traditional processes for the production of high quality natural fragrant oils, flavours and biological extracts. Advanced Phytonics Limited has developed this patented technology termed 'phytonics process'. The products mostly extracted by this process are fragrant components of essential oils and biological or phytopharmacological extracts which can be used directly without further physical or chemical treatment.

Quality Assurance: The Extraction Process and Solvent

The type of extraction procedure also plays a decisive role in determining the qualitative and quantitative composition of the extract.

The extraction of herbal drugs is illustrated in Fig.1.8 and factors affecting extraction are shown in Fig 1.9.

Some important points regarding the quality of the extracts need to be considered:

i. The more exhaustive the extraction, the better is the yield of the constituents from the herbal drugs.

ii. If maceration is facilitated by stirring and by use of comminuted material, the additional stirring and shearing forces may lead to better extraction.

iii. Other factors determining the quality of the extracts are extraction time, temperature and solvent volume.

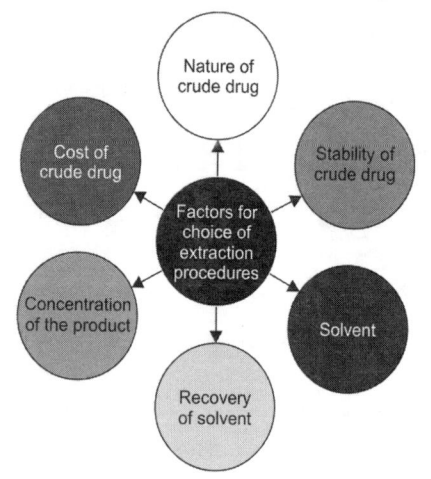

Fig. 1.9: Factors affecting choice of extraction procedures

v. The quality of the extracts and the spectrum of constituents obtained by maceration or digestion (i.e. maceration at higher temperature) are also influenced by the ratio of herbal drug to solvent. The quantity of extracted matter increases with the volume of extraction solvent. For example, maceration of *Salvia officinalis* flowers achieves almost exhaustive extraction and thus the full spectrum of constituents obtained with percolation can be achieved with a drug: solvent ratio of 1:20.

vi. The composition of an herbal extract depends on the type, concentration and elution strength of the solvent. The spectrum of constituents may vary considerably depending on the hydrophilic or lipophilic nature of the solvent.

Finished Herbal Products

Finished herbal products consist of herbal preparations made from one or more herbs. If more than one herb is used, the term mixed herbal product can also be used. Finished herbal products and *mixed herbal products* may contain excipients in addition to the active ingredients. Generally, however, finished products or mixed products to which chemically defined active substances have been added, including synthetic compounds and/or isolated constituents from herbal materials, are not considered to be herbal.

Herbal products and their applications are illustrated in Fig 1.11.

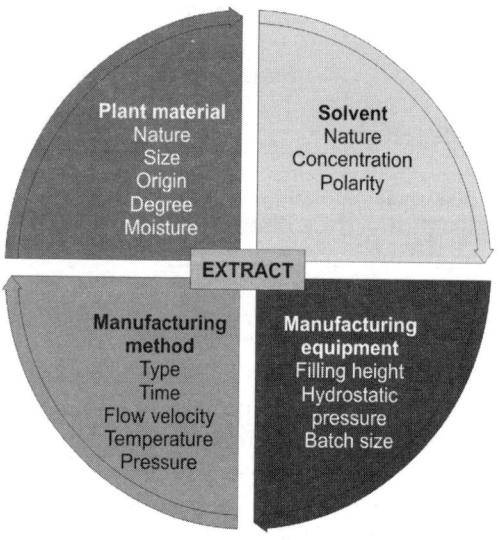

Fig. 1.10: Extract and factors affecting procedures

iv. Some drugs (e.g. *Hypericum spp.*) are extracted very slowly so that exhaustive extraction can only be achieved by percolation or multistage motion extraction. In many cases, the transfer of quality-relevant constituents from the herbal drugs to the extract (i.e. extraction rate) can be considerably improved by raising the temperature. Hypericin, pseudohypericin and biapigenin are extracted better at higher temperature and with longer extraction times.

IDENTIFICATION AND AUTHENTICATION OF HERBAL MATERIALS

The specifications for herbal starting materials, for herbal preparations and finished herbal products are primarily intended to define the quality rather than to establish full characterization, and should focus on those characteristics found to be useful in ensuring safety and efficacy. Consistent quality for herbal medicines (finished herbal products) can only be assured if the starting herbal materials are defined in a rigorous and detailed manner.

The methods of harvesting, drying, storage, transportation, and processing (for example, mode of extraction and polarity of the extracting solvent, instability of constituents, etc.) also affect herbal quality.

The matter of proper identification and appropriate quality—that is, lack of adulteration, sophistication, or substitution—is an extremely important one in the field of herbal medicine.

Also of great importance to the quality of an herb is the environmental conditions under which it is grown. Fertility of the soil, length of growing season, temperature, amount of moisture, and time of harvest are some of the significant factors.

1. In some cases more detailed information may be needed on aspects of collection or agricultural production. For instance, the selection of seeds, conditions of cultivation and harvesting are important aspects in producing a reproducible quality of herbal medicines. Their characterization (which also includes a detailed evaluation of the botanical and phytochemical aspects of the medicinal plant, manufacture of the herbal preparation and the finished herbal product) is therefore essential to allow the establishment of specifications which are both comprehensive and relevant.

2. Herbal materials
   ➲ The family and botanical name of the plant used according to the binomial system (genus, species, variety and the authority, i.e. the reference to the originator of the classification, e.g. Linnaeus). It may also be appropriate to add the vernacular name and the therapeutic use in the country or region of origin of the plant.
   ➲ Details of the source of the plant, such as country and/or region (also state and province, if applicable) of origin, whether it was cultivated or WHO GMP: Updated supplementary guidelines for the manufacture of herbal medicines collected from the wild and, where applicable, method of cultivation, dates and conditions of harvesting (e.g. whether there was extreme weather), collection procedures, collection area, and brand, quantity and date of pesticide

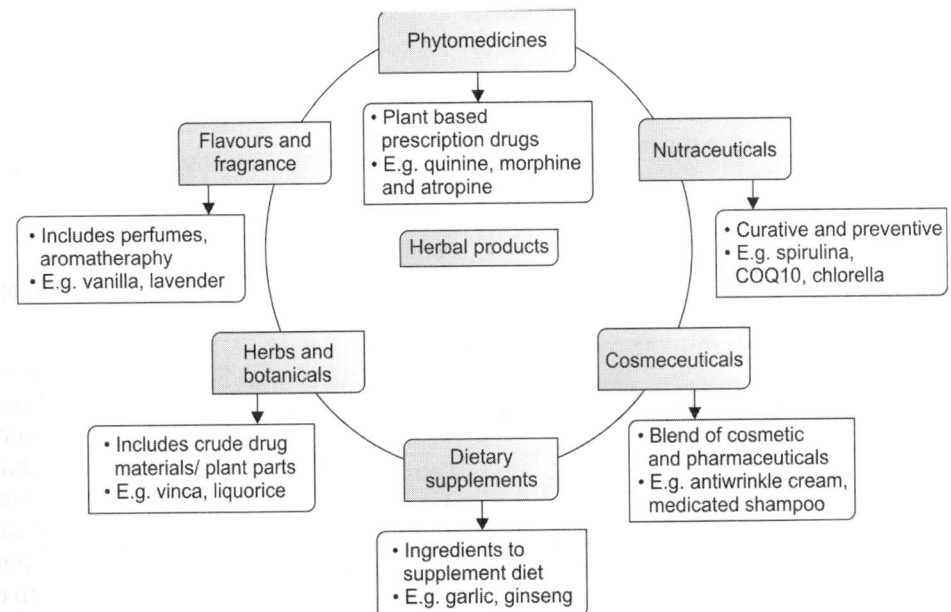

Fig. 1.11: Herbal products and their applications

application, as required by the WHO guideline on good agricultural and collection practices.

➲ Whether the whole plant or only a part is used. In the latter case, which part of the plant is used and its state, e.g. whole or reduced. For dried plant material, the drying system should be specified, if applicable.

➲ A description of the plant material based on visual (macroscopic) and/or micro-scopic examination.

➲ Suitable identity tests including, where appropriate, identification tests (such as TLC or other chromatographic finger-print) for known active ingredients or markers. A reference sample should be available for identification purposes.

➲ Details of the assay, where appropriate, of active constituents or markers. Limit tests such as dry residue of liquids, ash value (total ash, and ash insoluble in hydrochloric acid), water-soluble extractives, moisture/water content and loss on drying (taking into account the presence of essential oils, if any).

➲ Suitable methods for the determination of possible pesticide contamination and the acceptable limits for such contam-ination in herbal materials or herbal preparations used in the manufacture of herbal medicines.

➲ Tests for toxic metals and for likely contaminants, foreign materials and adulterants.

➲ Tests for fungal and/or microbiological contamination, fumigant residues (if applicable), mycotoxins, pest-infesta-tions, radioactivity and their acceptable limits.

➲ Other appropriate tests (e.g. particle size, swelling index and residual solvents in herbal preparations and biological fingerprints such as induced fluorescent markers).

➲ Uniformity of weight (e.g. for tablets, single-dose powders, suppositories,

capsules and herbal tea in sachets), disintegration time (for tablets, capsules, suppositories and pills), hardness and friability (for uncoated tablets), viscosity (for internal and external fluids), consis-tency (semisolid preparations), and dissolution (tablets or capsules), if applicable. Physical appearance such as colour, odour, form, shape, size and texture. Loss on drying, or water content.

➲ Identity tests, qualitative determination of relevant substances of the plants (e.g. fingerprint chromatograms).

➲ Quantification of relevant active ingre-dients, if they have been identified, and the analytical methods that are available.

➲ Limit tests for residual solvents.

Herbarium

A herbarium is a pressed collection or deposi-tory of dried plants specimens. The herbarium clearly displays the characteristic parts of each plant and is labeled with scientific and common names. An accompanying description of the species form, habitat and location allows for comparison of the herbarium specimen with plants found in the field. A herbarium is an invaluable reference for new volunteers and group members to identify species they find. Proper identification ensures that only the target weeds are removed. Creating a herbarium can also give the group a greater understanding and appreciation of the floral diversity that exists in your patch. Well-pressed herbariums create an important scientific record for flora at your patch. Herbarium specimens are carefully documented, well-preserved plant specimens. They consist of well-laid out, dried plant material that is attached, together with a label, to a sheet of paper.

Searching For Plants

Almost all natural environments are suitable for searching for plants for the herbarium, so you must not overlook places which could appear sterile and dry. Even in the cities it is possible to look for plants, just do not take specimens from the parks and gardens. At first you could rely on the richness of the flowers and plants which live on grasslands and prairies, but you will soon notice how easy it is to find interesting specimens during trips to the mountains, swamps, coast, woods or wherever the climate and the temperature are not too extreme for plant survival.

The most important part of every collected specimen is the flower, so the best seasons for picking up plants are spring and summer; but remember that certain species show their flowers in autumn or even winter, so do not neglect colder months for your excursions. As you can read in the books, a few plants have a very short blooming time, which you must strive to catch them at!

The most convenient specimens to pick up are those which seem quite dry, and lacking any trace of surface moisture. For that reason it is better not to look for plants during rainy days, or early in the morning. Also, the hottest hours during summer days should be avoided, as plants will not show their freshest appearance.

- How to learn to identify plants
- Get a good picture book of the plants in your area, preferably one that sorts the pictures by colour and flower shape. When you have identified your plant, read all about it.
- Watch out for wild flower hikes, possibly sponsored by your state's Native Plant Society, the Audubon Society, or local naturalists club.
- If there is a Forest Service, Park Service, or Bureau of Land Management office in your vicinity, ask the folks there about groups, opportunities, and books.
- Ask for advice at your nearest herbarium; these are often located in colleges, universities, or natural history museums.
- Check your local library for books about plants.
- Take a college course in plant taxonomy or systematic.
- See what you can find on the Web.
- PRACTICE! Study plants; then study more plants.

Essential Tools and Equipment

1. **Digger (trowel or pick):** In the field, digger is needed for digging roots.
2. **Secateur:** Secateur is required for cutting twigs of trees and shrubs for herbarium specimens.
3. **Vasculum:** Vasculum is a container made up of tin or aluminium sheet. It is somewhat oval on end and usually 45 to 60 cm long. The collected specimens are carried in a box called vasculum to avoid loss of moisture and distortions by drying and shrivelling up.
4. **Covering bags/packets:** Some material requires special preservation. Cones are placed, with their label, in plastic bags. Bryophytes are dried and stored in paper packets. Fungi are stored, after being completely dried, in plastic bags and boxes. Fleshy fruits may be stored, with their label, in alcohol or other preservatives. But for most plants, and most purposes, the combination of pressing, drying, and gluing to paperworks just fine. Although simple the technique is effective: Specimens made over 500 years ago are still being studied.
5. **Field notebook:** Taxonomy students carry a field notebook for recording every detail rather than depending upon the memory. These notes not only will help the identification of the specimens, but also can be compared and added to the current botanical knowledge. The herbarium could encourage the collection of many written data which can actually increase the botanical knowledge of certain geographical areas. This is a list of what you could record to add many valuable information to your herbarium:
   - *Name of locality and exact location:* Be precise, if possible include the longitude and latitude
   - Local name of plant, if any
   - *Habitat and ecology:* Vegetation type, associations with other plants. Plant habit: Describe the overall size and shape of the plant (tree, bush, epiphyte, etc.)

➢ *Stems and trunks:* Height and diameter; colour, texture, thickness and hardness; the presence of thorns and spines

➢ *Leaves:* Deciduous or evergreen; colour, texture and overall aspect; orientation; exudate or glands

➢ *Inflorescence and flowers:* Note of everything that could be undetected in prepared specimens; colour; hetero-stylous, monoecious or dioecious; different behaviour (open/closed).

➢ *Fruits and seeds:* Size, shape, colour, texture; smell

➢ *Underground organs:* Take some samples or describe them (size and shape, tap root, tubers, bulb etc.)

➢ Record any particular scent, especially of cut parts and flowers.

➢ *Sap or latex:* Note the colour, smell, consistency, etc.

➢ *Name:* Record the locally used name(s)

➢ Date of collection

➢ Soil characteristics

➢ Botanical name (if known)

➢ Field number of specimen

6. **Portable plant press:** This is equipment by means of which fresh specimens are pressed flat, without folds and become quickly dried. The collected specimens should be put into a strong bag made of cloth or polythene or similar material (plastic, etc.), the function of these containers being to protect plants from damage during your outing. If time of collection is in summer time or lasts for two or more days, it is better to bring a folder of approximately 45 × 30 cm or more. The folder must be made of cardboard or some other strong stuff, e.g. aluminium, and it must contain some old newspapers. The folder can be covered with cloth and it should be closed with straps or belts, and a handle or shoul-der-belt should be added for easy carrying. The picked specimens must be arranged inside the folder between a few layers of paper, so that every plant has some paper on both sides. The closed folder does not have to press the specimens too firmly

between the newspapers. Blotting paper can be used instead of newspapers, but the latter is much cheaper, as you do not have to buy it just for the purpose of the herbarium.

Taking Pictures

Taking colour pictures of each plant in its natural environment is also something which could substantially enrich the quality of your herbarium, not only aesthetically, but also from the scientific point of view. In that way the dried specimen can be placed together with one or more photographs, which are very helpful for bulky plants like trees or bushes, which obviously cannot be entirely included in a herbarium! Also the habitat of a plant can be well described with a photograph, taking care not to be too distant from the nearby bushes or trees.

Collection of Plant Specimens

The following thing should be kept in mind while collecting plant specimens for making herbarium:

1. The plant specimen should be either in flowering or fruiting condition, preferably both.

2. Herbaceous plants should be collected with underground parts as far as possible.

3. In case of woody plant a twig of about 25 cm will form a good specimen. Its help in comprehension of phyllotaxy and inflo-rescence of plant.

4. It is always good to collect at least four specimens of each plant.

Making Herbarium Specimens

A. **Pressing of specimens:**

1. The specimen should be carefully displayed on the pressing sheet (blotters or new print sheet).

2. The larger specimens which cannot fit easily on the sheet should be bent into V, N or W shape.

3. In case of aquatic plants on the sheet when they are removed from water, they should be taken on unprinted news sheet floated on the water and such

sheet with specimen should be placed in the pressing sheet.

B. **Drying of specimens:** For drying, the press containing specimens is placed in the sun. The press is opened after 24 hours, the specimens are rearranged, placed between the fresh blotters and then again tightly bound in the press. The wet blotters removed should be dried usually by placing them in the sun.

Mounting of Specimen

There are different ways to mount the specimens to the herbarium sheets:

Strapping: This method will let you to remove and examine the specimen every time is needed, but will allow a certain degree of movement which can cause some trouble. The specimens can be strapped with linen or cotton thread that will be knotted on the reverse side of the sheet, where it is better to add some gummed paper to avoid contact with underlying specimens.

Gluing: Glue is chosen to mount the specimens, should be water-based woodworking adhesive or library pastes or latex adhesive, which must be applied quickly, taking care of not using an excessive amount. Glued material should then be left under pressure overnight, covering each sheet with waxed paper and with drying paper. With aquatic plants only latex glue is the right solution for gluing the specimens, as these plants can take up water from the glue.

Pins: Some herbaria have their specimens mounted using small paper bands which fix the plant to the sheet with the help of pins. The strip is placed on the stem and the pin joins together the mounting sheet, the stem and the strip, passing below the specimen. For the preservation of herbarium sheet for long period after the mounting of plant, it is treated with $CuSO_4$ or mercuric chloride.

Labelling of Specimens

After mounting the specimen, a label is glued on the lower right hand corner of the sheet. The label provides information taken from the field notebook. The label should include at least the following data (Table 1.1):

1. A label heading indicating the name of institution with which specimen originated and the region of collection.
2. The name of family
3. The botanical name of the plant with authority
4. The locality of collection
5. The date of collection
6. The habitat
7. The field notes
8. The name of the collector
9. The collectors field number
10. The vernacular name and local uses, if any

Table 1.1: Protocol for herbarium preparation	
	Details of herbarium:
	Department of botany:
	Field number:
Specimen	Specimen name:
Photographs	Common name:
	Place of collection:
	Month and time of collection:
	Description of specimen:
Specimen name	Specimen collected by:
	Date of collection:
Taxonomical classification	Herbarium prepared by:
• Kingdom	Herbarium authenticated by:
• Division	
• Class	
• Order	
• Family	
• Genus	
• Species	

PROCESSING OF HERBAL RAW MATERIAL

Processing plays a role due to constituents of herbal raw materials, some of them are heat labile, need to be dried at low temperatures. While others are destroyed by enzymatic processes that continue for long periods of time, herb is dried too slowly. The most effective way to ensure herbal quality is to assay—that is, to establish by some means—the amount of active constituents in the plant material. If the chemical identity of the constituent is known, or a marker compound indicative of the activity of the herb can usually be isolated and quantified by appropriate physical or chemical methods. If it is unknown, if it is a complex mixture of constituents, or if no marker compound is available, biological assays such as that employed for digitalis must be utilized, at least initially. Once the potency of the herb is known, it can be mixed with appropriate quantities of material of greater or lesser potency to produce a product with defined activity. In terms of quality, the more expensive the plant material is, the more likely it is to be inferior. Finely powdered herbs or dosage forms such as tablets or capsules made from them are particularly susceptible to fraud by adulteration or substitution. The processing of herbal raw material is shown in Fig. 1.12.

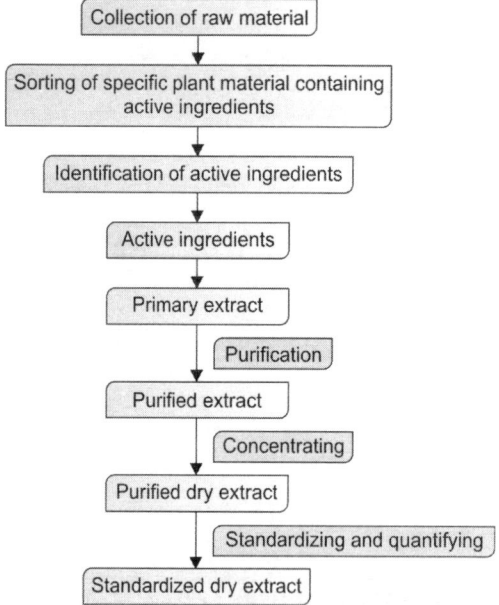

Fig. 1.12: Processing of herbal raw material

1. **Sorting and milling of crude herbs:** Sort all the herbs individually for any foreign matter. Mill these herbs separately using suitable mill. Herbs should be reduced to around mesh sieve.

2. **Steam distillation and decoction for volatile constituents and extraction of crude herbs:** Take specified quantity of milled crude herb powder in steam distillation

unit containing demineralised water or a specific solvent in 1:6 to 1:10 (depending on the nature of material) proportion. Steam distil volatile constituents if present (it may be noted that volatile constituent separation is possible only in case of aqueous extraction). Collect the distillate in a stainless steel container and close it tightly. Separate the liquid from slurry used for steam distillation and transfer to a suitable steam jacketed SS tank. Start steam spraying and circulation of the decoction. During this process samples of decoction are taken out at regular intervals to check the concentration of the extract in water (solvent). When the concentration level remains unchanged (less than 0.1% w/v), transfer the solution to a storage vessel after filtration (filter press/nylon cloth/sieve/centrifuge). Repeat the entire process if required (this stage is for syrup/liquid preparations) with another specific solvent.

3. **Settlement of filtered solution:** The filtrated solution from the above stage is allowed to stand between 12 and 18 hours for settlement of suspended particles if any at the bottom. Decant the supernatant liquid and send it for concentration.

4. **Concentration of extract:** Concentration is done in close distribution unit or open evaporating pan. In close distillation unit it is to be done under vacuum till honey like thick paste is obtained (similarly in open pan) with recovered solvent. In certain selected cases, this is achieved with help of specially designed evaporators also.

5. **Drying of the extract:** The concentrate obtained in stage (4) is dried in a vacuum tray dryer at 60°C with 30 mm pressure or spray dried.

6. **Pulverization of dry extract:** The extract obtained in stage (5) is pulverized in suitable mill to get 40/60 mesh powder (Temp. NMT 25°C/RH NMT 45%).

7. **Storage of extract:** Store the powder/liquid extract with appropriate preservatives (0.25% w/w Na. methyl

paraben for liquid and 0.02% w/w bromidiol for powder) in a cool dry place away from light at a temperature of NMT 25°C and RH NMT 45% (powder only).

Natural products played a vital role in improving the human health and due to their safety and efficacy these products are drugs of choice despite facing a tough competition from compounds obtained by chemical procedures. The most striking feature of natural products in connection to their long-lasting importance in drug discovery is their structural diversity that is still largely untapped. In recent decades development of science and technology is able to produce high-quality herbal medicines. The public of developed countries accepts of herbal medicine as a natural and gentle alternative to synthetic drugs and, from a global perspective, unit sales of herbal medicines are constantly growing.

A comprehensive approach to these problems, the state of the field of medicinal plants and herbal remedies, can be repaired. A better education of people is involved in the collection and cultivation of medicinal plants on the necessity of obtaining plant raw material of high quality. In particular, it should encourage the concept of organic production herbal products. Producers should be required to produce only quality-assured medicines. Improved harmonization of regulatory classification of herbal preparations in the world would inevitably lead to greater transparency and consistency of the market.

Quality control of the phytoproducts for human consumption and world market can be ensured by maintaining the quality of raw material adequacy of processing technology and quality of the finished products. Thus, the quality concept commences right from the choice of authentic and improved seeds (varieties) to the post harvest treatment of the raw material and to the process control for avoiding contamination. As such for developing phytoproducts, WHO's Good Manufacturing Practice (GMP) must be followed to satisfy the ISO 9000 certification. Recently, ISO 14000 certification has also become necessary to safeguard the environment. This means certifying that the product has been developed without inflicting ecological damage whatsoever.

GAP: Good Agro technological Practices. Large cultivation of medicinal plants relies upon strong and continuing research. Plant varieties with an abundance of desired constituents can be reproduced and improved upon under cultivation even in an entirely different area. For example, cultivation of American ginseng (*Panax quinquefolia*) in China. Attempt should be made to select appropriate region based on similar ecological conditions to introduce good cultivated variety, improve yield of the desired secondary metabolite and reduce the undesirable constituents.

Non-polluted cultivation: In order to protect the environment, to sustainably utilise the resources and to get a good quality of crude drug, non-polluted agrotechnology is rapidly

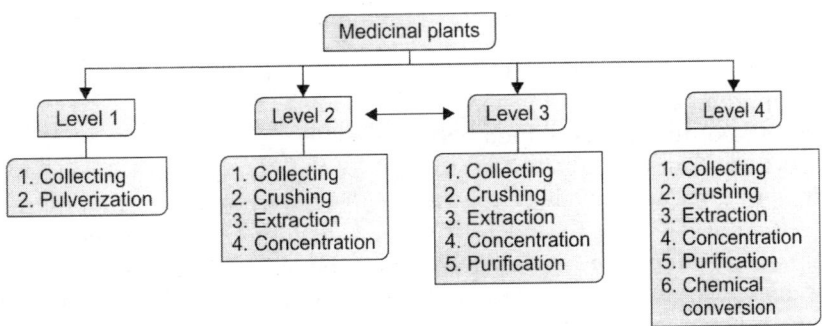

Fig. 1.13: Processing of medicinal plants

developed in recent years. These products are commonly called 'green crude drugs'. This involves biological control of insects and pathogens and use of botanical pesticides for the control of pest and diseases.

Postharvest technology: Right time harvesting, good processing, good storage, extraction or distillation, quality control.

PLANT METABOLITES

Plant metabolites are chemical compounds that are necessary for their basic functions, i.e. biochemical pathways for survival and propagation. Basic or primary metabolism refers to all biochemical processes for the normal anabolic and catabolic pathways which result in assimilation, respiration, transport, and differentiation, while secondary metabolisms generate diverse and seemingly less essential or non-essential byproducts. These secondary products give the colours, flavours, and smells to the plant. Plant metabolites of medicinal importance form an extensively diverse group of chemical compounds showing greater variation in solubility and stability. They can be broadly classified as follows:

1. Fixed oils, fats and waxes (lipids)
2. Phenols
3. Tannins
4. Proteins
5. Alkaloids
6. Carbohydrates
7. Glycosides
8. Volatile oils, and
9. Resins and resin combinations

Primary metabolites consist of many different types of organic compounds, including carbohydrates, lipids, proteins, and nucleic acids. They are available universally in the plant kingdom as they are the components or products of fundamental metabolic pathways or cycles such as glycolysis, the Krebs cycle, and the Calvin cycle. They are responsible for normal growth and reproduction of plants. Examples include energy rich fuel molecules, such as sucrose and starch, structural components such as cellulose, informational molecules such as DNA

(deoxyribonucleic acid) and RNA (ribonucleic acid), and pigments, such as chlorophyll.

In addition to having fundamental roles in plant growth and development, some of the primary metabolites are precursors (starting materials) for the synthesis of secondary metabolites.

Secondary metabolites mainly consist of three classes of compounds: Alkaloids, terpenoids, and phenolics. However, these classes of compounds also include primary metabolites, so whether a compound is a primary or secondary metabolite is a distinction based not only on its chemical structure but also on its function and distribution within the plant kingdom. Many thousands of secondary metabolites have been isolated from plants, and many of them have powerful physiological effects in humans and are used as medicines. They are major components of plant defense mechanism against herbivores, pest and pathogens. They also attract pollinators and seed dispersing materials. It produces product that aid in growth and development of plant but not required for plant to survive.

Lipids

The term *lipid* refers to fixed oils, fats, and waxes. They are esters of long-chain fatty acids and alcohols and closely related derivatives. They are stored in seeds, spores, and vegetative perennial organs such as bulbs. Fats and fixed oils are generally esters of long-chain fatty acids (such as stearic, palmitic, oleic acids) combined with trihydric alcohol, glycerol; hence, they are also called triglycerides. Waxes contain higher monohydric alcohol moieties such as cetyl, myristyl, and stearyl alcohols instead of the trihydric alcohol.

Phenols

Phenols are compounds in which one or more hydroxyl groups are directly attached to a carbon atom of an aromatic nucleus. Phenols are water soluble and mildly acidic in nature. Polyhydric phenols are powerful reducing agents. Phenolic acids are also abundant in plants as caffeic, ferulic, and coumaric acids.

Tannins

Tannins are chemically complex mixture of polyphenols widely distributed in the plant kingdom and localized in specific plant parts such as fruit, barks, leaves, stems, roots, etc. They are generally soluble in water, have astringent action, and usually bitter taste. Tannins precipitate proteins from solution, rendering them resistant to proteolytic enzymes.

Proteins

Proteins are nitrogenous organic substances occur in both the plant and animal kingdoms. Plants usually store proteins in the form of aleurone grains. Proteins are derived from amino acids, which are the building units.

Alkaloids

Alkaloids mean 'alkali-like,' referring to basic nitrogenous compounds of vegetable origin, possessing some marked physiological action. The names of alkaloids end in -ine to differentiate them from glycosides, which end in -in. Alkaloids occur in dicotyledons and less commonly in monocotyledons, gymnosperms, and cryptogams. Alkaloids are found mostly in fruits, stems, bark, roots, leaves, and seeds. Alkaloids are generally insoluble in water and soluble in ether or chloroform and other nonpolar solvents. They form water-soluble salts with acids. Basic chemical structures generally found are phenylalkylamine,

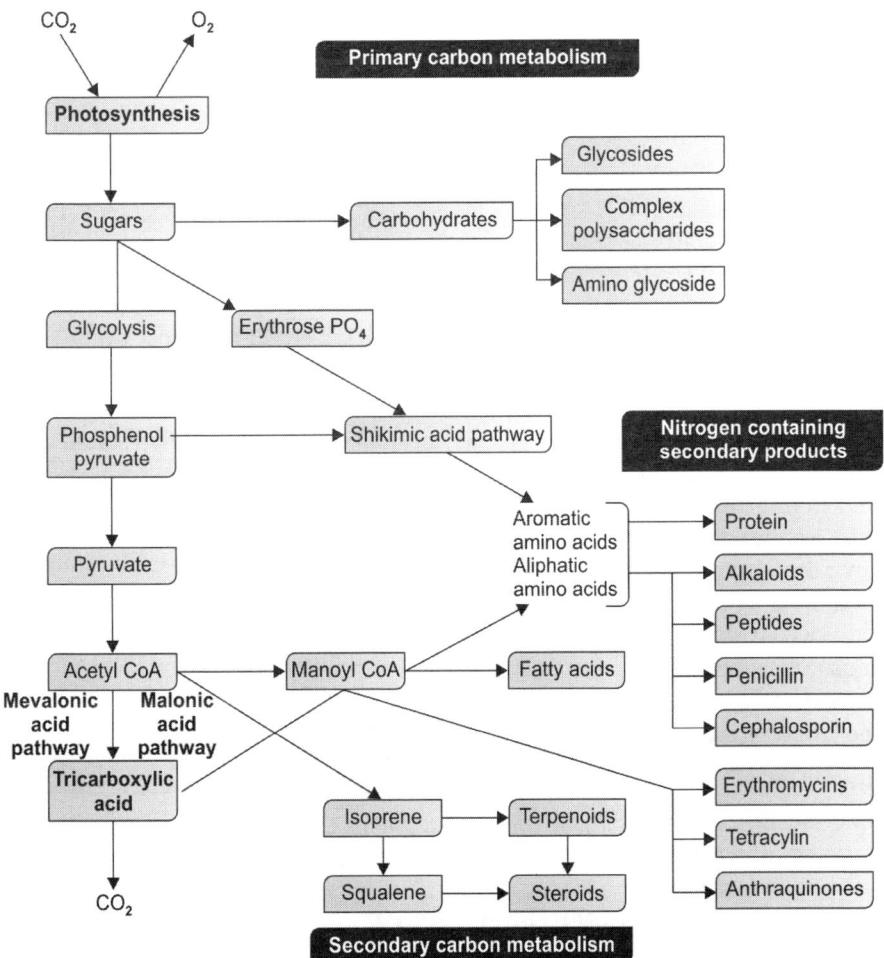

Fig. 1.14: Processing of medicinal plants

pyridine, piperidine, tropane, quinoline, isoquinoline, indole, carboline, imidazole, purine, phenanthrene, and steroidal. The physiological and pharmacological action of alkaloids varies widely. Examples are given in Table 1.2.

Table 1.2: Pharmacological classification of alkaloids

Activity	Alkaloids
Analgesic and narcotic	Morphine, Codeine
CNS stimulant	Strychnine, brucine, caffeine
Mydriatics	Atropine, homatropine
Myotics	Physostigmine, pilocarpine
Hypertensive	Ephedrine
Hypotensive	Reserpine, veratrine
Vermifuge	Pelletierine
Local anesthetic	Cocaine
Antimalarial	Quinine
Antiemetic	Emetine
Muscle relaxant	Curare
Antispasmodic	Papaverine
Uterine stimulant	Ergometrine
Antigout	Colchicines

Carbohydrates

Carbohydrates are compounds containing the elements carbon, hydrogen, and oxygen. They are either aldehydic or ketonic alcohols in which hydrogen and oxygen are present in the same ratio as in water. Carbohydrates are widely used in pharmaceutical preparations in numerous applications. They are broadly classified into three major groups:

1. True sugars
   a. monosaccharides
   b. oligosaccharides
2. Polysaccharides and
3. Derived carbohydrates

True Sugars

a. Monosaccharides.
   i. *Pentoses*: L-arabinose, D-xylose, D-ribose, and apiose.
   ii. *Hexoses*: D-glucose (dextrose), D-fructose (levulose), D-mannose, and L-galactose.

b. Oligosaccharides (less than 9 monosaccharide units). Those occurring naturally are usually di-, tri-, and tetrasaccharides
   i. *Disaccharides*: Non-reducing: Sucrose, trihalose
   Reducing: Maltose, lactose, turanose, cellobiose, gentiobiose, melibiose.
   ii. *Trisaccharides*: Raffinose (non-reducing).
   iii. *Tetrasaccharides*: Stachiose (non-reducing).

Polysaccharides (Non-sugars)

a. *Starch*: It is the principal food reserve of plants. It gives alpha-D glucose on complete hydrolysis, it is formed of amylose, which is a straight chain of alpha- 1,4-glycosidic bonds (more soluble in water) and amylopectin, which is branched presumably through an additional alpha-1,6-glycosidic bond (less soluble in water and more viscous in solution).

b. *Dextrins*: Obtained by incomplete hydrolysis of starch.

c. Glycogen, which is the reserve polysaccharide of the animal kingdom.

d. Inulin, a fructosan (molecular weight about 5000) consisting of a linear chain of B-(1, 2)-fructofuranose units.

e. Cellulose, the most widely distributed skeletal polysaccharide and most abundant and chemically resistant of all substances elaborated by living cells. It is a linear polysaccharide, consisting simply of 1, 4-linked B-D-glucopyranose units.

f. *Lichenin*: A cellulose-like polysaccharide that occurs as a cell wall constituent in lichens as Iceland moss. Unlike cellulose, lichenin is soluble in hot water to form a colloidal solution. It contains both B-1,4- and B-1,6-linkages.

g. *Dextran*: Used as a plasma substitute. It is an alpha–1, 6-linked polyglucan.

Derived Carbohydrates

They are polysaccharide complexes that yield in addition to monosaccharide, their sulfate esters, uronic acids, or amino sugars. They include hemicellulose, pectins, alginates, gums, mucilages, and some microbial polysaccharides. Gums are soluble in water; mucilages do not dissolve but form slimy masses.

Glycosides

Glycosides are non-reducing substances that, on hydrolysis brought about by reagents or enzymes, yield one or more reducing sugars among the products of hydrolysis. The non-sugar part of the molecule is called the aglycone or genin; the sugar component is called the glycone.

The glycosidic linkages: The usual linkage between the sugar and aglycone is an oxygen linkage, connecting the reducing group of a sugar and an alcoholic or phenolic hydroxy group of the aglycone.

O-glycosides are the most common ones found in nature.

S-glycosides and N-glycosides: In S-glycosides (e.g. sinigrin), the sugar is linked to the thiol (sulfhydryl) group of the aglycone. In N-glycosides (e.g. the streptidine moiety of streptomycin, glucosamine, or adenosine), the sugar is linked to the amino group of the aglycone.

C-glycosides (e.g. barbaloin) in which the sugar is linked to the aglycone by a carbon-to-carbon bond.

Classification

Glycosides are usually classified into the following groups using the chemical nature of the aglycone.
1. Phenol (e.g. arbutin)
2. Alcohol (e.g. salicin)
3. Lactone or coumarin (e.g. daphnin)
4. Flavone (e.g. rutin)
5. Anthraquinone (e.g. gluco aloe-emodin)
6. Aldehydes (e.g. glucovanillin)
7. Cyanophore (e.g. amygdalin)
8. Thiocyanate (e.g. sinigrin)
9. Steroid (e.g. digitoxin)
10. Saponin (e.g. digitonin)
11. Indoxyl (3-hydroxyindole) (e.g. indican)
12. Others in which are included neutral principles (e.g. crocin and picrocrocin, gentiopicrin and gentiamarin).

Function of glycosides in plants: They act as sugar reserves, regulating, detoxifying, and defensive roles.

Volatile Oils

Volatile oils are odorous principles found in various parts of the plant. They are products of plant metabolism. They are called volatile oils because they are volatile in steam and at higher temperatures evaporate. They are also called essential oils because they represent the 'essences' or odoriferous constituents of plants. Sources of volatile oils are given in Table 1.3.

Table 1.3: Sources of volatile oils

Sources	Part
Animal source	Liver of fish
Plant families	
Lamiaceae and Asteraceae	Specialized secretary structures glandular hairs
Lauraceae and Piperaceae	Modified parenchyma or oil cells, oil tubes (ducts)
Apiaceae	Vittae
Pinaceae and rutaceae	Internal lysigenous or schizogenous passages or glands
Umbelliferous fruits	Pericarp
Plants	
Rose	Petals
Cinnamon	Bark, leaves and glandular hairs
Mints	Stems and leaves
Orange	Flower petals and rind of the fruits.

Families

The chief families are: Pinaceae, Lauraceae, Rutaceae, Myrtaceae, Apiaceae, Lamiaceae, and Asteraceae.

Importance

They can be used for their therapeutic action; for example, local stimulants, carminatives, diuretics, mild antiseptics, local irritants, anthelmentics, or parasiticides. They can be also used as spices and for flavouring of foods, confections, beverages, pharmaceuticals, cosmetics, and tobacco.

Classification

1. *Hydrocarbon volatile oils:* Bitter orange, turpentine, juniper, cade, etc.
2. *Alcoholic volatile oils:* Mentha, coriander, geranium, rose, sandalwood, etc.

3. *Ester volatile oils:* Lavender, rosemary, sweet orange, neroli, etc.
4. *Aldehyde volatile oils:* Cinnamon bark, cassia bark, lemon, lemongrass, etc.
5. *Ketonic volatile oils:* Caraway, dill, spearmint, etc.
6. *Phenolic volatile oils:* Cinnamon leaf, clove, thyme, ajowan, horsemint, etc.
7. *Ethers:* Anise, star anise, fennel, parsley, nutmeg, etc.
8. *Oxides and peroxides:* Eucalyptus, cajuput, chenopodium, etc.
9. *Non-terpenoid and derived from glycosides:* Mustard, wintergreen, bitter almond, etc.

Resins and Resin Combinations

The term *resin* is applied to indicate a group of related solid or semisolid substances, complex mixtures of resin acids, resin alcohols, resinotannols, esters, and resenes. These substances are brittle secretions or exudations of plant tissues, either produced normally or as the result of pathogenic conditions. Resins, as a class, are hard, transparent or translucent brittle substances. They are generally heavier than water (sp. gr. 0.9–1.25).

Properties

They are amorphous (rarely crystallizable). On heating at comparatively low temperatures, resins soften and finally melt, forming sticky or adhesive fluids, without volatilization or decomposition. Resins are insoluble in water and hence have little taste. They are usually insoluble in petroleum ether, with a few exceptions (e.g. colophony, when freshly powdered, mastic).

Balsams are resinous substances that contain varying amounts of aromatic balsamic acids, viz. benzoic acid or cinnamic acid or both, or esters of these acids. They often contain small amounts of volatile oil as well.

Mucilages are viscous, usually white amorphous (when in a pure form) masses, that form colloidial, nonadhesive solutions with water. On hydrolysis, they form a mixture of pentoses, hexoses, and uronic acids. Most mucilages contain varying amounts of component sugars (i.e. glucose, xylose, arabinose,

galacturonic and glucuronic acids). Mucilage also occurs in the cells and tissues of many different plants; for example, in seaweeds, flowers, fruits, leaves, barks, roots, and seeds. Some plants containing mucilage are althea root (*Althea officinalle*), slippery elm bark (*Ulmus fulva*), Comfrey root (*Symphytum officinale*), and malva (*Malva sylvestris*).

TECHNIQUES FOR DETECTION OF PHYTOCHEMICAL GROUPS IN EXTRACTS

Carbohydrates

Molisch's test: 5 ml of sugar solution with 2 drops of Molisch's reagent (10 g α-napthol in 100 ml of 95% alcohol) mix and add concentrated sulfuric acid through sides of the sloping test-tube, a purple ring forming at the interface between the acid and test layer. The reaction forms five-member oxygen containing rings, known as furfural, further reacts with Molisch reagent to form coloured compounds.

Benedict's test assays for the presence of reducing sugars. Add 1 ml of the solution to be tested to 5 ml of Benedict's solution (solution of copper sulfate, sodium carbonate, and sodium citrate, pH 10.5), and shake test tube. Place the tube in a boiling water bath and heat for 3 minutes. Remove the test tube from the heat and allow them to cool. Formation of a green, red, or yellow precipitate is a positive for reducing sugars.

Barfoed's test is a test for monosaccharides Add 1 ml of the solution to be tested to 3 ml of freshly prepared Barfoed's reagent (copper acetate in dilute acetic acid, pH 4.6). Place test tubes into a boiling water bath and heat for 3 minutes. Cool it, formation of a green, red, or yellow precipitate is a positive test for reducing monosaccharides.

> **Note:** Do not heat the tubes longer than 3 minutes, as a positive test can be obtained with disaccharides if they are heated long enough.

Alkaloids

1. **Mayer reagent:** *Solution I:* Dissolve 1.36 g $HgCl_2$ in 60 ml water.

Solution II: Dissolve 5 g KI in 10 ml water.

Procedure: Combine the two solutions and dilute with water to 100 ml. Add a few drops to an acidified extract solution (diluted HCl or H_2SO_4), and if alkaloids are present, a white to yellowish precipitate will appear. Care should be taken not to agitate the test system, because the precipitate may be redissolved.

2. **Dragendorff reagent:** *Solution I:* Dissolve 8.0 g bismuth subnitrate [Bi $(NO_3)_3$. H_2O] in 30% w/v HNO_3.

Solution II: Dissolve 27.2 g KI in 50 ml water.

Procedure: Combine the solutions and let stand for 24 hours, filter, and dilute to 100 ml with deionized water. In acid solutions, an orange-brownish precipitate will appear. The alkaloids may be recovered by treatment with Na_2CO_3 and subsequent extraction with diethyl ether. This reaction may also be performed on a filter paper or on a TLC plate by adding a drop of the reagent onto a spot of the sample.

3. **Wagner reagent solution:** Dissolve 1.27 g I_2 (sublimed) and 2 g KI in 20 ml water, and make up with water to 100 ml.

Procedure: A brown precipitate in acidic solutions suggests the presence of alkaloids.

4. **Ammonium reineckate solution:** Add 0.2 g hydroxylamine to a saturated solution of 4% ammonium reineckate {NH_4 [Cr $(NH_3)_2(SCN)_4$].H_2O}, and acidify with dilute HCl.

Procedure: When added to extracts, a pink precipitate will appear if alkaloids are present. The precipitate is soluble in 50% acetone, which may also be used for compound recrystallization.

Glycosides

Borntrager's test for anthraquinone glycosides: Boil the powder with diluted HCl, filter, cool, shake with organic solvent, separate organic layer, shake with NH_4OH, the aqueous layer becomes rose pink or cherry red.

Modified Borntrager's test: In case of dianthrone, e.g. sennosoides: Boil the powder with alc. KOH and filter. Add diluted HCl to the filtrate and extract with ether. Oxidize with H_2O_2. Add NH_4OH to the ethereal extract and shake, a rose red colour is produced in the aqueous layer.

Keller Killiani test for cardiac glycosides: 0.1 mg of glycoside is dissolved in a mixture of 1 ml of 5% ferric sulphate and 99 ml of glacial acetic acid and to this 1–2 drop of conc. H_2SO_4 is added, it gives blue colour within 2–3 min constitutes a positive test.

Kedde's test for cardiac glycosides: Sample with Kedde's reagent (3, 5-dinitrobenzoic acid and NaOH) gives violet colour.

Baljet's test for cardiac glycosides: Sample with Baljet's reagent (picric acid and NaOH) gives orange or red.

Flavonoids

Shinoda test: To an alcoholic solution of the sample, add magnesium powder and a few drops of concentrated HCl. Flavones, flavonols, the corresponding 2, 3-dihydro derivatives, and xanthones produce orange, pink, red to purple colours with this test. By using zinc instead of magnesium, only flavanonols give a deep-red to magenta colour; flavanones and flavonols will give weak pink to magenta colours or no colour at all.

Lipids

H_2SO_4 test (Salkowski): Dissolve sample in a little chloroform and add equal volume of conc. sulphuric acid. A play of colours from bluish-red to cherry-red and purple is formed in the chloroform, whereas the acid assumes a marked green fluorescence.

Sterols

1. **Liebermann-Burchard test:** Combine 1ml acetic anhydride and 1ml $CHCl_3$, and cool to 0°C, and add one drop concentrated H_2SO4. When the sample is added, either in the solid form or in solution in $CHCl_3$, blue, green, red, or orange colours that change with time will indicate a positive reaction; a blue-greenish colour in particular is observed for sterols, with maximum

intensity in 15–30 min. (This test is also applicable for certain classes of unsaturated triterpenoids.)

2. **Salkowski reaction:** Dissolve 1–2 mg of the sample in 1ml $CHCl_3$ and add 1ml concentrated H_2SO_4, forming two phases, with a red colour indicating the presence of sterols.

Saponins

When shaken, an aqueous solution of a saponin containing sample produces foam, which is stable for 15 min or more.

Hemolysis test for saponins: Add sample to 1 drop of horse blood on glass slide, observe under microscope hemolytic zone appears.

Other Polyphenols

Vegetable tannins are loosely defined by a combination of structural and functional characteristics as polyphenolic compounds that precipitate protein.

1. **Ferric chloride:** Dissolve 5% (w/v) $FeCl_3$ in water or EtOH. Addition of several drops of the solution to an extract produces a blue, blue-black, or blue-green colour reaction in the presence of polyphenols. This is not a specific reagent for tannins, as other phenolic compounds will also give a positive result.

2. **Gelatin-salt test:** This test is used for the detection of tannins in solution, dissolve 10 mg of an extract in 6 ml of hot deionized, distilled water (filtering if necessary), and the solution is divided between three test tubes. To the first is added a 1% solution of NaCl, to the second is added a 1% NaCl and 5% gelatin solution, and to the third is added a $FeCl_3$ solution. Formation of a precipitate in the second treatment suggests the presence of tannins, and a positive response after addition of $FeCl_3$ to the third portion supports this inference.

Quality Control of Herbal Drugs

Quality can be defined as the status of a drug that is determined by identity, purity, content, and other chemical, physical, or biological properties, or by the manufacturing processes. Quality control is a term that refers to processes involved in maintaining the quality and validity of a manufactured product. The quality control of herbal drugs is illustrated in Fig. 1.15.

PARAMETERS FOR QUALITY CONTROL OF HERBAL DRUGS

Quality is conformance to requirement and meeting stated as well as implied needs of

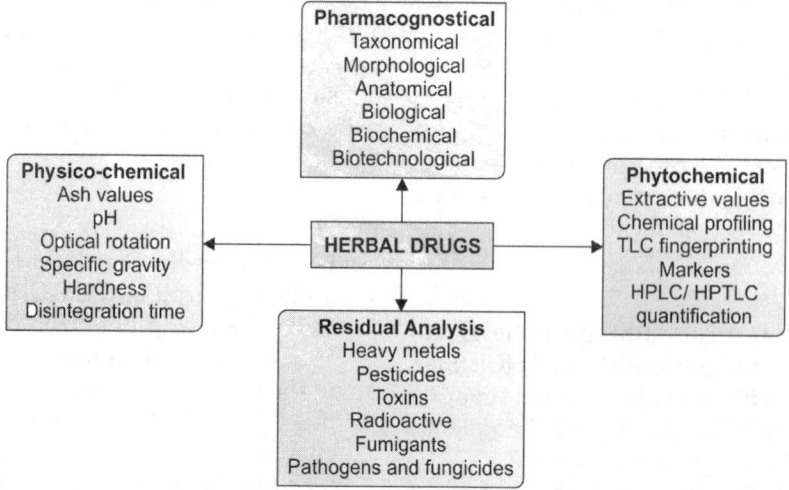

Fig. 1.15: Quality control of herbal drugs

customer. The word quality is derived from Latin *'qualis'* means *'of what kind'* and encompasses composition and properties of object. Quality is of paramount importance to herbal drugs; because of several reasons quality control is a herculean task. The quality of pharmaceuticals has been a concern of the World Health Organization (WHO) since its inception.

Determination of Foreign Matter

Herbal materials should be entirely free from visible signs of contamination by moulds or insects, and other animal contamination, including animal excreta. No abnormal odour, discolouration, slime or signs of deterioration should be detected.

Foreign matter is mineral admixtures not adhering to the herbal materials, such as soil, stones, sand and dust.

Procedure

1. Weigh a sample of herbal material, specified in the test procedures for the herbal material concerned.
2. Spread a thin layer and sort the foreign matter into groups either by visual inspection, using a magnifying lens (6× or 10×), or with the help of a suitable sieve, according to the requirements for the specific herbal material.
3. Sift the remainder of the sample through a No. 250 sieve; dust is regarded as mineral admixture.
4. Weigh the portions of this sorted foreign matter to within 0.05 g.
5. Calculate the content of each group in grams per 100 g of air-dried sample.

Macroscopic and Microscopic Examination

Macroscopic identity of herbal materials is based on shape, size, colour, surface characteristics, texture, fracture characteristics and appearance of the cut surface.

Microscopic inspection of herbal materials is indispensable for the identification of broken or powdered materials; the specimen may have to be treated with chemical reagents.

Visual Examination and Odour

Size: Measurement of the Length, Width and Thickness of Crude Materials

1. Graduated ruler is used to measure in millimetres.
2. Small seeds and fruits may be measured by aligning ten of them on a sheet of calibrated paper, with 1 mm spacing between lines, and dividing the result by ten.

Colour

1. Examine the untreated sample under diffuse daylight.
2. If necessary, an artificial light source with wavelengths similar to those of daylight may be used.
3. The colour of the sample should be compared with that of a reference sample.

Surface characteristics, texture and fracture characteristics

1. Examine the untreated sample.
2. If necessary, a magnifying lens (6x to 10x) may be used.
3. Wetting with water or reagents, as required, may be necessary to observe the characteristics of a cut surface.
4. Touch the material to determine if it is soft or hard; bend and rupture it to obtain information on brittleness and the appearance of the fracture plane—whether it is fibrous, smooth, rough, granular, etc.

Odour

1. If the material is expected to be innocuous, place a small portion of the sample in the palm of the hand or in a beaker of suitable size, and slowly and repeatedly inhale the air over the material.
2. If no distinct odour is perceptible, crush the sample between the thumb and index finger or between the palms of the hands using gentle pressure.
3. If the material is known to be dangerous, crush by mechanical means and then pour a small quantity of boiling water onto the crushed sample in a beaker.

4. First, determine the strength of the odour (none, weak, distinct, strong) and then the odour sensation (aromatic, fruity, musty, mouldy, rancid, etc.). A direct comparison of the odour with a defined substance is advisable (e.g. peppermint should have an odour similar to menthol, cloves should have an odour similar to eugenol).

Inspection By Microscopy

Once the material has been examined and classified according to external characteristics, inspection by microscopy can be carried out with the help of microscope equipped with lenses providing a wide range of magnification and a substage condenser, a graduated mechanical stage, objectives with a magnification of 4×, 10× and 40×.

Preliminary Treatment

Softening before preparation: Dried parts of a plant may require softening before preparation for microscopy, preferably by being placed in a moist atmosphere or by soaking in water.

- **For small quantities of material**, place a wad of cotton-wool moistened with water into the bottom of a test-tube and cover with a piece of filter-paper. Place the material being examined on the paper, stopper the tube and allow it to stand overnight or until the material is soft and suitable for cutting.
- **Larger quantities of material:** Use a desiccator for larger quantities of material, placing water into the lower part instead of the drying agent.
- Bark, wood and other dense and hard materials usually need to be soaked in water or in equal parts of water, ethanol and glycerol for a few hours or overnight until they are soft enough to be cut.
- Boiling in water for a few minutes may sometimes be necessary.
- Any water-soluble contents can be removed from the cells by soaking in water.
- Starch grains can be gelatinized by heating in water. In certain cases, material can be moistened with water for a few minutes to soften the surfaces and allow sections to be cut.

Preparation of Specimens

Powdered materials

1. Moisten the tip of a needle with water and dip into the powder, transfer the material that adheres to the needle tip into the slide containing one or two drops of water, glycerol/ethanol TS or chloral hydrate TS
2. Stir thoroughly, but carefully, and apply a cover-glass.
3. Press lightly on the cover-glass with the handle of the needle, and remove excess fluid from the margin of the cover-glass with a strip of filter-paper.
4. If the specimen is to be freed from air bubbles, boil carefully over a small flame of a microburner until the air is completely removed.
5. Care should be taken to replace the fluid that evaporates so that the space beneath the cover-glass is completely filled with fluid at the conclusion of the operation.

Analytical Standards

Determination of Leaf Constants

A number of leaf measurements are used to distinguish some closely related species not easily characterized by general microscopy.

Stomatal number: Stomatal number is defined as the average number of stomata per sq mm of epidermis. Fragments of leaf from the middle of the lamina were cleaned with chloral hydrate.

1. Peel off upper and lower epidermis separately by means of a forceps and mount in glycerine water.
2. Draw a square of known dimensions (1 sq mm) by means of a stage micrometer and camera lucida and count number of stomata on that area.
3. Observe type of stomata on the same preparation.
4. Determine ten and calculate the average. Observe under 10X (eyepiece) and 40X (objective).

Stomatal index: Stomatal index is the percentage which the numbers of stomata form to the total number of epidermal cells, each stoma being counted as one cell. Whilst stomata number varies considerably with the age of the leaf and due to changes in environmental conditions, stomatal index is relatively constant and, therefore, of diagnostic significance for a given species.

1. Count number of epidermal cells and stomata within the square.
2. Determine ten and calculate the average.
3. Observe under 10X (eyepiece) and 40X (objective).
4. Calculate stomatal index by using the following equation.

$$\text{Stomatal index (SI)} = (S/E+S) \times 100$$

where,

S = number of stomata per unit area

E = number of epidermal cells in the same unit area

Palisade ratio: Palisade ratio is defined as the average number of palisade cells beneath each epidermal cell.

1. Clear pieces of leaf about 2 mm square by boiling with chloral hydrate solution.
2. Trace epidermal cells and the palisade cells lying below them by camera lucida.
3. First a number of groups each of four epidermal cells were traced and their outlines made more conspicuous.
4. The palisade cells lying beneath each group focused and traced.
5. The palisade cells in each group counted, cells which were more than half covered by the epidermal cells were also counted; the figure obtained was divided by 4 to obtain palisade ratio of that group.
6. Twenty-five groups from different leaf samples were determined for the calculation of range and average.
7. Observe under 10X (eyepiece) and 40X (objective).

Vein-islet number: The vein-islet is the minute area of photosynthetic tissue encircled by the ultimate divisions of the conducting strands. Vein-islet number is defined as the number of vein-islets per sq mm of the leaf surface, midway between the midrib and the margin.

1. The leaf sample, after soaking in water, was treated successively with sodium hypochlorite to bleach, 10% hydrochloric acid to remove Ca oxalate and finally chloral hydrate.
2. Set up Camera Lucida by means of a stage micrometer the paper was divided into squares of 1 sq mm.
3. In the cleared preparation veins traced in four continuous squares, in a square of 2 mm × 2 mm.
4. Each vein-islet was numbered during counting. The range and average was determined in 10 sets of 2 mm × 2 mm area. Observed under 10X (eyepiece) and 4X (objective).

Veinlet termination number. Veinlet termination number is defined as the number of veinlet terminations per sq mm of the leaf surface. A vein termination is the ultimate free termination of a veinlet or branch of a veinlet. Veinlet termination was counted in the same preparation as for vein-islet number. The total number of vein-islets and veinlet terminations in four adjoining squares was divided by four in order to get the value in 1 sq mm. The range and average was determined in 10 sets of 2 mm × 2 mm area Observe under 10X (eyepiece) and 4X (objective).

The chromatographic techniques used in the isolation of various types of natural products can be broadly classified into two categories: Classical or older, and modern.

Classical or older chromatographic techniques include:

1. Thin-layer chromatography (TLC).
2. Preparative thin-layer chromatography (PTLC).
3. Open-column chromatography (CC).
4. Flash chromatography (FC).

Modern chromatographic techniques are:

1. High-performance thin-layer chromatography (HPTLC).
2. Multiflash chromatography
3. Vacuum liquid chromatography (VLC).
4. Chromatotron.
5. Solid-phase extraction
6. Droplet countercurrent chromatography (DCCC).

7. High-performance liquid chromatography (HPLC).

8. Hyphenated techniques (e.g. HPLC-PDA, LC-MS, LC-NMR and LC-MS-NMR).

Traditional herbal medicines make excellent leads for new drug development. New plant-derived medicines can come from three sources: Single active principles, active fractions, and validated prescriptions. Conventionally, for single active compounds, lead discovery and drug development involve highly efficient bioactivity-directed fractionation and isolation (BDFI) coupled with structural characterization, analog synthesis, and mechanism of action studies. Today, new scientific technologies, including biological screening methods, continue to improve this process. For multi-component herbal prescriptions standardization and quality control, including GAP (Good Agricultural Practice), GMP (Good Manufacturing Practice) and GCP (Good Clinical Practice), must be performed to guarantee high quality and consistency. To validate herbal efficacy and safety reliable chemical, pharmacological, as well as drug administration, distribution, metabolism, excretion, and toxicological (ADMET) studies are needed. Parameters of quality control of herbal drugs are enlisted in Table 1.4.

Table 1.4: Parameters for quality control of herbal drugs

S. No	Type of standards	Examples
1.	Structural standard	A. **Macroscopic examinations:** Evaluation on the basis of morphological characteristics i. *Macromorphological evaluation* ✧ *Bark*: Curvature, tranverse, in surface and fracture characteristics ✧ *Underground organs*: Shape, surface characters and transverse section ✧ *Leaves*: Surface appearance and texture (Glabrous, pubescent, hispid, punctate) and lamina structure ★ Shape: Cordate, round, obovate, ovate, lanceolate, oblong, oval and linear ★ Margin: Dentate, sinuate, crenate, serrate, entire ★ Incision: Partite, fid, sect ★ Composition: Paripinnate, imparipinnate, pinnate, palmate ★ Apex: Acute, acuminate, truncate, obtuse ★ Base: Cordate, decurrent, symmetrical, asymmetrical ★ Venation: Parallel, pinnate, palmate and reticulate. ✧ *Flowers*: Receptacle, calyx, corolla and inflorescence (Umbel, Panicle, Raceme and Capitulum) ✧ *Fruits*: Shape and size (simple, aggregate and collective), type (simple inhedehiscent fruit, succulent fruits) ✧ *Seeds*: Size, shape, colour, appearance and occurrence of any testa outgrowth. ✧ *Unorganised drug*: Solid (physical state, presence of vegetable debris, effect of heating) ✧ Liquid/semisolid (colour, fluorescence, viscosity, density and solubility) ✧ *Cytomorphological evaluation*: Examination and arrangements of cell types ★ Parenchyma, collenchyma and sclerenchyma ★ Epidermis and periderm ★ Xylem and phloem

Contd.

Table 1.4: Parameters for quality control of herbal drugs (*Contd.*)

S. No.	Type of standards	Examples

B. **Microscopic examinations**: To magnify the fine structure of minute objects.

Preliminary treatment: Dried parts of a plant may require softening in moist atmosphere, place a wad of cotton-wool moistened with water into the bottom of a test-tube and cover with a piece of filter-paper. Bark, wood and other dense and hard materials usually need to be soaked in water or equal parts of water, ethanol and glycerol for a few hours or overnight.

Preparation of specimens: Powdered materials, surface tissues of leaves and flowers, section

Use of clarifying agents like chloral hydrate TS, lactochloral TS, lactophenol TS, sodium hypochlorite TS, solvents for fats and oils (xylene R and light petroleum R)

Histochemical detection of cell walls and contents

Iodinated zinc chloride (for detection of cellulose cell walls), phloroglucinol TS (for lignified cell wall), sudan red TS (for suberized or cuticular cell walls), iodine/ethanol TS (for Aleurone grains), acetic acid (~60 g/l) TS or hydrochloric acid (~70 g/l) TS (for *calcium carbonate*), chloral hydrate TS (for calcium oxalate), potassium hydroxide (~55 g/l) TS (for *hydroxyanthraquinones*), 1-naphthol TS and sulfuric acid (~1760 g/l) TS (for inulin), Chinese ink TS/ thionine TS (for mulicage), iodine (0.02 mol/l) VS (starch) and ferric chloride (50 g/l) TS (for tannin).

Disintegration of tissues

Method 1. Nitric acid and potassium chlorate

Method 2. Nitric acid and chromic acid

Method 3. Caustic alkali method

Measurement of specimens

Use a microscope with an ocular micrometer and calibration of the ocular micrometer.

Microscopical examination

Microchemical testing

Microchemical precipitation

Micro sublimation

2. Analytical standards   **Quantitative analytical microscopy:** Determining purity and botanical source of powdered drug

Stomatal number

Vein islet number

Palisade ratio

Lycopodium spore method

Standardization parameters

Determination of ash: Ignition of medicinal plant materials

Total ash: Measure the total amount of material remaining after ignition. This includes both 'physiological ash', which is derived from the plant tissue itself, and 'non-physiological ash', which is the residue of the extraneous matter (e.g. sand and soil) adhering to the plant surface.

Acid-insoluble ash: Residue obtained after boiling the total ash with dilute hydrochloric acid, and igniting the remaining insoluble matter. This measures the amount of silica present, especially as sand and siliceous earth.

Water-soluble ash is the difference in weight between the total ash and the residue after treatment of the total ash with water.

Contd.

Table 1.4: Parameters for quality control of herbal drugs (*Contd.*)

S. No.	Type of standards	Examples

Determination of extractable matter: This method determines the amount of active constituents extracted with solvents from a given amount of medicinal plant material. Hot extraction and cold maceration

Determination of water and volatile matter: Limits for water content should therefore be set for every given plant material. This is especially important for materials that absorb moisture easily or deteriorate quickly in the presence of water

Preparation of material (cutting, granulating or shredding)

Azeotropic method (toluene distillation)

Loss on drying (gravimetric determination)

Determination of volatile oils: By steam distillation with clevenger apparatus

Determination of bitterness value: Bitter drugs are used therapeutically, mostly as appetizing agents. Their bitterness stimulates secretions in the gastrointestinal tract, especially of gastric juice, compared by that of a dilute solution of quinine hydrochloride.

Determination of haemolytic activity: Medicinal plants with caryophyllaceae, araliaceae, sapindaceae, primulaceae, and dioscoreaceae contain saponins. When added to a suspension of blood, saponins produce changes in erythrocyte membranes, causing haemoglobin to diffuse into the surrounding medium.

Determination of tannins: By hide powder method.

Determination of swelling index: The swelling index is the volume in ml taken up by the swelling of 1 g of plant material under specified conditions.

Determination of foaming index: The foaming ability of an aqueous decoction of plant materials and their extracts is measured in terms of a foaming index.

Determination of pesticide residues: Limits for pesticide residues should be established following the recommendations of the Food and Agriculture Organization (FAO) of the United Nations and the World Health Organization (WHO) which have already been established for food and animal feed. These recommendations include the analytical methodology for the assessment of specific pesticide residues.

Determination of arsenic and heavy metals

Limit test for arsenic: The amount of arsenic in the medicinal plant material is estimated by matching the depth of colour with that of a standard stain. The contents of lead and cadmium may be determined by inverse voltametry or by atomic absorption spectrophotometry.

Determination of microorganisms

Radioactive contamination: The amount of exposure to radiation depends on the intake of radio nuclides and other variables such as age, metabolic kinetics, and weight of the individual (also known as the dose conversion factor).

Culture media and strains of microorganisms

Culture media: Baird-Parker agar, brilliant green agar, buffered sodium chloride—peptone solution pH 7.0, casein-soybean digest agar, cetrimide agar, deoxycholate citrate agar, Enterobacteriaceae enrichment broth-Mossel, lactose broth, MacConkey agar, MacConkey broth, sabouraud glucose agar with antibiotics, soybean-casein digest medium, tetrathionate bile brilliant green broth, triple sugar iron agar, violet-red bile agar with glucose and lactose, xylose, lysine, deoxycholate agar.

S. No.	Type of standards	Examples
3.	Standard relating to physical constants	**Determination of density:** Pycnometer and oscillating U-tube.
		Determination of refractive index: Refractometer
		Determination of viscosity: Viscometer
		Determination of optical rotation: Polarimeter

2

Biodynamic Agriculture

- WHO guidelines on good agricultural and collection practices for medicinal plants
- Organic Farming

- Pest and pest management in medicinal plants: Biopesticides/bioinsecticides.
- Quality assurance in manufacture of herbal medicine

INTRODUCTION

According to **WHO guidelines**, during last two decades uses of traditional medicines, especially herbal medicines have been increased worldwide. Simultaneously, various analysis and studies have revealed a variety of reasons for the number of patients experiencing unfavourable consequences caused by the use of herbal medicines has also been increasing.

The major causes are insufficient attention paid to the **Quality Assurance and Control** of traditional medicine, particularly herbal. The reports revealed that adverse effects are due to poor quality of herbal medicines, including raw medicinal plant materials. The good

medicinal plant practices include GAP, GHP, GLP and GMP as shown in Fig. 2.1.

More than 90% of the formulations predominantly contain plant-based raw materials under the Indian Systems of Medicine that is, Ayurveda, Siddha, Unani, and Homoeopathy (AYUSH). The efficacy of these systems thus mainly relies upon the use of raw material of quality and standardized ingredients in the manufacture of medicines of these systems.

In view of the above situation, genuine measures are needed to promote the effective cultivation of medicinal plants and create awareness in the midst of people, peculiarly farmers, about the values focusing medicinal

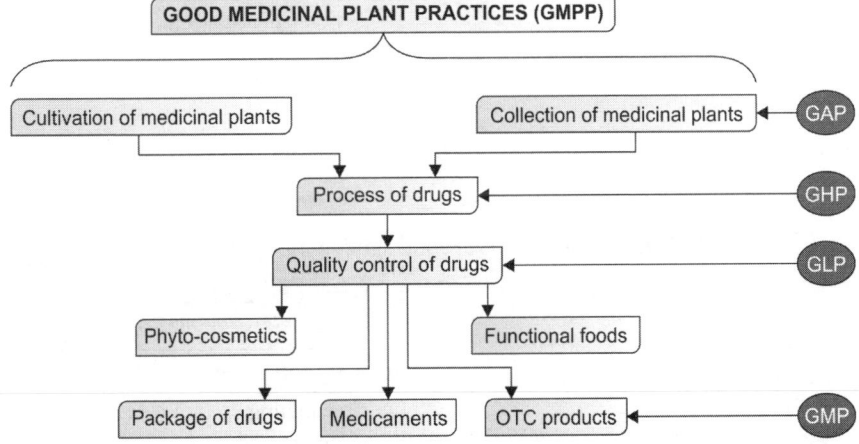

Fig. 2.1: Good medicinal plant practice

and economic factors so that these treasures of nature, i.e. plants can be used wisely as well as conserved.

Quality control directly impacts the safety and efficacy of herbal medicinal products. Good agricultural and collection practices for medicinal plants is only the first step in quality assurance, on which the safety and efficacy of herbal medicinal products directly depend upon, and will also play an important role in the protection of natural resources of medicinal plants for sustainable use.

Need for Good Agricultural Practices

In India, medicinal plants are mostly collected from wild resources. Therefore, the plant material collected from these wild sources is loaded with the problems of adulteration and misidentification. However, the plant material collected from such sources may also be contaminated by other species or parts. Such wild plant varieties mainly differ by presence of the active constituents from area to area. Therefore, only way to have quality raw material is cultivation of genuine, authentic variety of plants. But it is neither commercially viable nor easy to cultivate authentic variety of

these plants. Four pillars of good agricultural practices are described in Fig. 2.2. Benefits and challenges of GAP is described in Fig. 2.3.

The basic reason for their exploitation from wild sources is non-availability of proper techniques, soil, and authentic plantation material. The safety and quality of raw medicinal plant materials and finished products depend on various factors like genetic makeup, environmental conditions, collection and cultivation practices, harvest and post-harvest processing, transport and storage practices, and so on. Inadvertent contamination by microbial or chemical agents during any of the production stages can also lead to deterioration in quality.

Good agricultural practices are 'practices that address environmental, economic and social sustainability for on farm processes, and result in safe and quality food and nonfood agricultural products'.

The objective of GAP codes, standards and regulations include to a varying degree:

1. To ensure safety and quality of the produce in the food chain.
2. To modify supply chain governance to capture new market.

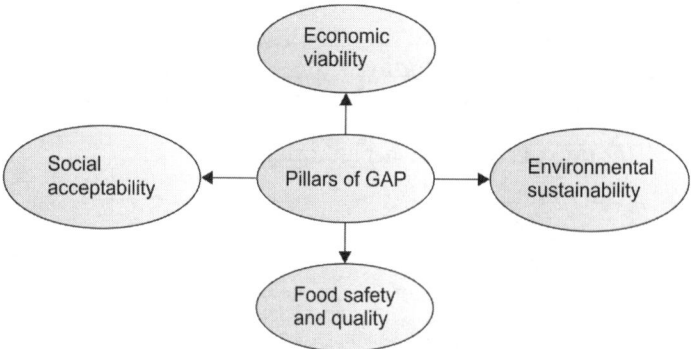

Fig. 2.2: Four pillars of good agricultural practices

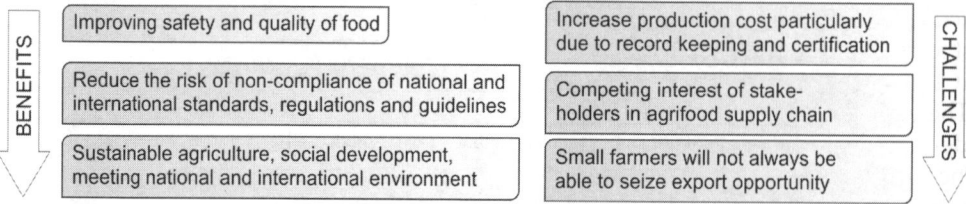

Fig. 2.3: Benefits and challenges of good agricultural practices

3. To improve the use of natural resources, maintain working conditions as well as worker health.

4. To create new market opportunities for farmers as well as exports.

WHO GUIDELINES ON GOOD AGRICULTURAL AND COLLECTION PRACTICES FOR MEDICINAL PLANTS

Good Agricultural and Collection Practices for Medicinal Plants (GACP) are a set of guidelines developed in 2003 by the World Health Organisation (WHO), aimed at improving the quality of medicinal plant material being used in herbal medicines in the market.

The main objectives of the GACP guidelines, as stated by the WHO, are as follows:

⊃ To contribute to the quality assurance of medicinal plant materials used as the source for herbal medicines and to improve the quality, safety and efficacy of finished herbal products;

⊃ To guide the formulation of national and/ or regional GACP guidelines and GACP monographs for medicinal plants and related standard operating procedures; and

⊃ To encourage and support the sustainable cultivation and collection of medicinal plants of good quality in ways that respect and support the conservation of medicinal plants and the environment in general.

The development of WHO guidelines on GACPs for medicinal plants is an important step to ensure quality of herbal medicines and ecologically sound cultivation practices.

The GACPs cover a wide spectrum of cultivation and collection activities, including site selection, climate and soil considerations, identification of seed, main post-harvest operations, and legal aspects. It is necessary to concentrate on standardizing the cultivation practices, collection practices, and post-harvest technologies for these plants adhering to GACPs.

The basic guidelines needed to be followed under GACPs for cultivation and harvesting of the medicinal plant are characterized below:

⊃ Selection of applicable site for cultivation of a selective medicinal plant.

⊃ Selection of time for cultivation.

⊃ Screen proper variety.

⊃ Follow organic farming.

⊃ Precaution should be taken while pruning and collecting desired mature parts of plant, without harming the mother plant.

⊃ To leave at least 30–40% for regeneration, do not try to collect whole population.

⊃ While collecting of plant parts, do not cut twinges and branches.

⊃ To use proper equipment for cutting, shearing, and peeling.

⊃ After collection, immediate drying should be done; complete drying should be ensured before packing and storage.

⊃ To dry aromatic herbs and delicate fruits in shade in order to preserve volatile constituents.

⊃ To remove dust and other undesirable matter in appropriate shifter.

⊃ Pack the herbs in suitable packaging material to avoid losses due to external factors.

⊃ Store the herbs in proper storage conditions to minimize loss on storage.

Following guidelines are considered for collection of leaves, flowers, fruits, seeds, floral parts.

1. To harvest only mature parts from healthy plants.

2. Do not collect all parts of the plant at a time.

3. Do not cut branches for collecting leaves, fruits, flowers, and so on.

4. To facilitate natural regeneration leave some floral parts on the plants.

5. Fleshy flowers preferably be dried in shade, may be dried in the sun.

6. Parts like stigma, anthers and buds should be collected at appropriate time.

7. To harvest the seeds once the fruits are completely mature.

For collection of underground part(s), bark, and whole plant, following guidelines should be adhered to:

⊃ To collect after the seeds are shed to facilitate regeneration.

⊃ To facilitate regeneration, do least digging for collection of underground parts and leave some underground part.

- To collect underground parts when the mother plant is fully matured.
- To cut large parts into smaller pieces and dry fleshy parts before packing and storing.
- Do not harvest bark from immature plant; instead, collect from the branches of main trunk.
- To harvest only mature branches for stem.

For collection of gums, oils, resins, galls, and so on:

- To make incisions only vertically on some portions of the tree and not horizontally.
- To treat the incisions after collection of the desired material.
- Do not collect the gum or resin from a tree continuously and collect them in precisely right season.
- Do not leave gum/resin exposed in the field. Pack them in appropriate containers or drums with polyethylene lining.

Good Agricultural Practices for Medicinal Plants (Fig. 2.4)

It describes general principles and provides technical details for the cultivation of medicinal plants. It also describes quality control measures, where applicable.

Identification/Authentication of Cultivated Medicinal Plants

Selection of medicinal plants

Plant identification is the process of matching a specimen plant to a known taxon. The authentication of species or botanical varieties can be done following authorities documents:

1. With reference to **National Pharmacopoeia** or any authoritative national documents the specification of species or botanical variety selected for cultivation should be same.

2. In absence of substantial national documents, specified botanical varieties in the pharmacopoeia should be considered. Other authoritative documents of other countries can be considered for selection of varieties of botanical species.

3. The newly introduced medicinal plants should be identified and documented as the source material used or described in traditional medicine of the original country.

Botanical Identity

Identification of a species is the most critical task which necessitates application of instinct, knowledge and skill. A correctly identified

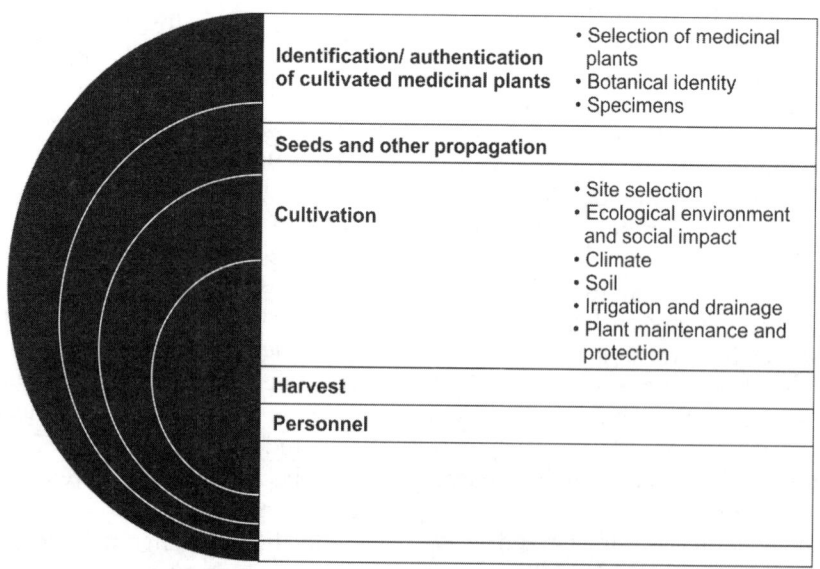

Identification/ authentication of cultivated medicinal plants	• Selection of medicinal plants • Botanical identity • Specimens
Seeds and other propagation	
Cultivation	• Site selection • Ecological environment and social impact • Climate • Soil • Irrigation and drainage • Plant maintenance and protection
Harvest	
Personnel	

Fig. 2.4: Good agricultural practices for medicinal plants

species is given recognition with the help of an appropriate name. The events of misidentification of plant species, inadvertent use of totally unrelated species or by closely related inferior quality species can hinder their medicinal use, the adverse effects of which may even kill a consumer. The medicinally useful plants and plant products must have their specific identity correctly ascertained with standardized circumscription and nomenclature for quality control and prevention of adulteration of drugs.

Seeds and Other Propagation Materials

Propagation material of plants such as seeds and cuttings are essential elements in establishing, expanding, diversifying and improving agriculture. The following points should be considered:

1. The suppliers of seed and other propagation materials should be specified and they should provide all relevant information related to identity, quality and performance of their products, as well as their breeding history, where possible.
2. The propagation or planting materials should be of the appropriate quality and be as free as possible from contamination and diseases in order to promote healthy plant growth.
3. Planting material should preferably be resistant or tolerant to biotic or abiotic factors.
4. Seeds and other propagation materials used for organic production should be certified as being organically derived. The quality of propagation material—including any genetically modified germplasm should comply with regional and/or national regulations and be appropriately labeled and documented, as required.
5. Care should be taken to exclude extraneous species, botanical varieties and strains of medicinal plants during the entire production process.

Cultivation

The principle of cultivation is to turn the soil into a fine tilth to provide the ideal environment for seeds to germinate. Cultivation was also a traditional form of weed control. Cultivation may be used in crusted soils to increase soil aeration and infiltration of water; it may also be used to move soil to or away from plants as desired. Cultivation among crop plants is best kept at a minimum; excessive cultivation can be harmful as it may cause root pruning and loss of soil water due to increased evaporation. Cultivation of medicinal plants requires intensive care and management. The following point should be considered for good plant husbandry appropriate rotation of plants selected according to environmental suitability should be followed, and tillage should be adapted to plant growth. Most of medicinal plants, even today, are collected from wild. It is necessary to initiate systematic cultivation of medicinal plants in order to conserve biodiversity and protect endangered species. In the pharmaceutical industry, where the active medicinal principle cannot be synthesized economically, the product must be obtained from the cultivation of plants. Systematic conservation and large scale cultivation of the

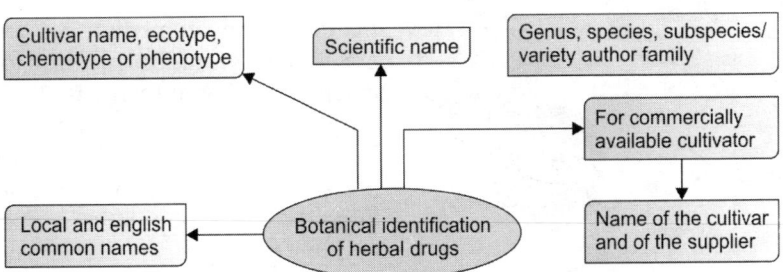

Fig. 2.5: Botanical identification of herbal drugs

concerned medicinal plants are thus of great importance. Efforts are also required to suggest appropriate cropping patterns for the incorporation of these plants into the conventional agricultural and forestry cropping systems.

Conservation agriculture referred to as resource-efficient/resource-effective agriculture should be aimed to conserve, improve and make more efficient use of natural resources through integrated management of available soil, water and biological resources combined with external inputs. It contributes to environmental conservation as well as to enhanced and sustained agricultural production.

Site Selection

The site selection plays a very important role in cultivation of plant material derived from the same species. These medicinal plants show remarkable differences in quality of plants due to influence of various factors like climate, type of soil, ecological and geographical variables, etc. These variations may be seen in physical appearance as well as in chemical constituents. Precautions should be taken to avoid risks of contamination by pollution of the soil, air or water by hazardous chemicals. The factors affecting cultivation of medicinal plants are illustrated in Fig. 2.6.

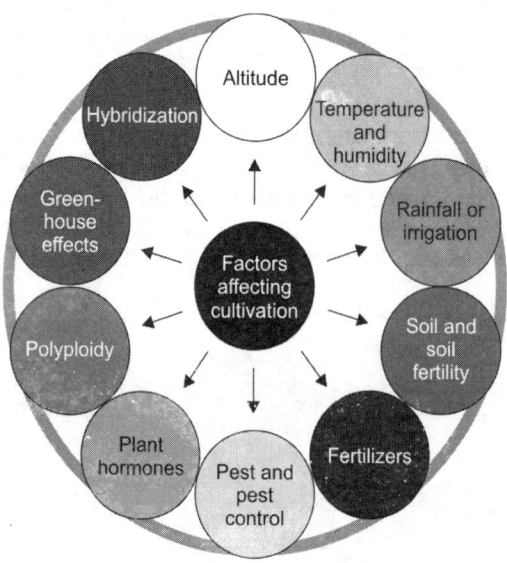

Fig. 2.6: Factors affecting cultivation of medicinal plants

Ecological Environment and Social Impact

The cultivation of medicinal plants may affect the ecological balance and, in particular, the genetic diversity of the flora and fauna in surrounding habitats. The quality and growth of medicinal plants can also be affected by other plants, other living organisms and by human activities. The introduction of non-indigenous medicinal plant species into cultivation may have a detrimental impact on the biological and ecological balance of the region. The social impact of cultivation on local communities should be examined to ensure that negative impacts on local livelihood are avoided. In terms of local income-earning opportunities, small-scale cultivation is often preferable to large-scale production, in particular, if small-scale farmers are organized to market their products jointly. If large-scale medicinal plant cultivation is or has been established, care should be taken that local communities benefit directly from, for example, fair wages, equal employment opportunities and capital reinvestment.

Climate

The climate plays a major role in cultivation, it indeed influences the physical, chemical and biological qualities of medicinal plants. The various climatic conditions include length of day, rainfall (water supply) and field temperature, duration of sunlight, average rainfall, average temperature, including daytime and nighttime temperature differences. These factors also influence the physiological and biochemical activities of plants.

Soil

Soil is the unconsolidated mineral or organic material on the immediate surface of the earth and serves as a natural medium for the growth of land plants. A soil consists of mineral matter, organic matter and pore space, which is shared by air, water and life forms. In addition to the above constituents, the soil also contains a large and varied population of micro-organism and macro-organisms. Soil is crucial for plant and life. It supports plant roots and provides essential nutrients for plant growth. Optimal soil conditions, including soil type, drainage, moisture retention, fertility and pH, will be dictated by the selected medicinal plant species and/or target medicinal plant part.

Soil fertility is a complex quality of soils that is closest to plant nutrient management. It is the component of overall soil productivity that deals with its available nutrient status, and its ability to provide nutrients out of its own reserves and through external applications for crop production. It combines several soil properties (biological, chemical and physical), all of which affect directly or indirectly nutrient dynamics and availability. Soil fertility is a manageable soil property and its management is of utmost importance for optimizing crop nutrition on both a short-term and a long-term basis to achieve sustainable crop production. Soil productivity is the ability of a soil to support crop production determined by the entire spectrum of its physical, chemical and biological attributes. Soil fertility is only one aspect of soil productivity but it is a very important one. For example, a soil may be very fertile, but produce only little vegetation because of a lack of water or unfavourable temperature. Even under suitable climate conditions, soils vary in their capacity to create a suitable environment for plant roots.

Irrigation and Drainage

Water is the preliminary requirement for medicinal plants, so irrigation and drained should be maintained and controlled as per need of the medicinal plants varieties during its various stages of growth. Water used for irrigation purposes should comply with local, regional and/or national quality standards. Need to ensure that plant under cultivation should get adequate quantity of water neither over-watered nor under-watered.

Harvest

The detailed and relevant information about harvesting of medicinal plants and species is available in national pharmacopoeias, published standards, official monographs and major reference books.

According to WHO guidelines on good agricultural and collection practices (GACP) for medicinal plants:

- Medicinal plants should be harvested during the optimal season or time period to ensure the production of medicinal plant materials and finished herbal products of the best possible quality.
- The time of harvest depends on the plant part to be used.
- The concentration of biologically active constituents varies with the stage of plant growth and development.
- The best time for harvest (quality peak season/time of day) should be determined according to the quality and quantity of biologically active constituents rather than the total vegetative yield of the targeted medicinal plant parts.
- During harvest, care should be taken to ensure that no foreign matter, weeds or toxic plants are mixed with the harvested medicinal plant materials.
- Medicinal plants should be harvested under the best possible conditions, avoiding dew, rain or exceptionally high humidity. If harvesting occurs in wet conditions, the harvested material should be transported immediatcly to an indoor drying facility to expedite drying so as to prevent any possible deleterious effects due to increased moisture levels, which promote microbial fermentation and mould.
- Cutting devices, harvesters, and other machines should be kept clean and adjusted to reduce damage and contamination from soil and other materials. They should be stored in an uncontaminated, dry place or facility free from insects, rodents, birds and other pests, and inaccessible to livestock and domestic animals.

The harvested raw medicinal plant materials should be transported promptly in clean, dry conditions. They may be placed in clean baskets, dry sacks, trailers, hoppers or other well-aerated containers and carried to a central point for transport to the processing facility.

All containers used at harvest should be kept clean and free from contamination by previously harvested medicinal plants and other foreign matter. If plastic containers are used, particular attention should be paid to any possible retention of moisture that could lead to the growth of mould. When containers are not in use, they should be kept in dry conditions, in an area that is protected from insects, rodents, birds and other pests, and inaccessible to livestock and domestic animals. The post-harvest technology of medicinal plants are shown in Fig. 2.7.

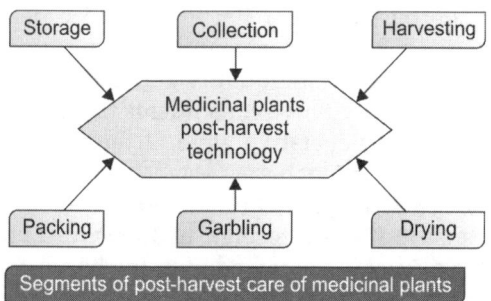

Fig. 2.7: Post-harvest technology of medicinal plants

Good Collection Practices for Medicinal Plants

Collection practices should ensure the long-term survival of wild populations and their associated habitats. Management plans for collection should provide a framework for setting sustainable harvest levels and describe appropriate collection practices that are suitable for each medicinal plant species and plant part used (roots, leaves, fruits, etc.).

Permission to Collect and Selection of Medicinal Plants For Collection (Fig. 2.8)

1. Collectors of medicinal plants and producers of medicinal plant materials and herbal medicines should prepare botanical specimens for submission to regional or national herbaria for authentication.
2. The voucher specimens should be retained for a sufficient period of time, and should be preserved under proper conditions.
3. The name of the botanist or other experts who provided the botanical identification or authentication should be recorded.
4. If the medicinal plant is not well known to the community, then documentation of the botanical identity should be recorded and maintained.

Collection

Collection practices should ensure the long-term survival of wild populations and their associated habitats.

Medicinal plant materials should be collected during the appropriate season or time period to ensure the best possible quality of both source materials and finished products. It is well-known that the quantitative concentration of biologically active constituents varies with the stage of plant growth and development. This also applies to non-targeted toxic or poisonous indigenous plant ingredients.

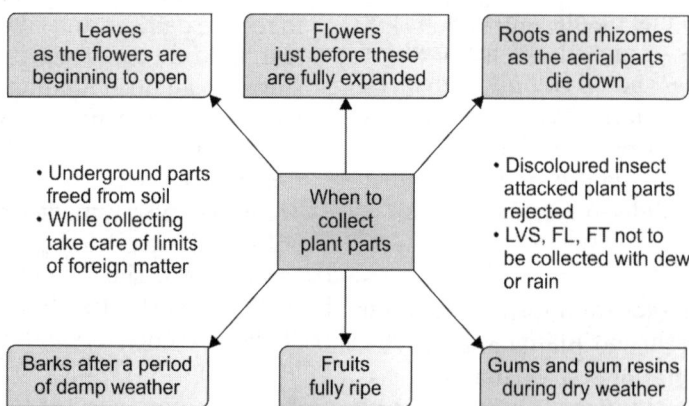

Fig. 2.8: Collection of plant parts

The best time for collection (quality peak season or time of day) should be determined according to the quality and quantity of biologically active constituents rather than the total vegetative yield of the targeted medicinal plant parts. These will vary widely from species to species. For example, while collecting roots of trees and bushes, the main roots should not be cut or dug up, and severing the taproot of trees and bushes should be avoided. Only some of the lateral roots should be located and collected.

When collecting species whose bark is the primary material to be used, the tree should not be girdled or completely stripped of its bark; longitudinal strips of bark along one side of the tree should be cut and collected. Medicinal plants should not be collected in or near areas where high levels of pesticides or other possible contaminants are used or found, such as roadsides, drainage ditches, mine tailings, garbage dumps and industrial facilities which may produce toxic emissions. In addition, the collection of medicinal plants in and around active pastures, including riverbanks downstream from pastures, should be avoided in order to avoid microbial contamination from animal waste. In the course of collection, efforts should be made to remove parts of the plant that are not required and foreign matter, in particular toxic weeds. Decomposed medicinal plant materials should be discarded. In general, the collected raw medicinal plant materials should not come into direct contact with the soil. If underground parts (such as the roots) are used, any adhering soil should be removed from the plants as soon as they are collected.

Collected material should be placed in clean baskets, mesh bags, other well-aerated containers or drop clothes that are free from foreign matter, including plant remnants from previous collecting activities.

After collection, the raw medicinal plant materials may be subjected to appropriate preliminary processing, including elimination of undesirable materials and contaminants, washing (to remove excess soil), sorting and cutting. The collected medicinal plant materials should be protected from insects, rodents, birds and other pests, and from livestock and domestic animals. If the collection site is located some distance from processing facilities, it may be necessary to air or sun-dry the raw medicinal plant materials prior to transport. If more than one medicinal plant part is to be collected, the different plant species or plant materials should be gathered separately and transported in separate containers. Cross-contamination should be avoided at all times. Collecting implements, such as machetes, shears, saws and mechanical tools, should be kept clean and maintained in proper condition. Those parts that come into direct contact with the collected medicinal plant materials should be free from excess oil and other contamination.

ORGANIC FARMING

Organic farming refers to the method by which agricultural products like food and fibre are cultivated and processed. Organic farmers aim to produce healthy food from a balanced, living soil. Organic agriculture is sustainable, keeping soils productive and alive, and helping to minimize contamination of the earth's water supplies.

Organic agriculture is a holistic production management system, which promotes and enhances agro-ecosystem health, including biodiversity, biological cycles, and soil biological activity. It emphasizes the use of management practices in preference to the use of off-farm inputs, taking into account that regional conditions require locally adapted systems.

Organic farming excludes the use of chemical fertilizers and pesticides, plant growth regulators, and livestock feed additives. Genetically modified organisms (GMOs) are not allowed in organic farming. As far as possible, organic farmers depend on crop rotation, green manure, compost, mulching, biological pest control, and mechanical cultivation to maintain productive soil and control pests.

Organic farming is based on the limited use of off-farm inputs and on management practices that restore, maintain, and enhance the environment. It is not only concerned with a product, but also with the whole system used to produce and deliver the product to the consumer. Organic agriculture practices cannot by themselves ensure that agricultural products are completely free of all contaminants. However, it is sometimes impossible for agricultural activities to avoid pollution from air, soil, water and other sources.

Organic farming is a technique, which involves cultivation of plants and rearing of animals in natural ways. This process involves the use of biological materials, avoiding synthetic substances to maintain soil fertility and ecological balance, thereby minimizing pollution and wastage. Organic farming make use of pesticides and fertilizers if they are considered natural and avoids the use of various petrochemical fertilizers and pesticides.

Organic farming is a method of crop and livestock production that involves much more than choosing not to use pesticides, fertilizers, genetically modified organisms, antibiotics and growth hormones.

Organic production is a holistic system designed to optimize the productivity and fitness of diverse communities within the agro-ecosystem, including soil organisms, plants, livestock and people. The principal goal of organic production is to develop enterprises that are sustainable and harmonious with the environment.

As per the definition of the United States Department of Agriculture (USDA) study team on organic farming—'organic farming is a system which avoids or largely excludes the use of synthetic inputs (such as fertilizers, pesticides, hormones, feed additives, etc) and to the maximum extent feasible rely upon crop rotations, crop residues, animal manures, off-farm organic waste, mineral grade rock additives and biological system of nutrient mobilization and plant protection'.

FAO suggested that 'organic agriculture is a unique production management system which promotes and enhances agro-ecosystem health, including biodiversity, biological cycles and soil biological activity, and this is accomplished by using on-farm agronomic,

biological and mechanical methods in exclusion of all synthetic off-farm inputs'.

Organic farming promotes the use of crop rotations and cover crops, and encourages balanced host/predator relationships. Organic residues and nutrients produced on the farm are recycled back to the soil. Cover crops and composted manure are used to maintain soil organic matter and fertility. Preventative insect and disease control methods are practiced, including crop rotation, improved genetics and resistant varieties. Integrated pest and weed management, and soil conservation systems are valuable tools on an organic farm.

Advantages of Organic Farming

Easy transition: One of the main advantages of organic farming is the easy transition that is mean to switch to this kind of farming from the conventional farming. There is no complexity involves in such transition for the farmer.

Production boost: The organic method of farming is the usage of crop rotation, compost pits, and manure. In traditional farming, use of pesticides and insecticides fertilizers which do not enhance the fertility of soil and to some extent these things adversely affect it.

Saving: Saving is another advantage of organic farming. There is no need to spend a lot on chemical pesticides and industrial for

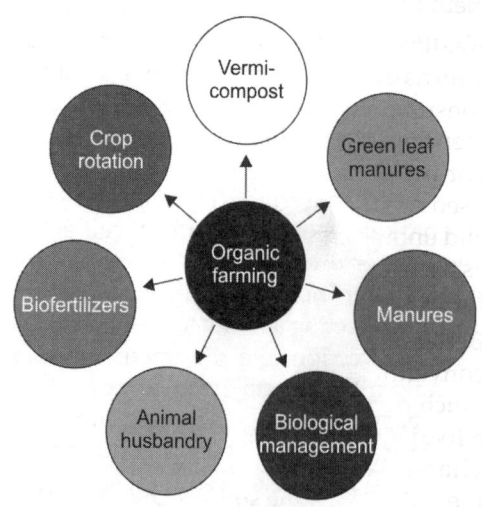

Fig. 2.9: Organic farming

organic farming. According to a study, this type of farming reduces the production costs of the farmer.

Soil nourishment: Soil nourishment is the vital advantages of organic farming. Farmer does not use the chemical in organic farming and therefore microorganisms, which are responsible for nourishment of soil, remain alive. On the other hand, in traditional farming the use of pesticides and chemical fertilizers kill them and soil does not get the essential nourishment.

Biodiversity promotion: In organic farming method care about animals is not needed. Animals can graze with freedom and live of farm. This method is based on the concept of biodiversity promotion idea, so no need to restrict animal and other organism. The best advantage of organic farming is to provide great freedom to everyone, i.e. farmer, animal, micro-organisms and many more.

Revenue generation: Another advantage of organic farming is more revenue generation. The demand of organic food is more than that of its supply and this factor boosts up the price of organic food. Therefore, when the farmers sell the organic foods in the market, then they earn more income. High income is an important advantage of organic farming due to which many farmers turn toward this method.

Healthy alternative: Organic food is a healthy alternative of traditional food. When the consumers start consuming this type of food then they notice positive change in their health. For producing organic food, a farmer never used synthetic substances which have toxic and unhealthy residual. Surely, it is considered as the biggest advantage of organic farming by the health conscious people.

Better nutrition: As compared to a longer time conventionally grown food, organic food is much richer in nutrients. Nutritional value of a food item is determined by its mineral and vitamin content. Organic farming enhances the nutrients of the soil which is passed on to the plants and animals.

Free of poison: Organic farming does not make use of poisonous chemicals, pesticides and weedicides. Studies reveal that a large section of the population fed on toxic substances used in conventional agriculture have fallen prey to diseases like cancer. As organic farming avoids these toxins, it reduces the sickness and diseases due to them.

Enhanced taste: The quality of food is also determined by its taste. Organic food often tastes better than other food. The sugar content in organically grown fruits and vegetables provides them with extra taste.

Longer shelf-life: Organic plants have greater metabolic and structural integrity in their cellular structure than conventional crops. This enables storage of organic food for a longer time.

Four Principles of Organic Farming

- **Principle of health:** Organic agriculture contributes to the health and well-being of soil, plants, animals, humans and the earth. It is the sustenance of mental, physical, ecological and social well-being. For instance, it provides pollution and chemical-free nutritious food items for humans.
- **Principle of fairness:** Fairness is evident in maintaining equity and justice of the shared planet both among humans and other living beings. Organic farming provides good quality of life and helps in reducing poverty. Natural resources must be judiciously used and preserved for future generations.
- **Principle of ecological balance:** Organic farming must be modeled on living ecological systems. Organic farming methods must fit the ecological balances and cycles in nature.
- **Principle of care:** Organic agriculture should be practiced in a careful and responsible manner to benefit the present and future generations and the environment.

The general principles of organic production include the following:

- Protect the environment, minimize soil degradation and erosion, decrease pollution, optimize biological productivity and promote a sound state of health.

⊃ Maintain long-term soil fertility by optimizing conditions for biological activity within the soil.

⊃ Maintain biological diversity within the system.

⊃ Recycle materials and resources to the greatest extent possible within the enterprise.

⊃ Provide attentive care that promotes the health and meets the behavioural needs of livestock.

⊃ Prepare organic products, emphasizing careful processing, and handling methods in order to maintain the organic integrity and vital qualities of the products at all stages of production.

⊃ Rely on renewable resources in locally organized agricultural systems.

Need of Organic Farming

With the increase in population our compulsion would be not only to stabilize agricultural production but also to increase it further in sustainable manner. The scientists have realized that the 'Green Revolution' with high input use has reached a plateau and is now sustained with diminishing return of falling dividends. Thus, a natural balance needs to be maintained at all cost for existence of life and property. The obvious choice for that would be more relevant in the present era, when these agrochemicals which are produced from fossil fuel and are not renewable and are diminishing in availability. It may also cost heavily on our foreign exchange in future.

The key characteristics of organic farming include:

⊃ Protecting the long-term fertility of soils by maintaining organic matter levels, encouraging soil biological activity, and careful mechanical intervention.

⊃ Providing crop nutrients indirectly using relatively insoluble nutrient sources which are made available to the plant by the action of soil micro-organisms

⊃ Nitrogen self-sufficiency through the use of legumes and biological nitrogen fixation, as well as effective recycling of organic materials including crop residues and livestock manures.

⊃ Weed, disease and pest control relying primarily on crop rotations, natural predators, diversity, organic manuring, resistant varieties and limited (preferably minimal) thermal, biological and chemical intervention.

⊃ The extensive management of livestock, paying full regard to their evolutionary adaptations, behavioural needs and animal welfare issues with respect to nutrition, housing, health, breeding and rearing.

⊃ Careful attention to the impact of the farming system on the wider environment and the conservation of wildlife and natural habitats.

Organic Farming Practices

Crop Rotation

Crop rotation involves planting different crop species at different times and locations on the same field. Rotating crops improve the tilth or structure of the soil. This practice reduces soil erosion and pest build up, promotes soil fertility and spreads out financial risk in case a crop fails. Crop rotations result in an increase in soil microbial activity, which may increase nutrient availability, including phosphorus. Yields are usually 10 to 15% higher with the practice of crop rotation than monoculture.

Cover Cropping

A cover crop is any crop grown to provide a cover for the soil. They can be annual, biennial, or perennial herbaceous plants grown in a pure or mixed stand during all or part of the year. This practice helps loosen compacted soil through root growth, improves water filtration, and prevents soil erosion by wind and water. Cover crops also help suppress weeds by keeping the sun from reaching weed seeds and reduce insect pests and diseases.

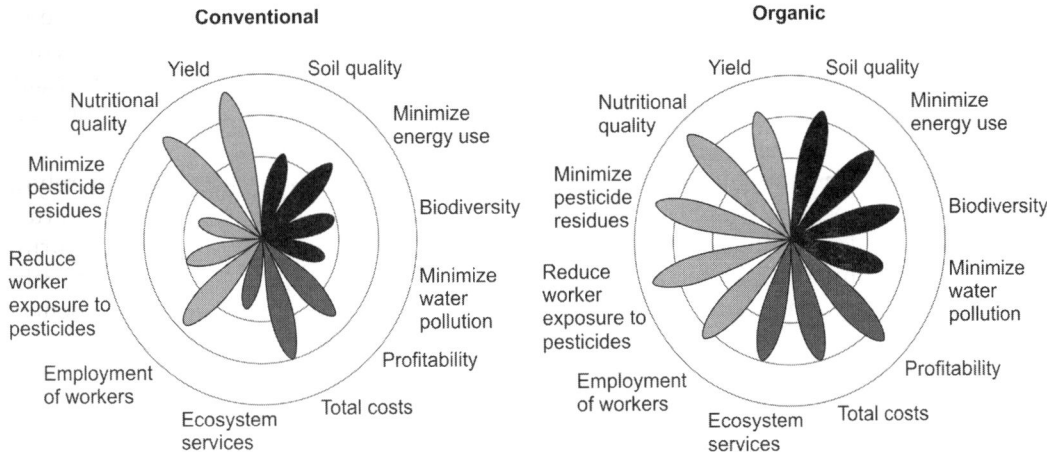

Fig. 2.10: An assessment of organic farming relative to conventional farming illustrates that organic systems better balance the four areas of sustainability: Production, environment, economics, and social well-being.

Green Manures

A cover crop that is tilled into the soil while it is still green is referred to as a green manure. It helps to add organic matter and nutrients to the soil. When a green plant is incorporated into the soil, it contains high amounts of nitrogen and moisture and becomes a food source for soil microorganisms and earthworms. Additional advantages from using green manures include the suppression of weeds and soil borne diseases.

Animal Manures

Manure can be applied to the field in either a raw or composted form. Raw manure contributes nutrients to the soil, adds organic matter, and encourages biological processes in the soil. Composting of manure is best, since the heat created during composting may kill most of the contaminants, thus the risk of pathogens related to food safety is minimized or eliminated. Composting reduces biomass volume, thus facilitating ease of transportation.

Weed Management

Crop rotations, removing weeds before seed set and reproduction, and not allowing weeds onto the farm, can also be used to reduce weed populations. Mulches help suppress weeds by preventing light from reaching them or by drastically decreasing the amount or quality of light reaching the weed seed or leaf. Certain mulches with naturally occurring chemicals can help prevent the germination of weed seeds.

Pest Management

Maintaining an ecological balance is the main goal under the organic system instead of complete eradication of pests. Ecological balance is maintained through the use of beneficial insects, predatory or parasitic mites, and spiders to keep pest populations down. 'Beneficial' insects include lady beetles and various wasps, as well as certain nematodes that are used for insect control. Where severe infestations occur farmers can use non-toxic pesticides that are not as harsh as conventional pesticides. These non-toxic pesticides include soaps, pheromones (used as bait for traps and to disrupt mating cycles), botanical plant extracts such as neem, and sulfur for control of foliar diseases and in some cases, mites.

Livestock Management

Livestock feed must be completely organically produced, including pasture and forage, contain no urea or manure, and should have no animal slaughter by-products. Provide suitable housing, pasture conditions, and sanitation practices to animals to reduce the occurrence and spread of diseases and parasites. Reduce the occurrence and spread of parasites and diseases by providing suitable housing, pasture conditions, and sanitation practices to animals. Move animals regularly to fresh pasture and use other preventative methods rather than routinely dosing the animals with drugs to control parasite in farm animals. Livestock may not be treated with antibiotics, any animal drug, and any animal drugs used to promote growth, including hormones. Animals must be provided with access to the outdoors, shade, shelter, exercise areas, fresh air, and direct sunlight based on the type of animal, stage of production, climate, and the environment.

PEST AND PEST MANAGEMENT IN MEDICINAL PLANTS

Pests are injurious to human health and/ or farmers economic efforts. Pesticides are mixtures of chemicals that are used for killing, repelling, mitigating or reducing pest damage. Pests organisms include insects, rodents, nematodes, fungi, weeds, birds, bacteria, viruses, etc., which damage the crops and reduce yield.

Classification of Pesticides

Pesticides may be classified according to:
 a. The target pest species (Fig. 2.11).
 b. Their chemical constitution (Fig. 2.12)
 c. Their site of action
 a. **Classification based on target pest species:** The following explains the classification of pesticides based on target organisms.
 b. **Classification based on chemical nature:** A classification based on the chemical composition or structure of the pesticide is the most useful for analytical chemists, for example:
    ➲ *Chlorinated hydrocarbons and related pesticides*: Hexachlorocyclohexane (HCH) or benzene hexachloride (BHC), lindane, methoxychlor
    ➲ *Chlorinated phenoxyalkanoic acid herbicides*: 2,4-D, 2,4,5-T
    ➲ *Organophosphorus pesticides*: Carbophenothion (carbofenotion), chlorpyrifos

and methylchlorpyrifos, coumaphos (coumafos), demeton, dichlorvos, dimethoate, ethion, fenchlorphos (fenclofos), malathion, methylparathion, parathion
 ➲ *Carbamate insecticides*: Carbaryl (carbaril)
 ➲ *Carbamoyl benzimidazoles*: Benomyl, carbendazim
 ➲ *Dithiocarbamate fungicides*: Ferbam, maneb, nabam, thiram, zineb, ziram
 ➲ *Amino acid herbicides*: Glyphosate
 ➲ *Inorganic pesticides*: Aluminium phosphide, calcium arsenate
 ➲ *Miscellaneous*: Bromopropylate, chloropicrin, ethylene dibromide, ethylene oxide, methyl bromide, sulfur dioxide
 ➲ *Pesticides of plant origin*: Tobacco leaf extract, pyrethrum flower, and pyrethrum extract; derris and lonchocarpus root and rotenoid
 c. **Classification based on site of action:** By segmenting insecticides/acaricides and fungicides separately, insecticides/ acaricides can be classified on the basis of their routes of entry into the body system of the target pest. They can be grouped as follows:
    i. Stomach poisons
    ii. Contact poisons
    iii. Systemic poisons
    iv. Fumigants
    i. **Stomach poisons:** Stomach poisons enter the body of the pest through the mouth during feeding into the digestive tract from where these are absorbed into the systems. Stomach poisons are more effective against chewing insects and useful in controlling insects with siphoning or sponging types of mouth parts (for example, housefly). Examples: Dieldrin, sulfur, lead arsenate, etc.
    ii. **Contact poisons:** These poisons enter the body directly through the cuticle by contact with the treated surface of the foliage, stem, etc. These poisons act on the nervous system of the pest. These may also be applied directly on to the body of the pest as a spray or dust. Examples: Benzene hexachloride,

dichloro diphenyl trichloro ethane, endrin, quinalphos, carbamates, etc. Some of the known pesticides derived from plants also have contact action. Examples: Pyrethrum, rotenone, sabadilla, nicotine, etc.

iii. **Systemic poisons:** These poisons are applied on the plants' surface such as the foliage, green parts of the stem, and near the roots from where these are translocated into the plant tissues. Most of the systemic poisons act as stomach poisons, or both as stomach and contact poisons. The parts of the plant where these poisons have been translocated become lethal to the pests feeding on

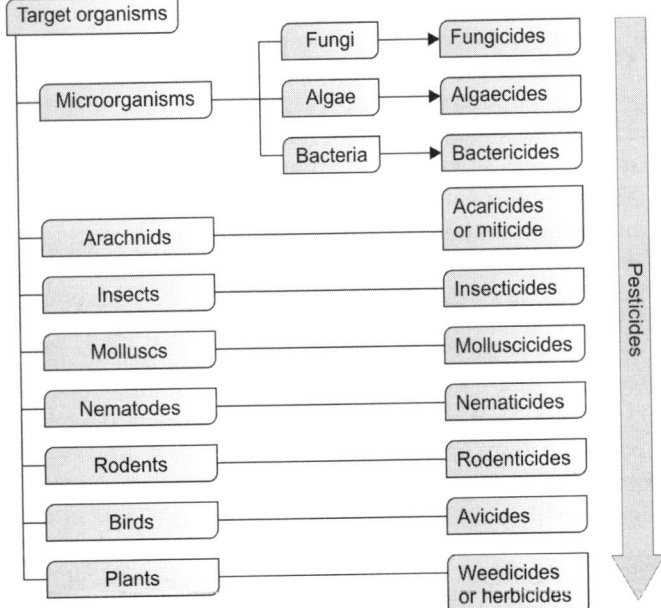

Fig. 2.11: Classification based on target pest species

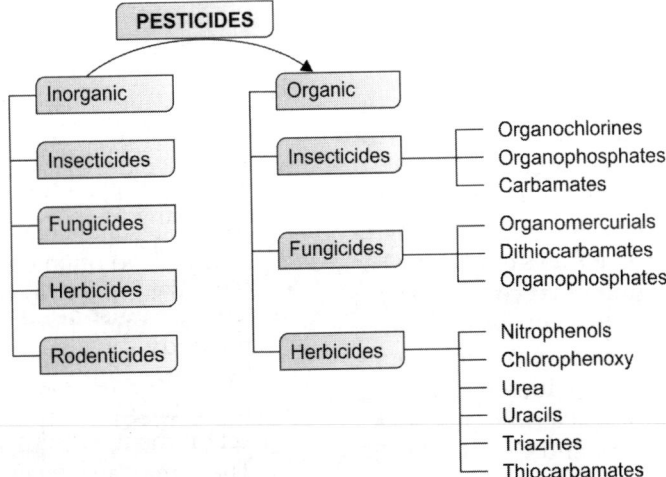

Fig. 2.12: Classification based on chemical nature

these parts of the plants. Systemic poisons are more effective against sucking pests. They have a selective action with a little effect on the predators and parasites directly, unless acting through the food chain. Translocation of these poisons takes place mostly through xylem vessels. Examples: Demeton-o-methyl, phosphamidon, monocrotophos, phorate. carbofuran. dimethoate, mevinphos, aldicarb, etc.

iv. **Fumigants:** Fumigants are volatile poisons and enter the body of the pests through the respiratory system. These are widely used in controlling stored grain pests. All types of pests can be killed by fumigants irrespective of the types of mouthparts provided a gas-tight atmosphere is ensured (i.e. fumigants are nonselective). Even for soil pests such as nematodes, fumigation is effective. Examples: Dichlorvos. hydrogen cyanide, methyl bromide, paradichlorobenzene, ethylene dichloride, carbon tetrachloride, naphthalene, nemagon, aluminum phosphide, etc.

BIOPESTICIDES/BIOINSECTICIDES

Biopesticides are certain types of pesticides derived from such natural materials as animals, plants, bacteria, and certain minerals. For example, canola oil and baking soda have pesticidal applications and are considered biopesticides.

Microbial pesticides consist of a microorganism (e.g. a bacterium, fungus, virus or protozoan) as the active ingredient. Microbial pesticides can control many different kinds of pests, although each separate active ingredient is relatively specific for its target pest. For example, there are fungi that control certain weeds, and other fungi that kill specific insects. The most widely used microbial pesticides are subspecies and strains of Bacillus thuringiensis (Bt.) Each strain of this bacterium produces a different mix of proteins, and specifically kills one or a few related species of insect larvae. While some Bts control moth larvae found

on plants, other Bts are specific for larvae of flies and mosquitoes. The target insect species are determined by whether the particular Bt produces a protein that can bind to a larval gut receptor, thereby causing the insect larvae to starve.

Plant-Incorporated-Protectants (PIPs) are pesticidal substances that plants produce from genetic material that has been added to the plant. For example, scientists can take the gene for the Bt pesticidal protein, and introduce the gene into the plant's own genetic material. Then the plant, instead of the Bt bacterium, manufactures the substance that destroys the pest. The protein and its genetic material, but not the plant itself, are regulated by EPA.

Biochemical pesticides are naturally occurring substances that control pests by non-toxic mechanisms. Conventional pesticides, by contrast, are generally synthetic materials that directly kill or inactivate the pest. Biochemical pesticides include substances, such as insect sex pheromones that interfere with mating as well as various scented plant extracts that attract insect pests to traps. Because it is sometimes difficult to determine whether a substance meets the criteria for classification as a biochemical pesticide, EPA has established a special committee to make such decisions.

Advantages of Biopesticides

1. Biopesticides are usually inherently less toxic than conventional pesticides.
2. Biopesticides generally affect only the target pest and closely related organisms, in contrast to broad spectrum, conventional pesticides that may affect organisms as different as birds, insects, and mammals.
3. Biopesticides often are effective in very small quantities and often decompose quickly, thereby resulting in lower exposures and largely avoiding the pollution problems caused by conventional pesticides. When used as a component of Integrated Pest Management (IPM) programs, biopesticides can greatly decrease the use of conventional pesticides, while crop yields remain high.

Applications

Biopesticides are biological or biologically-derived agents, which are usually applied in a manner similar to chemical pesticides, but achieve pest management in an environmentally friendly way. With all pest management products, but especially microbial agents, effective control requires appropriate formulation and application. Biopesticides for use against crop diseases have already established themselves on a variety of crops. A major growth area for biopesticides is in the area of seed treatments and soil amendments. Fungicidal and biofungicidal seed treatments are used to control soil borne fungal pathogens that cause seed rots, damping-off, root rot and seedling blights. They can also be used to control internal seedborne fungal pathogens as well as fungal pathogens that are on the surface of the seed. Many biofungicidal products also show capacities to stimulate plant host defence and other physiological processes that can make treated crops more resistant to a variety of biotic and abiotic stresses.

QUALITY ASSURANCE IN MANUFACTURE OF HERBAL MEDICINE

The appropriate quality assurance system should be applied for the manufacture of herbal medicine. Various analytical tools are available for quality assurance includes atomic absorption (AA), gas chromatography (GC), mass spectroscopy (MS), high performance liquid chromatography (HPLC), capillary electrophoresis (CE) to characterize sample of herbal medicine. The quality assurance is the mandatory perquisite to check identity, purity of starting material, maintenance of storage and purity.

Quality and Stability of Herbal Preparations

Standardization of herbal medicines is the process of prescribing a set of standards or inherent characteristics, constant parameters, definitive qualitative and quantitative values that carry an assurance of quality, efficacy, safety and reproducibility (Fig. 2.13).

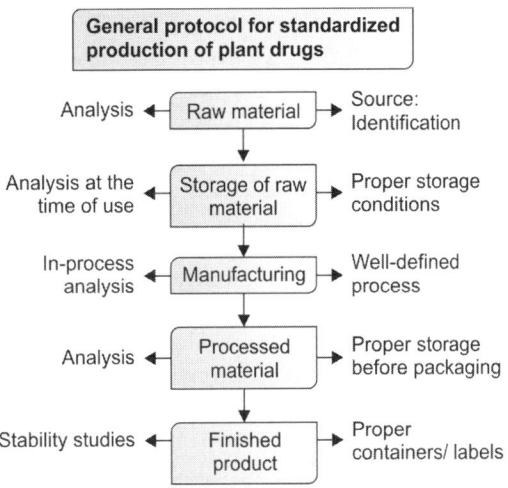

Fig. 2.13: General protocol for standardized production of plant drugs

It is the process of developing and agreeing upon technical standards. Specific standards are worked out by experimentation and observations, which would lead to the process of prescribing a set of characteristics exhibited by the particular herbal medicine.

Hence standardization is a tool in the quality control process.

Several factors which influence the quality of herbal drugs include:

1. Herbal drugs are usually mixtures of many constituents.

2. The active principle(s) is (are) in most cases unknown.

3. Selective analytical methods or reference compounds may not be available commercially.

4. Plant materials are chemically and naturally variable.

5. Chemo-varieties and chemo-cultivars exist.

6. The source and quality of the raw material are variable.

The methods of harvesting, drying, storage, transportation, and processing (for example, mode of extraction and polarity of the extracting solvent, instability of constituents, etc.) also affect herbal quality.

Quality control and the standardization of herbal medicines also involve several other steps:

1. Source and quality of raw materials,
2. Good agricultural practices and
3. Good manufacturing practices.

These practices play a pivotal role in guaranteeing the quality and stability of herbal preparations.

The quality of a plant product is determined by the prevailing conditions during growth, and accepted good agricultural practices (GAP) can control this. These include seed selection, growth conditions, fertilizers application, harvesting, drying and storage. In fact, GAP procedures are integral part of quality control.

Safety and quality assurance measures are needed to overcome these problems and to ensure a steady, affordable and sustainable supply of medicinal plant materials of good quality. In recent years, good agricultural practices have been recognized as an important tool for ensuring the safety and quality of a variety of food commodities, and many Member States have established national good agricultural practice guidelines for a range of foods. However, quality control for the

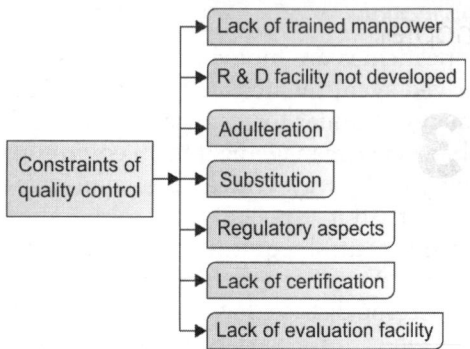

Fig. 2.14: Constraints in quality control

cultivation and collection of medicinal plants as the raw materials for herbal medicines may be more demanding than that for food production. The constraints in quality control of herbal medicines are enlisted in Fig. 2.14.

It was recommended that WHO should give high priority to the development of globally applicable guidelines to promote the safety and quality of medicinal plant materials through the formulation of codes for good agricultural practices and good collection practices for medicinal plants. It was envisaged that such guidelines would help to ensure safety and quality at the first and most important stage of the production of herbal medicines.

3 | Indian Systems of Medicine

- Basic principles involved in ayurvedic system of medicine
- Basic principles involved in siddha system of medicine
- Basic principles involved in unani system of medicine
- Basic principles involved in homeopathy system of medicine
- Preparation and standardization of ayurvedic formulations, viz. aristas and asawas, ghutika, churna, lehya and bhasma.

BASIC PRINCIPLES INVOLVED IN AYURVEDIC SYSTEM OF MEDICINE

Ayurveda, the 'Science of life,' or longevity, is more than 5,000 years old holistic alternative science from India. Ayurveda often called **Mother of all Healing** and is aimed at the physical, mental and spiritual well-being of human beings.

According to tradition, Ayurveda is one of the great gifts of the sages of ancient India to mankind, the teachings of Ayurveda were recollected by Brahma, the Lord of Creation, as he awoke to begin the task of creating the universe. It stems from the ancient Vedic culture and was taught from many thousands of years in an oral tradition from accomplished masters to their disciples.

Ayurveda is the original contribution of India (Bharatha) to the world and treats man as a whole—which is a combination of body, mind and soul. Ayurveda transcends the period of this universe, stretching beyond the concept of time itself, having no beginning and no end. Brahm taught this knowledge to *Daksa Prajapati* (the protector of all beings), whom in turn taught it to the *Asvini Kumaras* (the twin holy physicians), who in turn taught it to *Indra* (King of the Gods).

Ayurveda is a complete medical system. It places a great emphasis on prevention and encourages maintenance of health in all its aspects; physical health, mental balance, spiritual well-being, social welfare, environmental considerations, dietary and lifestyle habits, daily living trends, and seasonal variations in lifestyle, as well as treating and managing specific diseases. Ayurveda teaches respect for nature, appreciation of life and the means to empower the individual. It is holistic medicine at its best.

History of Ayurveda

Ayurvedic system is that Brahma reminded it to Prajapati, who handed it down to *Atreya Punarvasu*, etc. In the Rig Veda there is reference to the first divine physician Rudra and of how the *Aswini Kumaras* cured *Chyavana* of senility. The *Atharva Veda* is considered to have originated later than the Rig Veda, and contains a description of diseases and the cure of them. Those are basis of Ayurvedic learnings and practice even today. **Charaka samhita**, *Susruta samhita* and *Astangahrdaya* are the most important and popular among these samhitas, those are compiled approximately between 1500 BC to 500 AD. In these texts all eight clinical branches of Ayurveda are described together with its fundamental principles.

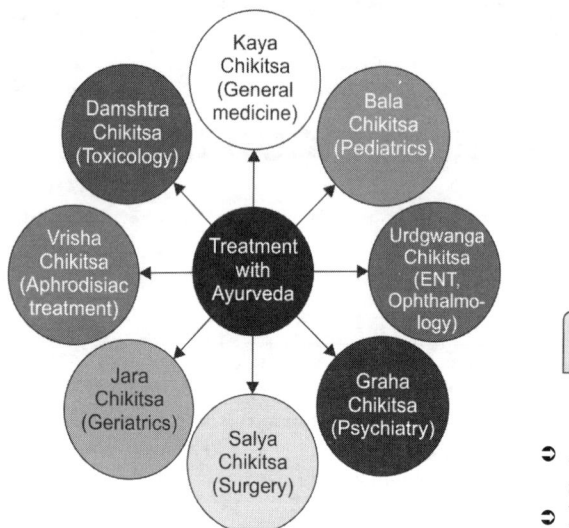

Fig. 3.1: Eight segments of treatment with ayurveda

Principles of Ayurveda

All material forms including body are composed of Panchamahabhutas (five subtle elements), namely *Prithivi* (earth), *Jala* (water), *Agni* (fire), *Vayu* (air) and *Akasha* (ether/space).

- ➲ The earth element represents mass in the material.
- ➲ Water provides the capacity of union of more than one principle.
- ➲ Fire provides heat which remains always in latent form with every material phenomenon.

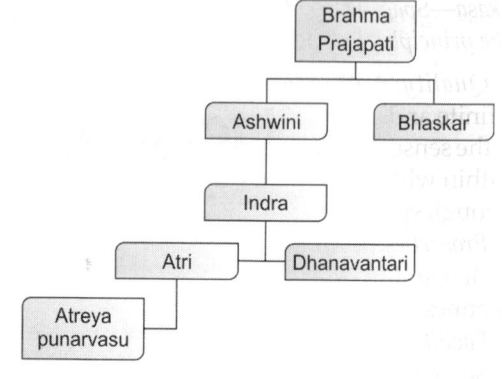

Fig. 3.2: History of ayurveda

- ➲ Air provides movements and ether provides space.
- ➲ Every material phenomenon, no matter how small it is, is composed of these elements. This remains always in some motion, which is characteristic of air element. This particle is surrounded by some space which is ether element. The segments and principles are given in Figs 3.1 and 3.3.

The Samkhya Philosophy and The Pancha-mahabhuta: The Five Primordial Elements

Samkhya means 'enumeration'. This refers to the categorization of evolution into a set of 24 principles (*tattvas*). According to Samkhya philosophy, *Prakriti* or nature is responsible for all manifestation and diversity. *Prakriti* is an eternal reality and the first cause of the universe.

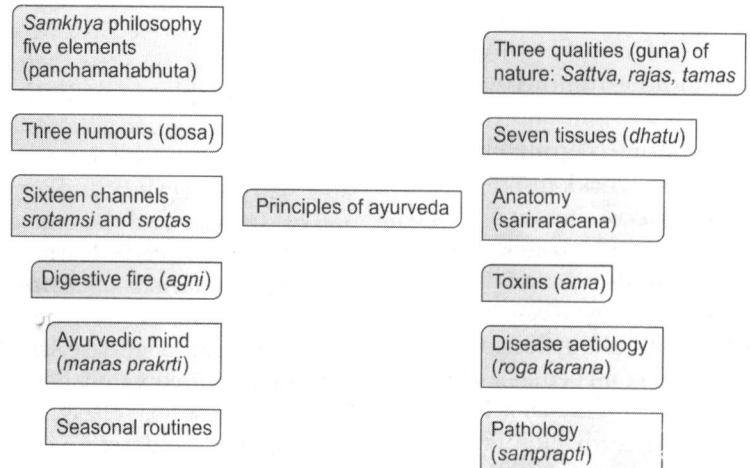

Fig. 3.3: Principles of ayurveda

Akasa—Space/Ether:
The principle of all pervasiveness

Quality: Expansive, light, subtle, clear, infinite and all-encompassing space. It relates to the sense of sound and the ear. It is the arena within which 'life' takes place. Sound travels through space.

Properties: Soft, light, subtle, porous, profuse

Action: Provides natural space, looseness, openness

Facilitates: Hearing sound

Sense organs: Skin

Substance: Light, abundant, and ethereal substance

Example: Hollow and light foods

Vayu—Air: The principle of motion

Quality: Like the wind, light, mobile, clear, rough, dry and erratic. It relates to the sense of touch, the nerves and the skin.

Properties: Light, clear, mobile, cool, dry, porous and subtle

Action: Offers motion or movement, evaporation, and dryness

Facilitates: Touching

Sense organs: Skin

Substance: Dry and airy substances

Example: Biscuits, cookies, cabbage, beans, and apples

Tejas—Fire: The principle of illumination

Quality: Hot, sharp, fluid, penetrating, luminous, light ascending and dispersing. It relates to the sense of sight and the eyes. Light and perception travel through the eyes due to the metabolic activity of light-sensitive photons in the eyes.

Properties: Rough, hot, sharp, dry, subtle, weightless, and controls the luster of the body

Action: Produces heat and light; assists in digestion and growth; aids eyesight

Facilitates: Sight

Sense organs: Eyes

Substance: Anything combustible and spicy

Example: Chilies, ginger, pepper, clove, cumin

Jala/Ap—Water: The principle of cohesion

Quality: Fluid, heavy, wet, lubricating, cool, soft, cohesive and stable. Relates to the sense of taste and the tongue. Flavours and tastes are only perceptible when the tongue is wet.

Properties: Cool, moist, and heavy fluid, sweet and pungent, sour and salty taste. Action—gives glossiness, increases fluid content, offers softness and coolness

Facilitates: Tasting

Sense organs: Tongue

Substance: Anything liquid, fluid or watery

Example: Drinks, soups, melons, cucumber

Prthvi—Earth: The principle of cohesion

Quality: Thick, dense, solid, hard, heavy and stable. Relates to the sense of smell and the nose. Earthy and dense objects give off smells.

Properties: Heavy, static, compressed, rough, cathartic, and slow

Actions: Offers firmness and strength, gives nutrient, and offers softness and coolness to the skin.

Facilitates: Smelling

Sense organs: Nose

Substance: Anything solid and heavy

Examples: Fried foods, cheese, cakes, banana

The Universal Constituents: Guna

The three qualities (*guna*) of nature: *Sattva, rajas, tamas.*

Prakrti is held together in a balanced state of tension by three universal constituents (*guna*). These three aspects combine in variable proportions to create manifest phenomena.

- *Sattva* refers to qualities of balance, equality, and stability. It is light (*laghu*) and luminous (*prakaśika*) and holds the capacity for happiness. It is conscious and intelligent, moving inwards and upwards.
- *Rajas* generate activity, change, and disturbance. It is mobile (*cala*) and excitable (*upastambhaka*). It is the motivator and expressor. It has a centrifugal force causing dispersion and disintegration. This movement away from the centre causes pain.
- *Tamas* is the immobile, still, and stuck quality. It is heavy (*guru*) and causes obstruc-

tion or lack of perception (*varana*). It moves down and is responsible for degeneration. Through the force of tamas there is delusion and confusion. *Tamas* has a bad reputation for being a negative, downward-bearing energy. To perceive it negatively is to misinterpret its role.

The *gunas* exist 'for a single purpose, like that of a lamp'. That they possess contradictory properties does not give any one quality priority over another. They come together for the single purpose of liberation (*moksa*), the ultimate goal of all *darsana*(s) and conscious existence. They are one force, with different aspects unfolding to be mutually 'supportive', 'productive', and 'subjugative.' They help each other and keep each other in check. They are accountable to each other; maintaining, encouraging, or restraining. Their varied proportions explain the variety in nature.

Dosas: The Three humours (Table 3.1)

Dosa is the ayurvedic term that generically describes our inherited traits, individual characteristics and tendencies. This refers to such things as the body frame, eye colour, digestive capacity, emotional balance as well as disease tendencies.

Dosa is described and translated in many different ways—'constitution', 'functional principle', 'humour'. There is no single word that accurately translates the meaning of breadth implied to '*dosa*' when it is used in different situations. 'Constitution' implies one's fixed and life-long inherited health, 'functional principle' implies an invisible catalytic active, and 'humour' is often used because of the European cultural familiarity with the Greek humoral system of medicine. 'Humour' comes from the Latin '*umere*' meaning 'moist' and again refers to the constitutional make up as well as something that can increase or decrease in volume as well as quality.

These three principles, namely Vata, Pitta and Kapha are most important phenomena in Ayurveda, as these produce good and ill effects on the entire system depending on their normal or abnormal state.

Table 3.1: Health effects of doshas		
Vata (air and space)	*Balance*	*Imbalance*
• It refers to movement of space and air within the body, by passing information particles and gases pass through the body. • It includes brain, nervous system, joints, colon and larger intestinal tract.	• Inspiration • Emotional balance • Good digestion • Good complexion • Clear mind and • Enthusiasm	• Insomina • Poor memory • Cough fatigue • Diarrhoea • Constipation • Sexual disorders • Arthritis
Pitta (fire and moisture)	*Balance*	*Imbalance*
• It refers to transformation, moisture and fire within the body. • It includes metabolism, digestion, liver, gall bladder and small intestine.	• Good digestion • Good eyesight • Sweating • Strong heart • Motivation	• Indigestion, addictions, anemia, heart attack, acne, skin cancer
Kapha (earth and water)	*Balance*	*Imbalance*
• It refers to strength, structure, earth, water within the body. • It includes bones, immune system, reproductive system, cognitive function and joint lubrication.	• Immune responses • Lymphatic movement • Fluid joint movement • Protecting brain	• Obesity • Food sensitivity • Slow digestion • Swelling • Headache • Irritability

Vata: This is kinetic principle, responsible for all the movements in body. The word Vata has its origin from Sanskrit root 'Va' denoting movements. This principle is characterized by lightness, dryness, roughness, nonsliminess, coldness, mobility and fineness. Thus it produces and maintains these qualities in body. When provoked it abnormally increases these qualities to cause a disease. It performs respiration, body movements, circulation, excretion sensations (conveying the sensory impulses), speech, foetal developments and all others that require any kind of movement. Though Vata is active throughout the body, but at certain regions in the body its actions are prominent such as colon and low back. These regions are known as its seat. **Vata** constricts and causes tightening, spasm and constriction in the channels and tissues; e.g. asthma, where the bronchioles are tight and the restricted airways cause wheezing, shortness of breath and coughing.

Pitta: This is a thermal principle. The word Pitta gets its origin from Sanskrit root 'Tapa' denoting 'heat'. This is characterized by slight oiliness or moisture, heat, liquidity, sourness, pungentness and sharpness. Thus in its normal state this produces and maintains these qualities in the body. When provoked it causes abnormal increase in these qualities and produce a disease. Pitta is responsible for digestion, catabolism, energy, heat, vision, valour, anger, hunger, thirst and intelligence. Its activities are prominent in stomach, intestine and umbilical region. **Pitta** expands and causes inflammation and swelling in the channels and tissues; e.g. colitis, where the intestinal lining is inflamed and swollen causing digestion to be irritated.

Kapha: This is a hydroic and uniting principle originated from Sanskrit root 'Ka' denoting 'water'. Shleshma' another synonym of this is originated from Sanskrit root 'Shlish' denoting 'embracing'. This is characterized by oiliness, coldness, heaviness, sweetness, stability, sliminess or stickiness and softness. Thus in its normal state it produces and maintains these qualities in the body and when provoked it may cause abnormal increase in these qualities and may produce a disease. It is responsible for anabolism, strength, potency, stability, lubrication, nourishment, tolerance and contentment. Its activities are prominent in chest, throat, head, joints and upper stomach. *Kapha* accumulates and causes adhesions and wastes to build up in the channels and tissues; e.g. atherosclerosis, where fatty deposits of plaque build up on the arterial lining which obstructs and blocks blood flow.

The Seven Tissues (Dhatu) (Fig. 3.4)

The *dhatus* represent the essence of the whole concept of that particular tissue. These are basic essential structural components, namely *Rasa* (plasma, leucocytes and thrombocytes), *Rakta* (red blood cells), *Mamsa* (muscle tissue), *Medas* (fat tissue), *Asthi* (bone and cartilage), *Majja* (marrow and brain), *Shukra* (male reproductive substances).

Sixteen Channels (Srotamsi and Srotas)

These are the spaces where the substances are transported or exchanged. These may be very gross, very small, of varying shapes. All the vessels, hollow spaces, tubular structures and all extra and intracellular spaces are the Srotas. The Srotas may be innumerable but for practical purposes thirteen types of Srotas have been emphasized. Seven Srotas are meant to transport seven Dhatus, those are in transforming phase. Three are meant to transport three Malas. Remaining three are for Prana (respiration), Anna (food) and Udaka (water).

16 channels that carry air (*pranavahasrotas*), food (*annavahasrotas*), water (*ambuvahasrotas*), faeces (*puri-savahasrotas*), urine (*mutravahasrotas*), sweat (*svedavahasrotas*), milk (*stanyavahasrotas*), menstrum (*artavavahasrotas*), and the mind (*manovahasrotas*).

Anatomy (Sariraracana)

Ayurvedic anatomy is based purely on observation and clinical experience. It traces an intricate body that has connecting principles from the smallest atom to the interrelationship of the whole being (Table 3.2).

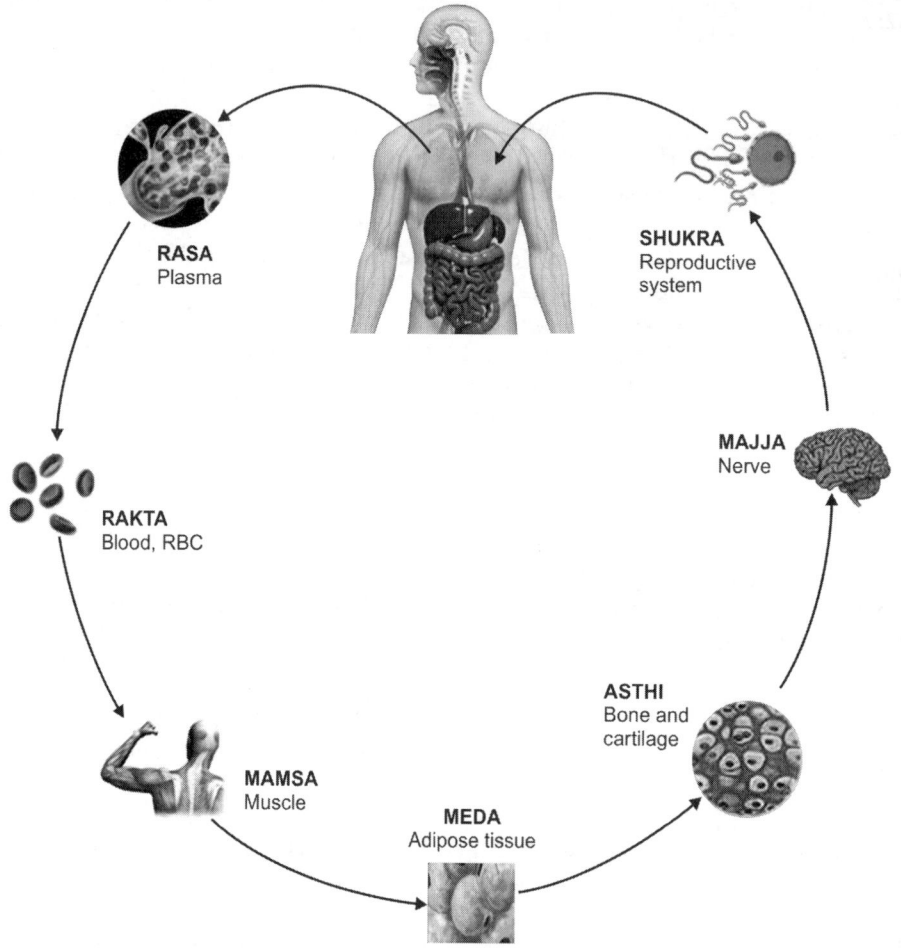

Fig. 3.4: Seven dhatus of ayurveda

The Digestive Fire: Agni

Agni is seen as the metaphor for all metabolic functions in the body. It includes the digestive function, sense perception, cellular metabolism and mental assimilation. *Agni* is involved in many functions: Absorption, assimilation, metabolism, digestion, perception, taste, touch, hearing, vitality, clarity, alertness, regular appetite, chemical combustion. It gives *ojas* or immunity, a sparkle in the eyes and lustre to the whole body.

Agni is the ayurvedic word for fire or 'little fire.' As the sun is the 'big fire,' the little fire is that which burns in our bodies and digests the food we eat. Digestion is an essential piece of ayurvedic medicine. Proper digestion gives us

energy via assimilation of nutrients. Through this assimilation process, we receive our life force, our prana. On a deeper level, agni is the medium through which the body, mind and consciousness are bridged together.

This principle acts at three levels and therefore described as three types: First type Jathargni acts for initial digestion of food. Second type Bhutagni acts after initial digestion to separate five elemental fractions in the food. The ultimate product in the process in 'Ojas', the vital essence or sustainor of the life. During this process some byproducts and wastes are also produced those have significant role in health as well as disease. Some general ways to help increase agni:

Table 3.2: Ayurvedic anatomy

Sarira	Body	That decays
Tvac	Skin	Seven layers
Asaya	Viscera or hollow organs	Where food, wastes and liquids are contained
Nadis	Nerves	Spread out from the brain and spinal cord
Dhamanis	Arteries	Carrying blood away from the heart
Kesikas	Hairlike	Capillaries linking the arteries and veins.
Hrdaya	Heart	*Rasa* and *rakta*, is affected by their state of vitality
Pephra	Lungs	Responsible for purifying blood of impurities
Pliha	Spleen	Seat of blood where red blood cells are produced
Yakrt	Liver	Channels carrying blood
Kloma	Pancreas	
Grahani	Small intestine	Pitta digests food
Pakvasaya	Large intestine	
Basti	Urinary bladder	
Vrkka	Kidneys	
Yoni	Female genital tract	Including the uterus
Garbhasaya	Uterus	
Anda/ Antarphala	Ovaries	

1. **Follow a daily routine:** A daily routine helps to reduce stress and it gets you more in touch with your body. When the body is at ease, it will become hungry at *natural* intervals.

2. **Meditate regularly:** Stress is very disruptive to the digestion process. If our bodies are exposed to chronic stress, it can ultimately affect assimilation of minerals and vitamins, and even, disrupt the hormonal process.

3. **Pranayama:** Specifically, kapalbhati breathing (or breath of fire). Our agni is directly affected by our oxygen intake. Pranayama or yogic breathing exercises, allow the deep tissues to be refreshed. Including pranayama in a daily routine is highly suggested. Kapalabhati breathing is especially helpful in supporting digestion as it tones the digestive organs, improving agni and the appetite.

4. **Participate in daily exercise:** Although ayurveda suggests different types of exercise and intensity depending on your dosha, in general, daily exercise at an 80 percent effort is suggested.

5. **Dietary cleanse:** Cleansing detoxes, repairs and rejuvenates the tissues, thereby supporting agni and it is ever important work.

Toxins: Ama

Ama is the unmetabolised waste that is not utilized by the body. It can be formed from foods that are absorbed but then not used, or that are undigested and create fermentation and imbalance all three *dosa*. Ama means unripe, uncooked, immature and undigested. It takes the form of *kapha*: Sticky, heavy, viscous, slimy, unctuous, wet, cold and is sweet. It causes blockage of the channels (*srotorodha*), mucus congestion, loss of strength, lack of movement and reverse flow of *vata*, accumulation of wastes, oedema, low digestive fire, bloating, constipation, itchy anus, thick tongue coating, sluggish and slippery pulse, lack of enthusiasm and stagnation in the tissues.

The Ayurvedic Mind: Manas Prakrti

The Ayurvedic concept of mind is both broad and illuminating. Not only does it include mental activity but also a consciousness that is housed in the heart, 'the heart is indispensable for normal mental and physical activities as the entire waking consciousness rests there'. Mind is built from different aspects. *Buddhi* is intellect and is really like a mirror reflecting universal consciousness as it cognizes and clarifies. It is the digestive system of the mind as it discriminates between different aspects of mental 'nutrition'. *Sadhaka pitta* corresponds to *buddhi*. *Manas* are that which conceptualises, analyses and interacts between our inner subconsciousness and our experience of the outer world.

It includes memory and the ability to recall (*smrti*) events. *Tarpaka kapha* relates to memory. *Ahamkara* is our 'I' maker and identity former that personalizes every experience. There is also *citta* that is considered to be consciousness and awareness. *Prana* connects these different aspects into something that is known as *antah-karana*, the inner active.

Disease Aetiology (Roga Karana)

The cause of disease involves many different aspects from the imbalance of the *dosa*, to an imbalanced digestive fire (*agni*), to the accumulation of ama, to the obstruction of the channels (*srotas*) and the deficiency of the *dhatu*. Internally, the movement of disease is from the mind to the body where the attitudes of greed, fear, anger, grief, arrogance, jealousy and hatred become somatised in the tissues. Ayurveda clearly states that 'desire' (*raga*) is a feeling that generates pathological 'heat' in the mind which generates these other emotions. Desire creates an obsessive attachment to various objects and this locks us into a cycle of grasping and unfulfillment. When stimulated, strong emotions create an agitating 'friction' that irritates digestion, the nervous system and then the tissues, which can then cause a range of diseases. For example, in the pathology of fever (*jvara*), accumulated heat leaves its residence in the stomach and invades the rasa tissues and disease-causing heat spreads throughout the system.

Seasonal influences (*parinama*) such as climate change, geographic peculiarities or merely the annual cycle of seasonal variation can disturb the *dosa* and cause disease.

These may involve:

- *Atiyoga*: Excessive indulgence
- *Hinayoga*: Inadequate indulgence
- *Mithyayoga*: Inappropriate indulgence.

Other causes are:

Inherited: These are the tendencies that we are born with. It is as though we have a constitutional threshold which, depending on various factors, may or may not manifest; e.g. psoriasis, diabetes or heart disease.

- **Trauma:** Accidents affecting the body and mind.

- **Divine:** Intervention on a subtle level from the divine realm, e.g. magical spells.
- **Environmental:** Availability of food, water and shelter has an obvious impact on health.
- **Karmic:** Disease has resulted from actions in another life.

Pathology and The Six Stages of Disease: Samprapti

The health of the system is optimized when the *dosa* are flowing out of the body and the *dhatu* are nourished. The stages enumerated below describe how this healthy process becomes imbalanced.

Accumulation (Caya)

Any of the causes of disease listed above can cause the *dosa* to accumulate at their site: *Kapha* gathers in the stomach with signs of sluggish digestion, lethargy, paleness, heavy limbs and heavy head. *Pitta* accumulates in the small intestine with signs of acidity in the stomach, yellowing of the eyes, urine and stool, sensations of heat, irritability, bitter taste in the mouth and loose and smelly stools. *Vata* collects in the large intestine with signs of bloating, gas, constipation, pebble-like stool, dryness, cramps, coldness, anxiety and insomnia. At this stage the disease is relatively easy to remove.

Aggravation (prakopa)

Prakopa is further aggravation of the symptoms mentioned above. The increased severity of doshic irritation starts to aggravate the viscera (*amas´aya*) that are containing the *dosa*. The aggravated *dosa* is still relatively easy to remove via the digestive pathway.

Spreading (prasara)

The disorder reaching maximum capacity in their respective sites the accumulated and aggravated *dosa* now cross their threshold and spill over into other parts of the body. They rebel in any direction that they can force themselves. Via the *rasa* and *rakta* tissues they spread to other associated locations. *Kapha* spreads to the lungs causing a wet cough, breathing difficulties and vomiting, to the joints causing swelling and the bowel causing mucus in the stool. *Pitta* spreads to the skin causing inflammatory skin problems, eyes causing redness, stomach causing nausea and bowels causing burning diarrhoea. *Vata* spreads to the skin causing dryness, joints causing cracking and pain, air passages causing a dry cough and the intestines causing further pain and obstructed motions. The *dosas* are still relatively easy to clear from the system even at this stage.

Relocation (stha-na sam sraya)

The irritated *dosa* now fixes in a set location, usually associated with an area of weakness or one of the areas of the body that the particular *dosa* is associated with, e.g. *kapha* in the lungs, stomach, joints, mucous membranes and fluid parts of the body; *pitta* in the liver, eyes, skin, intestinal lining or glands; *vata* in the ears, joints, bones, skin or colon. This is when the premonitory signs of disease start; the weak cough and slight wheeze that can develop to full-blown asthma. The *dosas* are now difficult to clear and require deep cleansing techniques and *pancakarma* to be removed.

Manifestation (vyakti)

The disease now manifests as an identifiable disease such as diabetes, asthma or diverticulosis. The disease is set and cure is often difficult.

Expression of unique characteristics of the disease (BHEDA)

Once a disease is fixed at a site it takes on a life of its own and its dominant features are reflected by the primary causative *dosa*. For example, eczema caused by *vata* is dry, fissured and itchy; by pitta is red, inflamed, bleeding and hot; and that caused by kapha is wet, suppurating, itchy and oedematous.

BASIC PRINCIPLES INVOLVED IN SIDDHA SYSTEM OF MEDICINE

Siddha system of medicine is a complex system of science as it has included in the works of medicine, an extensive set of pharmacopoeia and Alchemy. As per Siddha concept, human body is the replica of Universe; food and drugs irrespective of their origin are made of five basic elements, namely earth, water, fire, air and ether. The proportion of the elements present in the drugs vary and their preponderance or otherwise is responsible for their actions and therapeutic results. According to basic siddha concept the *Pancha bhootham* (five elements), *Arusuvai* (six tastes) and *Uyirthathu* (three humours) are interlinked. That is, predominance of fire and water element expresses salty taste, fire and air element expresses pungent taste, both are having hot potency. Similarly, the earth element with water element produces sweet tasted substance which can vitiate Iyya humour. In siddha system chemistry had been found well developed into a science auxiliary to medicine. Moreover, the knowledge in this system is not static and is inherently dynamic in nature and evolves in response to challenges posed by the environment. The practitioners of siddha applies several procedures divided into processes such as calcinations, sublimation, distillation, fusion, separation, conjunction or combination, fermentation, purification, incineration of metals, liquefaction and extraction for the preparation of formulations. The term siddha means achievement. The saintly personalities known as—Siddhars. Siddha system of medicine owes its origin to the Dravidian culture. It is mainly therapeutic in nature. The principle and doctrines of this system, both fundamental and applied, have a close similarity to Ayurveda, hence like Ayurveda this system also believes that all objects in universe are made up of five basic elements, viz. earth, water, sky, fire and air. The diagnosis is made through pulse reading, body colour, voice, examination of urine and tongue. The medicines mentioned in pharmacopeia of siddha mainly include the mercury, sulphur, iron, copper, bitumen, arsenic and vegetable poisons.

Siddhars have recommended certain basic guidelines to be followed for healthy living which includes observation of certain regimen as mentioned in '*Pini anugaa vidhi*' literally meaning rules that help prevent disease. Their concept of 'Kaayakarpam' for prevention of diseases is highly admirable as it makes one's body resistant to infections. Their concepts pertaining to Habitat, Seasons, Diet (*Thinai/ Nilam, Naal ozhukkam, Kaala ozhukkam, Unavu*) are preventive as well as adaptive.

Pini Anugaa Vidhi (Prevention of Diseases)

'Thinna mirandulae sikka adakkaamar...'
　　　　　　　　　　—Therayar

'Paal unbhom; ennai perin veneerir kulippom…'
　　　　　　　　　　—Therayar

The above verses illustrate the do's and don'ts in all our activities. These preventive measures against illness are summarized below:

   i. Drink boiled water
  ii. Take meals twice a day
 iii. Take diluted buttermilk and melted ghee
 iv. Take sufficient quantity of milk and milk products
  v. Never eat root tubers except yam
 vi. Never consume food that was prepared the previous day
 vii. Always have food after feeling hungry
viii. Always consume sour curd
 ix. Practice walking after a good diet
  x. Drink water at the end of meals
 xi. Use hot water while taking oil bath.
 xii. Never suppress any natural urge
xiii. Never sleep during daytime
xiv. Always indulge in healthy sexual acts
 xv. Take emetic medication once in six months
xvi. Take purgative medication every four months in a year
xvii. Take snuff medications eight times in a year
xviii. Shave hairs weekly
xix. Take oil bath once in every four days
 xx. Apply eye medications once in three days
xxi. Never smell fragrance during midnight
xxii. Never reside close to dust and articles related to dust
xxiii. Never sleep under a tree shade or near a burning lamp

These rules when followed strictly, keep away death. These simple preventive principles have an in-depth scientific value though they were designed much before the advent of modern science. These rules have been followed as routine custom through several generations.

Kaaya Karpam (Gerontology)

'Udambar azhiyil uyirar azhivar…'
　　　　　—Thirumandiram by Thirumoolar

The above quote states that maintaining a healthy body is essential as it holds a healthy mind which is required to attain salvation. Adoption of preventive techniques to maintain one's body health helps to retain youthfulness and attain spiritual perfection.'Kaaya Karpam' (rejuvenation and longevity) was practiced as a preventive measure against illness. Practicing Kaaya Karpam also provides acquired immunity (*seyarkai vanmai*) to our body. *Kaaya Karpam* acts in 2 ways, i.e. prevention against disease and restoration of health during illness. Thus, it is preventive as well as constructive. *Kaaya Karpam* is studied under three categories, viz.

   i. Mooligai karpam
  ii. Thathu and seeva karpam
 iii. Yoga karpam
   i. **Mooligai karpam:** This deals with drugs used in siddha for *Kaaya Karpam* (rejuvenation and longevity) which have plant origin, e.g. fruits of *Phyllanthus emblica* (amla).
  ii. **Thathu and seeva karpam:** This deals with minerals and animal products used as Kaaya Karpam preparations. This also includes 'Muppu' (A combination of three salts)—a very unique preparation in Siddha.
 iii. **Yoga karpam (Yogic practices):** *Yogasanam, Pranayamam, Iyamam,* and *Niyamam* fall under this category.

Siddhars have described several yogic postures which are aimed at developing and maintaining the wellness of the body and soul. Saint Thirumoolar has detailed several yogasanas (yogic postures) in his valuable work titled 'Thirumandiram'.

Concepts Regarding Habitat and Season

Siddha science which visualizes man as a microcosm, believes that planetary changes and natural rhythms that result in six seasons/ year (*perum pozhuthu*) and six periods/day (*siru pozhuthu*) also result in corresponding physiological changes in other creatures living in macrocosm, viz. the Universe.

> '*Andathil ullathae Pindam,*
> *Pindathil ullathae Andam ...*'
> —Satta Muni Gnanam

This verse means that the environment is same within and outside our body which indicates that the body physiology must be tuned according to the habitat and the prevailing season as an adaptive and preventive measure for one's health.

Accordingly, Siddhars designed basic regimen in harmony with the habitat (Nilam) and seasons (Pozhuthu).

BASIC PRINCIPLES INVOLVED IN UNANI SYSTEM OF MEDICINE

The Unani system of medicine originated in Greece, Hippocrates is known as the father of this system of medicine. The theoretical framework of Unani medicine is based on his teachings. There were other Greek scholars who followed in his footsteps to enrich this system considerably. In the 9th century, the Arabic and Persian physicians imbibed Unani system of medicine.

This system was developed during the Arab civilization. It is known as—Unani Tibb system of medicine. The system is based on the concept of four humors put forth by Hippocrates. According to this concept the cause of sickness is the harmony or disharmony of the four humors. The four humors present in body are blood, phlegm, yellow bile, and black bile. According to Galens concept the temperament of individual may be sanguine, phlegmatic, choleric, or melancholic, any change in temperament causes change in health state of individual. The humor are assigned temperament, thus the blood is hot and moist, phlegm is cold and moist, yellow bile is hot and dry and black bile is cold and dry. Thus the Unani Tibb system temperament of individual is considered as the basis of pathology, diagnosis and treatment of disease.

According to the principles of Unani medicine, disease is a natural process, its symptoms are the reactions of the body to the disease, and the primary function of the Unani physician is to aid the natural forces of the body. Unani medicine is based on the 'Humoral Theory', which presupposes the presence of four Humors—Dam (blood), Balghum (phlegm), Safra (yellow bile) and Sauda (black bile)—in the body. The temperaments (mizaj) of people are expressed by the words sanguine, phlegmatic, choleric and melancholic, according to the amount of each of these four humors prevalent in the human body respectively. The humors themselves are assigned temperaments—blood is hot and moist, phlegm is cold and moist, yellow bile hot and dry, and black bile cold and dry. There is a unique humoral constitution in every person representing his state of health. To maintain a healthy balance, there is a power of self-preservation or adjustment called Quwwat-e-Mudabbira (medicatrix naturae). A weakening of this power causes imbalance in the humoral composition and causes disease. What the Unani physician actually tries to do is to prescribe a medicine, which helps the body to regain this power and thereby restore the humoral balance. Correct diet and digestion is integral to this system. The Unani system of medicine emphasizes on diagnosing a disease through nabz (pulse), baul (wine), baraz (stool), etc. Besides, it gives due importance to the surroundings and the ecological conditions on the state of health of humans. The six essential prerequisites (called Asbab-e-Sitta Zarooriya) for the prevention of diseases in the Unani system are air, food and drinks, bodily movement and response, psychic movement and response, sleep and wakefulness, and excretion and retention. Various types of treatment are employed in Unani system. These include regimental therapy (Ilaj-bit-Tadbeer), dietotherapy (Ilaj-bit-ghiza), pharmacotherapy

(Ilaj-bit-Dawa) and surgery (Jarahat). The regimental therapy comprises venesection, cupping, diaphoresis, diuresis, Turkish bath, massage, cauterization, purging, emesis, exercise, leeching, etc. Dietotherapy tries to treat certain ailments by administration of specific diets or by regulating the quantity and quality of food. Pharmacotherapy deals with the use of naturally occurring drugs, mostly herbal, though drugs of animal and mineral origin are also used. In Unani medicine, single drugs or their combinations in raw forms are preferred over compound formulations. The naturally occurring drugs used in this system are usually free from any side effects while drugs that are toxic in crude form are first processed and purified in many ways before use so as to make them free of any kind of side effects.

BASIC PRINCIPLES INVOLVED IN HOMEOPATHY SYSTEM OF MEDICINE

The Law of Similars

The 'law' or 'principle' of similars (or similarity) constitutes the main acquisition of homeopathy and the basis for its understanding, though today, as we shall see, it is no longer regarded as a universal 'law' valid in all cases. According to this principle, which already figured in certain medical and philosophical systems of antiquity (Hippocrates, St. Augustine, Paracelsus), but which was rediscovered mainly by the German physician Samuel Hahnemann (1755–1853), a disease can be cured by administering the patient a substance which, in healthy human subjects, causes symptoms similar to those of the disease (hence the dictum 'similia similibus curentur'). In practice, this means that:

a. Every biologically active substance (drug or remedy) produces characteristic symptoms in healthy bodies which are susceptible to being in some way perturbed by that substance.
b. Every sick body expresses a series of characteristic symptoms which are typical of the pathological alteration of that particular subject.

c. The healing of a sick body, characterized by the progressive disappearance of all symptoms, may be obtained by targeted administration of the drug which produces a similar symptom picture in healthy bodies.

For example, the homeopath, starting from the observation that bee venom causes a characteristic wheal with pain and erythema mitigated by the application of cold compresses, administers bee extract in a homeopathic presentation (diluted and dynamized) to cure patients presenting urticaria with wheals and pain similar to those of bee stings, albeit of different etiology. In its early formulations, the remedy is prescribed not only on the basis of the diagnosis, this being of secondary importance, but also by seeking with the utmost care the correspondence between the symptomatological picture of the disease and the symptom picture caused by a given substance in healthy subjects. If the match is substantial or perfect (the remedy is a 'simillimum' or 'most similar medicine'), the administration even of only a minimum dose of the remedy triggers a reaction in the patient which leads, often after an initial aggravation of the disease, to healing. The healing, then, would appear not to be a direct suppressive effect of the substance administered ('law of opposites'), but the result of the subject's reaction, due, according to classic homeopathy, to the action of the so-called 'vital force'. For the purposes of identifying the remedies most suited to the individual circumstances, the homeopathic pharmacopoeia has been gradually built up right from the early days of homeopathy on the strength of tests of a 'toxicological' type, performed by administering small doses of a whole variety of substances to healthy volunteers and painstakingly recording the symptomatological results as soon as a reaction is observed. These experiments, called drug provings, have been collected in the so-called materia medicas (encyclopedias of drug effects), which have been and are being continually updated and contain data on hundreds of different mineral, vegetable, and animal substances. The materia medicas have been and continue to be checked, modified, and updated also on the basis of the experience gained with patients. In fact, for a particular remedy to be introduced and used in the homeopathic pharmacopoeia, it is not enough for it to be capable of causing symptoms in a healthy subject; it must show proven ability to cure patients presenting the symptoms detected during the provings. Another aspect which should be stressed, in as much as it is a recurrent feature of the literature, is the fact that, in this patient, thorough analysis of the symptoms (called repertorization), a great deal of importance is attributed to the more unusual symptoms, which may reveal a particular type of individual reactivity, as well as to those in the psychological sphere, which are regarded as no less important than the somatic symptoms. Correct repertorization, in fact, requires an analytical and at the same time a holistic all-embracing approach to the sick person. According to homeopathic methodology, it is only in this way that the correct choice of drug indicated for each patient can be made. The concept of the choice of drug on the basis of the law of similars can be illustrated here with an example. Three patients with influenza are treated with three different remedies: The first patient presents chills, is anxious and restless, and wants to be covered up and drink fresh water; his eyes and nose are producing an irritating mucous runny discharge causing reddening of the nose and upper lip; he also presents gastrointestinal symptoms (vomiting and diarrhea). The remedy indicated for this patient is Arsenicum album (arsenic). The second patient with influenza in the same epidemic feels tired and lethargic, experiences chills, and complains of occipital headache; he wants something to warm his back, wants to stay stock-still in bed, and not make any kind of physical effort. In this case the remedy indicated is Gelsemium (yellow jasmine). The third person has influenza with a feverish temperature and the most striking symptom is achiness throughout the entire body, as if all his bones were broken. The remedy indicated in his case is Eupatorium perfoliatum (boneset). All three patients have contracted the same influenza virus, but their individual reactions to the disease are different and thus their treatment has to be differentiated. To the homeopathic practitioner, a symptom like fever says very little, in that it is a very nonspecific reaction of the inflammatory process, but he will take great care to analyze the types of fever and the concomitant symptoms as a guide to establishing the right remedy: Fever with heat sensations, reddening of the skin, perspiration, a very high pulse rate, a throbbing headache, mydriasis, and photophobia indicates that the patient needs Belladonna (deadly nightshade). Fever of sudden onset after a cold, with anxiety even to the point of fearing death, reddening of the skin (without perspiration), and a strong, hard pulse, but also with miosis, intense thirst, and an aversion to blankets, indicates Aconitum (monkshood) as the remedy of choice. It is thus particular details and subtle differences which guide the doctor in his choice.

PREPARATION AND STANDARDIZATION OF AYURVEDIC FORMULATIONS VIZ ARISTAS AND ASAWAS, GHUTIKA, CHURNA, LEHYA AND BHASMA

Ayurvedic medicines are widely practiced in modern India and are becoming popular day by day throughout the world as compared with allopathic medicines because it has no side effects. Ayurvedic treatment is non-invasive and non-toxic, so it can be used safely as an alternative therapy or along-side conventional therapies. There are number of plants, herbs present in nature which are useful in classical formulations.

According to the ancient ayurvedic texts, the main goal of ayurveda is prevention as well as promotion of the body's own healing capacity. Ayurveda mainly concentrates on the main cause of disease and cures it from root level. Ayurveda has been used to treat different disorders like acne, allergies, asthma, anxiety, arthritis, chronic fatigue syndrome, colds, colitis, constipation, depression, diabetes, flu, heart disease, hypertension, immune problems, inflammation, insomnia, nervous disorders, obesity, skin problems, and ulcers.

Ayurvedic Formulations

The evolutionary phases of dosage forms followed by ayurveda starting from crude plant material are mentioned in the following paragraphs. Different ayurvedic herbal drug preparations mentioned in ayurvedic literature are mentioned Fig. 3.5.

Swarasa (fresh juice): The evolution of liquid orals started from the administration of freshly obtained juices of plant material. To obtain fresh juices, green herbs are crushed and the juice is expressed by squeezing the crushed material. The product is referred to as swarasa.

Kalka (wet bolus): In this method, the crushed fresh plant material is administered as such, without expressing the juices.

Kwatha (decoction): One part of coarsely powdered herb is boiled with 16 times its weight of water in an earthen pot over a mild fire until the liquid is reduced to one-fourth or one-eighth of the original quantity, depending upon the nature of the plant material.

Hima (cold infusion): The plant material is dried and coarsely powdered. As and when required, the powder is soaked in plain water for a defined period. Then it is filtered, the marc is squeezed, and the combined filtrate is used.

Phanta (hot infusion): As a further advancement of hima, the phanta method was adopted. This method uses boiled water for obtaining a hot infusion.

Solids: Anjana, churna, mansa potli, utkarika, kshara, gutika, guda, dhumravarti, puplika, prithuka, mandura, modaka, rasakriya, vati, varti, shashkuli, saktu, bhasmas, rasaushadhis.

Semisolids: *Oral:* Odana (rice preparation), kalka, krishara, avaleha.

Topical: Lepa, upnaha (poultice), tilapishta, patrasveda, madhucchishta (beeswax).

Liquids: *Oral:* Taila, ghrita, asava/arishta, arka, kwatha, kshirapaka, takra, phanta, hima,

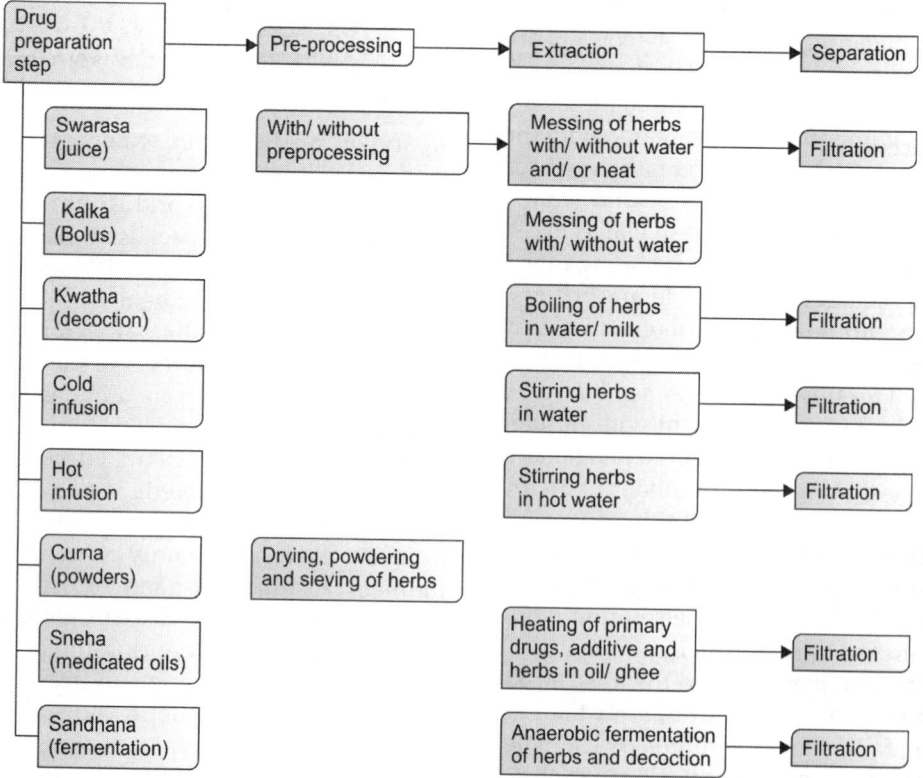

Fig. 3.5: Different ayurvedic herbal drug preparation mentioned in ayurvedic literature

swarasa, peya, phanita, manda, manasa rasa, yusha, vesavara, vilepi, madya

Topical: Ashchyotana, karna purana.

Fumes: *Dhumrapana, dhupana.*

Asava and Arishtas

Asava and Arishta are alcoholic preparations. Former is made with decoctions of herbs in boiling water while later is prepared by directly using fresh herbal juices or decoction to undergo fermentations. These are unique liquid dosage forms that contain self-generated alcohol.

Arishtas are made with decoctions of herbs in boiling water while asavas are prepared by directly using fresh herbal juices. These are unique liquid dosage form that contains self-generated alcohol. Arishtas are classical ayurvedic preparations typically used as digestive and cardiotonic. The arishta (fermented decoction) and Asava (fermented infusion) are considered as a unique and valuable therapeutics in ayurveda, due to their medicinal value, sweet taste and easy availability. The manufacturer and sell of arishtas and asavas occupies an important place in the ayurvedic pharmaceutical industry.

Asava-Arishta formulations are better known as hydro-alcoholic formulations, self-generated alcohol during this biomedical fermentation process can reach in between 4–12% v/v, and due to its improved aromatic properties and palatability these formulations has better patient acceptability. These traditionally fermented formulations has several merits over other ayurvedic medicines, like due to self-generated alcohol has better preservation quality with ageing.

Benefits of Asava-Arishta Formulations

1. Self-generated alcohol and hydrolyzing enzymes released by yeasts aids extraction of phytochemicals from raw herbals
2. Self-generated alcohol gives pleasing organoleptic properties and dramatically improves palatability of the preparation
3. Palatability improvement ensures patient compliance and hence clinical outcome

4. Alcohol is considered as 'Yogvahi' meaning facilitate faster and even distribution of drug in body
   ➤ Self-generated alcohol improves bio-availability of drug molecules
5. Self-generated alcohol acts as a preservative, asava-arishta preparation last for several years, without special storage conditions
6. Preservation benefits availability of herbs independent of seasonal availability of the botanical drugs
   ➤ Microbial transformation may reduce toxicity of phyto ingredients
7. Microbial transformation increases chemical diversity in the formulation, which is crucial for its clinical action over the raw drug
8. Biochemical transformation makes the drug available in its metabolized or activated form, which translates into quick action.

Examples: Dasamoolaarishtam, Amruthaarishtam, Kutajaarishtam, Draakshaarishtam, Abhayaarishtam, Balarishtam, Devadaarvaarishtam, Asokaarishtam, Jeerakaarishtam, Khadirashtam, Karpoorasavam, Pippalyaaadi asavam, Punarnavaasavam, Usiraashtam Aravindaarishtam, Patrangaasavam.

Method of Preparation of Arishta

The basic pieces of equipment required for the preparation of Arishta are—earthen pot, sufficiently large and strong with a glazed exterior or glaze, porcelain jar of suitable size, a lid of correct size to close the vessel, a cloth ribbon to seal the vessel, a paddle-like stirrer, a clean cloth of fine and strong texture for filtering, a vessel for boil the drugs. The major components are divided into four types according to their specific role in the process. This includes the main herb from which decoction is taken out as the case may be. They yield drugs which are pharmacologically and therapeutically much important in the given medicine and the name of these medicines is derived from these herbs denoting their importance. The flavouring agents are herbs besides contributing to the flavour of the medicine have their own pharmacological action too. The fermentation initiator provides inoculums for the fermentation to start. The medium of sugar is required for fermentation.

If the drug is dry and is to be used in the preparation of asava, it is coarsely crushed and added to the water to which the prescribed quantities of honey, jaggery or sugar are added. If it is an Arishta, a decoction is obtained by boiling the drugs in the specified volume of water. The water used should be clean, clear and potable.

When the extract is obtained, the sugar, jaggery and/or honey are added and completely dissolved. Sometimes any one or more of these sugary substances omitted if so directed in the recipe. In the case of sugar, it should be pure, white cane sugar. The jaggery should be of sweet taste and at least one year old. The honey should be genuine. The flavouring agents are coarsely powdered and added to the sweetened extract. Too fine a powdered of the flavouring agent is undesirable as it causes sedimentation in the prepared medicine and its filtration is difficult. The earthen pot intended for keeping the medicine to ferment is tested for the weak spots and cracks and similarly a lid is also chosen. The internal surfaces of the pot and the lid are wiped with the clean dry cloth and cow's ghee is smeared to surface to prevent oozing out of the contents when poured and kept for fermentation. The pot should be perfect before ghee is smeared and if it be moist, ghee will not stick and penetrate the pours. When the pot or the jar is ready, the sweetened and flavoured drug extract is poured into it up to the capacity. This unfilled space provides room for the fermenting liquid when it rises up frothing and evolving a large amount of gases. Otherwise, the medium may damage the container and flow out. Now the inoculum is to be added to initiate fermentation. As we know the process of fermentation necessitates the presence of fermenting microorganisms known as yeast. In the preparation of alcoholic medicaments in the ayurvedic systems, the inoculums of yeast come from the flowers which contain the wild species of yeast. Finally, the vessel is closed and sealed. Sealing is done by winding around a long ribbon of cloth smeared with clay on one surface. When sealing the blank surface of the ribbon should line the rim of the vessel and lid and the clay side should be external. After sealing, the vessel is placed in a dark place without much circulation of air. The vessel is left undisturbed for a month and then opened. The medicine is filtered and taken for use.

Merits of The Process

The benefits of fermented herbal products which are reproduced below:

- Fermentation removes most of the undesirable sugars from plant material, makes the product more bio-available and eliminates side effects such as gas and bloating.
- Fermentation extracts a wider range of active ingredients from the herb than any extraction method since the menstruum undergoes a gradient of rising alcohol levels.
- Yeast cell walls naturally bind heavy metals and pesticide residues and, therefore, act as a natural cleansing system.
- Not only does fermentation remove contaminants, it can also lower the toxicity of some of the toxic components in plants.
- Fermentation actively ruptures the cells of the herb, exposing it openly to the menstruum and bacteria have enzymes that break down cell walls to further assist in the leaching process. Fermentation also creates an active transport system that moves the dissolved constituents from the herbal material to the menstruum.

Application of Asava/Arishta Technology in New Drug Discovery

The ayurvedic dictum with regard to *asava arishtas* that 'older is better' needs to be scientifically evaluated. The process of preparing *asava arishtas* appears to involve:

1. Slow hydro-alcoholic extraction at room temperature of crude plant material particles floating in the liquid. Since the particle size of the plant material floating in the liquid is small, the effectiveness of

extraction may be higher because of the larger surface area.

2. During the process, if the product is kept for a prolonged period, the probability of development of analogues of some of the pure chemical compounds of the plant material is high.

With a view to enhance the success rate of isolation of pure 'druggable' compounds from medicinal plants, it is advised to start from 2- to 3-year-old self-fermented preparations than from solvent extracts. The chances of successful isolation of effective therapeutic compounds using this approach may be high and need to be evaluated.

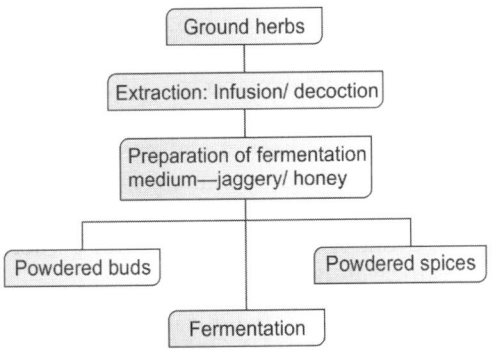

Fig. 3.6: Method of preparation of arishta

Standardization of Asava/Arishta

It generally involves the following parameters.

1. **Organoleptic parameters:**
   a. Color of sample
   b. Odor of sample
   c. Taste of sample
   d. Determination of pH of sample
2. **Physical parameters:** These parameters are for standardization of drug material:
   a. Determination of foreign organic matter
   b. Determination of ash value
      ⊃ Total ash value
      ⊃ Acid-insoluble ash
      ⊃ Water-soluble ash
      ⊃ Sulfated ash
   c. Determination of extractive value:
      ⊃ Alcohol-soluble extractive value
      ⊃ Water-soluble extractive value
   d. Determination of moisture content

e. Determination of physical constants:
   ⊃ Melting point
   ⊃ Boiling point
   ⊃ Refractive index
   ⊃ Optical rotation
f. Determination of specific gravity
g. Determination of solid content
h. Determination of alcohol content

3. **Chemical parameters:** Chemical parameters involve the following parameters in chemical evaluation:
   a. *Alkaloids:* Dragendorff's test
   b. *Glycosides:* Molish test
   c. *Flavonoids:* Shinoda test
   d. *Phenolic:* Lead acetate test
   e. *Tannins:* Ferric chloride test
   f. *Steroids:* Salkowski reaction
   g. *Amino acids:* Ninhydrine test
   h. *Carbohydrates :* Fehling's test, Benedict test

4. **Toxicological parameters:** These involve following parameters:
   a. Pesticides residue
   b. Heavy metal
   c. Microbial contamination

Avaleha or Lehya

Avaleha or Lehya is a semi-solid preparation of drugs, prepared with addition of jaggery, sugar or sugar-candy and boiled with prescribed juices or decoction.

The Lehya should neither be hard nor a thick fluid. When pulp of the drugs is added and ghee or oil is present in the preparation, this can be rolled between the fingers.

These preparations generally have:

1. Kasaya or other liquids,
2. Madhur dravya (sweetening agents) like jaggery, sugar, sugar candy and honey
3. *Prakshepa dravyas (additives):* These are herbals added to the Avaleha to increase its potency, palatability or to improve organoleptic properties. There are two types of prakshepa dravya: Kasthoushadhis (herbal) and rasoushadhis (metallic).
   a. Powders or pulps of certain drugs
   b. Sneh dravyas (fats) like ghee, oil

Method of Preparation

1. Jaggery, sugar or sugar-candy is dissolved in the liquid and strained to remove the foreign particles and boiled over a moderate fire.
2. It should be removed from fire, when pressed between fingers, it becomes thready (Tantuvat), or when it sinks in water without getting easily dissolved.
3. Powdered drugs are then added in small quantities and stirred continuously to form a homogenous mixture.
4. Ghee or oil is added and mixed well.
5. Finally, honey is added when the preparation becomes cool and mixed well.

Storage: The Lehya should be kept in glass or porcelain jars. It can also be kept in a metal container which does not react with it. Normally, the Lehya should be used within one year.

The Lehya should be kept in glass or porcelain jars. It can also be kept in a metal container, which does not react with it. Normally, Lehyas should be used within one year.

Examples: Dashamulaharitaki, Bilvadileha, Vasavaleha, Citraka Haritaki, Chyavanaprasa, Kusmandaka Rasayana, Vyaghri Haritaki, Kalyanaka Guda, Ashvagandhadi Lehya, etc

Tailas

Tailas are also known as medicated oils forming a group of drugs in ayurvedic system of medicine with the principle is to extract the therapeutic compounds into oil.

Preparation: The method of preparation requires heating of oil with prescribed kashayas (decoction) and Kalkas (powdered drugs) according to formula. They are generally used for Abhyanga (external application).

It consists of:
1. Drava [Any liquid medium as prescribed in the composition]
2. Kalka [Fine paste of the specified drug]
3. Sneha dravya [Tailas]
4. Gandha dravya [Perfuming agents]

The medicated Tailas will have the odour, colour and taste of the drugs used in the process. If a considerable amount of milk is used in the preparation, the Tailas will become thick and may solidify in cold seasons. Tailas are preserved in good quality of glass, steel or polythene containers. These medicated preparations retain the therapeutic efficacy for 16 months.

Churnas

Churna is defined as a fine powder of drug or drugs in Ayurvedic system of medicine. Drugs mentioned in Patha, are cleaned properly, dried thoroughly, pulverized and then sieved. The churna is free flowing and retains its potency for one year, if preserved in airtight containers. The churna consisting of fine powder of herbs in appropriate ratio was subjected to standardization by means of various physical, chemical and microbiological methods.

Powders are solid dosage form of medicament meant for internal and external uses. They are available in crystalline or amorphous form. Powder of a single drug is called simple and that of a compound formulation is called compound powder.

Storage: The packed materials should be stored in cool, dry and dark conditions.

Standardization of Churnas

It generally involves the following parameters:
1. Determination of sieve size
2. Loss on drying/moisture content
3. TLC
4. Total ash
5. Acid-insoluble ash
6. Water-soluble ash
7. Extractive value in water, alcohol and other solvents
8. Phytoconstituents
9. Microbial contaminations
10. Heavy metal limit test for mercury, arsenic, cadmium, and lead
11. Microscopic analysis

Lepas

Lepas are semi-solid preparations intended for external application to the skin or certain mucous membranes for emollient, protective, therapeutic or prophylactic purposes where a degree of occlusion is desired. They usually consist of solutions or dispersions of one or more medicaments in suitable bases. The base should not produce irritation or sensitization of the skin, nor should it retard wound healing; it should be smooth, inert, odourless, physically and chemically stable and compatible with the skin and with incorporated medicaments. The proportions of the base ingredients should be such that the ointment is not too soft or too hard for convenient use. The consistency should be such that the ointment spreads and softens when stress is applied.

Standardization of Lehyas

- ⊃ Loss of drying
- ⊃ Ash values
- ⊃ Extractive values
- ⊃ pH
- ⊃ Thin layer chromatography

Bhasmas

The bhasmas are the powder of substances obtained by calcinations. The preparation of Bhasmas include the following stages shown in Fig. 3.7:

1. **Purva karma:** Sodhana (purification).
2. **Pardhana karma:** Marana (incineration/calcination).
3. **Paschat karma:** Amritikarna, Lohitikarna.

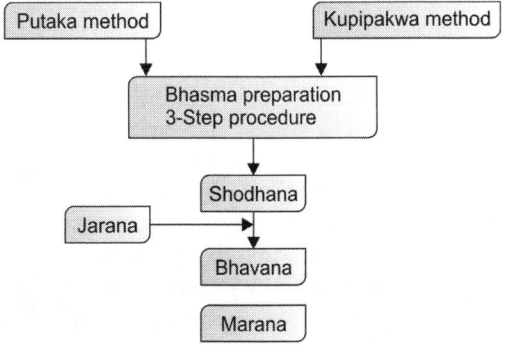

Fig. 3.7: Procedure for preparation of Bhasmas

Sodhana (Purification)

It is prepared from purified minerals, metals, marine and animal products. The following changes are observed: After purification, the materials become free from impurities and become fine as well.

Marana (Incineration/calcination)

The purified drug is mixed with Kasaya of drugs, and it is ground with motar and pestle for specified period of time. The cakes are prepared and their size and thickness depend on heaviness of the drug. The cakes are dried on the sunlight and placed in Sarava (shallow earthen plate) and closed with other plate and sealed with clay smeared cloth and dried. The pit is dug in open space and sealed plates and cow dung are filled in the pit. Fire is put on all the sides and when burning is over, allowed to cool. The earthen pot is removed and seal is opened and contents are taken out. The medicine is ground into fine powder in a Khalva (motar and pestle). The process of triturating is repeated as many times for proper fineness and quality.

Putapaka Method

In this method, bhasma is prepared from three-step procedures (Shodhana, Bhavana and Marana).

Shodhana: Metals or minerals are made by hammering into coarse powder, then subjected to shodhana (purification). Then heated to red hot or melted and quenched in particular liquid media for specified times.

Shodhita materials are then mixed with specific drugs for incineration and are levigated by liquid media for specified time.

Bhavana is a process of wet grinding in which material are ground with particular liquid media for a specified period.

From levigated doughy mass, chakrikas (pellets) are prepared and taken in earthen crucibles faced together and junction is sealed by mud smeared clothes. The material is subjected to heating and heating of materials continue to this apparatus called Putapaka. Burning is continued for specified time and materials is cooled down, opened to get incinerated powder.

Procedure is repeated to get final bhasma.

Low melting point metals (tin, lead and zinc) intermediate process Jarana (polling) is performed. Metal is melted and mixed with plant drug powders and rubbed by a iron ladle with inner surface of pot until metals become in complete powder form.

Kupipakwa Method

Bhasma is prepared by four steps shodhana, kajjali preparation, bhavana and kupipaka. The metals like gold, silver and copper are subjected to amalgamation with mercury, and then purified sulphur is mixed and triturated till black, lustreless, fine and smooth mass is prepared. This procedure is called Kajjali preparation. Prepared Kajjali is levigated by particular liquid media for certain period. It is allowed to complete dryness and filled in glass bottle (Kachkupi) covered by 7 layers of mud smeared cloth. Bottle is then subjected to sand bath (Valukayantra) for indirect and homogenous heating for a certain period. After self-cooling bottle is broken, sublimed product is collected from neck and Bhasma is collected from the bottom of bottle and ground to powder form.

Standardization of Bhasmas

It is shown in Fig. 3.8.

a. Determination of foreign organic matter
b. Determination of ash value:
  ➲ Total ash value
  ➲ Acid-insoluble ash
  ➲ Water-soluble ash
  ➲ Sulfated ash
c. Determination of extractive value:
  ➲ Alcohol-soluble extractive value
  ➲ Water-soluble extractive value
d. Determination of moisture content
e. Determination of physical constants:
  ➲ Melting point
  ➲ Boiling point
  ➲ Refractive index
  ➲ Optical rotation
f. Determination of specific gravity
g. Determination of solid content
h. Determination of alcohol content

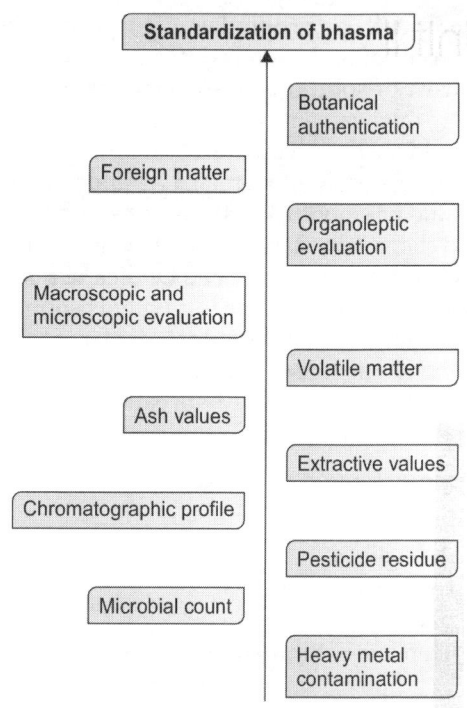

Fig. 3.8: Standardization of bhasma

Ayurveda has an advantage of being a holistic approach that works on the whole body. It does not just rely on traditional medicine which only masks the problems we face in life for the most part. We need harmony with nature and health in our soul, body, senses, and mind. Ayurveda looks at all these areas through therapies. We can heal ourselves of many ailments when we understand our body and how it is out of balance.

Medications in Ayurveda only come from pure natural sources and do not use the chemicals we are so used to with traditional medicines. With this type of medicine we do not have the side effects that normally occur with traditional medicine which is often worse than the condition. We moderate our lifestyle and work on a whole body healing when we use Ayurveda. It has been in practice for thousands of years and has shown to work for people over that time. Ayurveda is an alternative to harsh chemicals and other medications that we use to treat conditions today.

Unit II

Introduction to Nutraceuticals and Herbal Interactions

☞ Nutraceuticals

☞ Herbal-Drug and Herb-Food Interactions

Chapter

4   Nutraceuticals

NUTRACEUTICALS

Let food be your medicine

The old proverb 'an apple a day will keep the doctor away' is now replaced by 'a Nutraceutical a day may keep the doctor away'.

Hippocrates advocated that

'Let food be thy medicine and medicine be thy food' (460–377 BC).

Hippocrates emphasized the relationship between nutrition and human health, and conceptualized the use of appropriate foods for health and their therapeutic benefits.

The DSHEA formally defined 'dietary supplement' using several criteria.

A dietary supplement is:

- ➲ a product (other than tobacco) that is intended to supplement the diet that bears or contains one or more of the following dietary ingredients a vitamin, a mineral, a herb or other botanicals, amino acids or a dietary substance for use by man to supplement the diet by increasing the total daily intake or a concentrate, metabolite, constituent, extract, or combinations of these ingredients.

- ➲ intended for ingestion in pill, capsule, tablet or liquid form.

- ➲ not represented for use as a conventional food or as the sole item of a meal or diet.

- ➲ labelled as a 'dietary supplement'.

The term nutraceutical was coined from nutrition and pharmaceutical in 1989 by *Stephen De felice*, founder and chairman of Foundation for Innovation in Medicine, an American organization which encourages medical health. According to him 'a nutraceutical is any substance that is a food or a part of food and provides medical or health benefits, including the prevention and treatment of disease'. Nutraceuticals are products and their derivatives that occur in nature and are constituents of plants and animal, including humans. These constituents confer a health benefit above and beyond basic nutrition or basic fortification. Nutraceuticals are the active ingredients in functional food or nutritional supplements that deliver a health benefit.

Some examples are n-3 long-chain fatty acids in milk to reduce cardiovascular risks, probiotics in yogurt to improve growth of beneficial intestinal flora, phytosterols in margarine to reduce cholesterol uptake, and folic acid in flour to reduce homocysteine, a risk factor for cardiovascular disease. Combinations of essential nutrients and nutraceuticals may strengthen the health promoting potential by synergy and could be expected to contribute to risk reduction of chronic diseases, ageing, etc.

Nutraceutical is a term coined to describe substances which are not traditionally recognized nutrients but which have positive physiological effects on the human body. They do not easily fall into the legal category of food and drug and often inhabit a grey area between the two. Risk of toxicity or adverse effect of drugs led us to consider safer nutraceutical and functional food based approaches for the health management. This resulted in a worldwide nutraceutical revolution. The nutraceutical revolution will lead us into a new era of medicine and health, in which the food industry will become a research, oriented one similar to the pharmaceutical industry.

'A nutraceutical is a food or a part of a food for oral administration with demonstrated safety and health benefits beyond the basic nutritional functions to supplement diet, presented in a non-food matrix or nonconventional food formats, in such a quantity that exceeds those that could be obtained from normal foods and with such frequency as required to realize such properties, and is labelled as a 'nutraceutical'.'

A nutraceutical is any substance that is a food or a part of a food and provides medical or health benefits, including the prevention and treatment of disease. Such products may range from isolated nutrients, dietary supplements and specific diets to genetically engineered designer foods, herbal products, and processed foods such as cereals, soups and beverages.

A nutraceutical is a product isolated or purified from foods that is generally sold in medicinal forms not usually associated with food. A nutraceutical is demonstrated to have a physiological benefit or provide protection against chronic disease.

A nutraceutical is, 'any nontoxic food component that has scientifically proven health benefits, including disease treatment and prevention'.

Nutraceuticals are isolates that provide concentrated nutrients in the form of pills, tablets, liquids, or powders for direct consumption or for use as ingredients in functional foods. Nutraceuticals include micro- and macronutrient isolates, herbs and botanicals, and isolated reagents (e.g. hormones).

Nutraceutical are commodities derived from foods, but are used in the medicinal form of pills, capsules, portions and liquids and again render demonstrated physiological benefits.

Nutraceutical is any substance that may be considered a food or part of a food and provides medical or health benefits, encompassing, prevention and treatment of diseases.

Nutraceuticals have been proven to offer physiologic benefits or to reduce the risk of chronic disease, or both, beyond their basic nutritional functions.

Nutraceuticals are food or food ingredients that have defined physiological effects. These products, in general terms, cover health promotion, 'optimal nutrition' the concept of enhanced performance both physically and mentally and reduction of disease risk factors.

Nutraceutical can be formulations or foods, taken orally in addition to the normal diet over prolonged periods at concentrations below RDA norms to prevent nutrition related disorders, provide structure/function support and fulfil special physiological needs of the body.

Formulations or foods with health benefits that are taken orally in addition to the normal diet and can even be taken over prolonged periods in concentrations which are lower than the Recommended Daily Allowance (i.e. below the therapeutic range) to supplement the diet to help prevent nutrition related disorders; provide structure/function support that may help prevent specific diseases like diabetes, cancer, obesity through beneficial and proven effects that go beyond the known nutritional effects; and fulfil special physiological needs of the body such as pregnancy, lactation, sports, infancy and sedentary lifestyle. Further to this definition, functional foods, dietary supplements and functional beverages categories have been considered under the purview of 'Nutraceutical.

Nutraceuticals are bioactive natural compounds that have health promoting or disease preventing properties.

Nutraceutical is the term used to describe a medicinal or nutritional component that includes a food, plant or naturally occurring material, which may have been purified or concentrated, and that is used for the improvement of health, by preventing or treating disease.

Nutraceuticals are chemicals found as a natural component of foods or other ingestible forms that have been determined to be beneficial to the human body in preventing or treating one or more diseases or improving physiological performance. Essential nutrients can be considered as nutraceutical if they provide benefit beyond their essential role in normal growth or maintenance of human body.

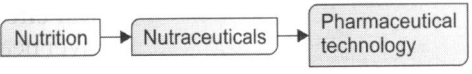

Fig. 4.1: Nutraceuticals

Categories of Nutraceuticals (Table 4.1)

Nutraceuticals are non-specific biological therapies used to promote wellness, prevent malignant processes and control symptoms. These can be grouped into the following categories:

➲ **Nutrient:** A feed constituent in a form and at a level that will help support the life of an animal. The chief classes of feed nutrients are proteins, fats, carbohydrates, minerals and vitamins.

➲ **Dietary supplement:** A product that contains one or more of the following dietary ingredients: Vitamin, mineral, herb or other botanical, amino acid (protein) and also includes the diet as concentrates, constituents, extracts or metabolites of these compounds.

➲ **Nutraceutical:** Any nontoxic food component that has scientifically proven health benefits, including disease treatment and prevention.

➲ **Herbals** are as old as human civilization and they provide a complete storehouse of remedies to cure acute and chronic diseases.

India has the oldest written tradition for the nature's remedies called 'Ayurveda' which possess many effective means of ensuring health care. Numerous nutraceuticals are present in medicinal herbs of key components.

Product Classes

Vitamins

Vitamins are essential organic compounds that are not synthesized in the human or animal organism. They must be consumed with the diet either as such or as a precursor, a so-called pro-vitamin, which can be converted to the vitamin, e.g. β-carotene is a pro-vitamin that is converted biochemically to vitamin A.

13 compounds or groups of compounds have been classified as vitamins (for humans):

Water-soluble	Fat-soluble
Vitamin B_1 (thiamin)	Vitamin A (retinols)
Vitamin B_2 (riboflavin)	Vitamin D (calciferols)
Vitamin B_6 (pyridoxal group)	Vitamin E (tocopherols)
Vitamin C (L-ascorbic acid)	Vitamin K (phylloquinone)
Pantothenic acid	
Biotin	
Folic acid	
Niacin	

Table 4.1: Nutraceuticals play in the continuum between food and pharmaceuticals				
Food ⟹	Functional foods and nutritional supplements	Core nutraceuticals	Medical nutrition	Pharma-ceuticals ⟸
Target group	Healthy people seeking to preserve wellness	People with common health problems	Special nutritional needs	
Examples	Probiotic yoghurts	Cholesterol lowering products	Infant feeding problem	
	Vitamin and mineral supplements	Products to slow progression of diabetes and other disorders.	Nutrition solutions Clinical nutrition products	
Channels	Supermarkets internet	Supermarkets internet	Pharmacies	

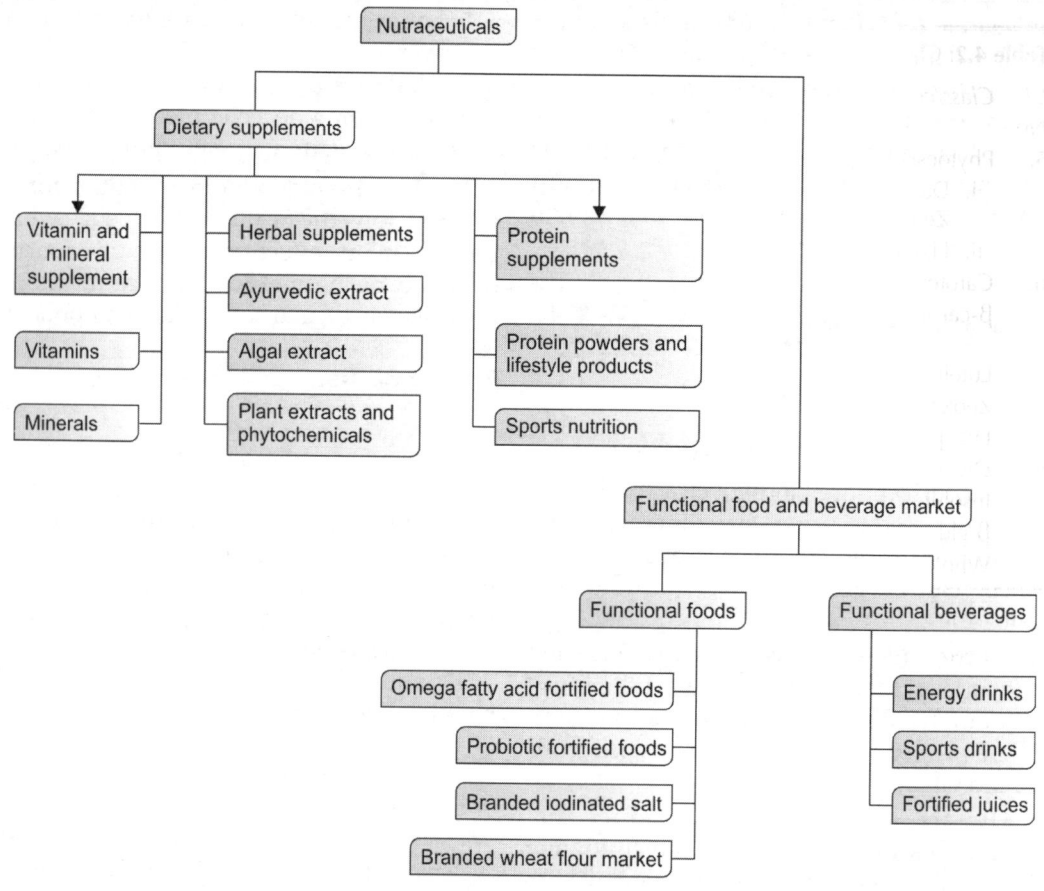

Fig. 4.2: Classification of nutraceuticals

Table 4.2: Classes and components of phytonutrients

S. no.	Class/components	Sources	Potential benefits
1.	Fatty acids	Milk and meat	Improve body composition, reduce cancers
2.	Polyphenols		
	i. Flavonones	Citrus fruits	Neutralizes free radicals, reduce risk of cancer
	ii. Flavones	Fruits, vegetables, soya bean	
	iii. Catechins/Tannin	Tea, babul pods, mustard cake and rape seeds	
	iv. Anthocyanidine	Fruits	
	v. Pro-anthocyanidine	Cocoa, chocolate, tea, rape seed	Reduce cardiovascular disorders
3.	Saponins	Soya beans, chick pea	Lower cholesterol, anti-cancer
4.	Probiotics/Prebiotics/Synbiotics		
	Lactobacillus	Yogurt	Improve GI health
	Fructo oligosaccharides	Whole grains, onions, combination of probiotics and prebiotics	

Contd.

Table 4.2: Classes and components of phytonutrients (Contd.)

S. No.	Class/components	Sources	Potential benefits
5.	Phytoestrogen		
	i. Daidzein, Zenistein	Soya bean, flax, maize, lentils	Reduce menopause symptoms, maintain bone health
	ii. Lignans	Flax, rye, vegetables	Reduce cancer and heart diseases
6.	Carotenoids		
	β-carotene	Oat, maize fodder, carrots, vegetables and fruits	Neutralizes free radicals
	Luteine	vegetables	Healthy vision
	Zeoxanthine	Eggs, citrus, corn	
	Lycopene	Tomatoes	Reduce prostate cancer
7.	Dietary fiber		
	Insoluble fiber	Wheat bran	Reduce breast, colon cancer
	β-glucan	Oats	Reduce cardiovascular disorders
	Whole grain	Cereal grains	

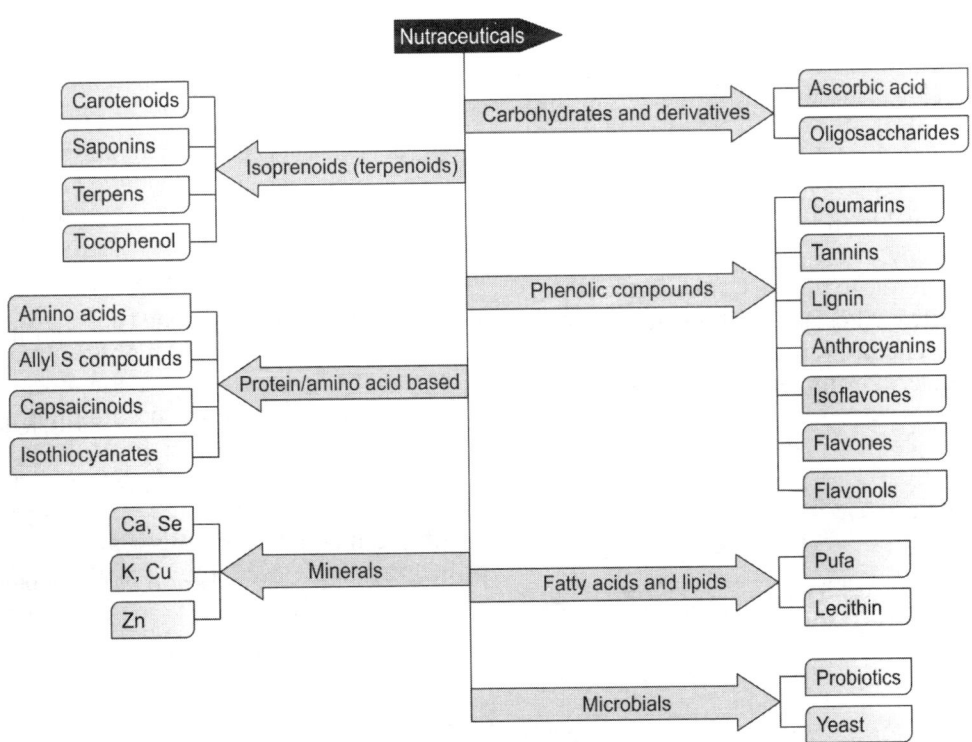

Fig. 4.3: Categorization of nutraceuticals

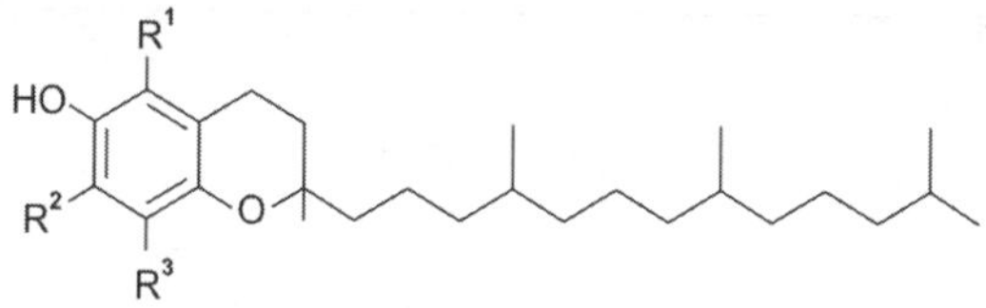

R¹ = R² = R³ = CH₃: α-tocopherol
R² = H, R¹ = R³ = CH₃: β-tocopherol
R² = H, R² = R³ = CH₃: γ-tocopherol
R¹ = R² = H, R³ = CH₃: δ-tocopherol

Fig. 4.4: Tocopherol

Vitamin E: Vitamin E is a group of compounds based on 6-chromanol. Differences between α-, β-, γ-, δ-tocopherol are given in the number of methyl groups on the chromane ring.

Vitamin E is thought to function primarily as a chain-breaking antioxidant that prevents the propagation of free radical reactions in this manner protecting membrane lipids and blood lipids (e.g. LDL cholesterol) against oxidative damage. vitamin E is believed to help prevent diseases associated with oxidative stress, such as cardiovascular disease, cancer, chronic inflammation, and neurologic disorders.

Vitamin K₁ (Fig. 4.5): Vitamin K is the term for 2-methyl–1, 4-naphthoquinone. Vitamins K are lipophilic compounds, heat resistant, stable in air, but sensitive to alkali and light. Vitamin K₁ is localized in chloroplasts of green leafy vegetable and is also found in plant oils, e.g. from soya beans, or olives. Vitamin K has a significant role to play in human health that is beyond its well-established function in blood clotting. Vitamin K may also positively affect Ca balance, a key mineral in bone metabolism.

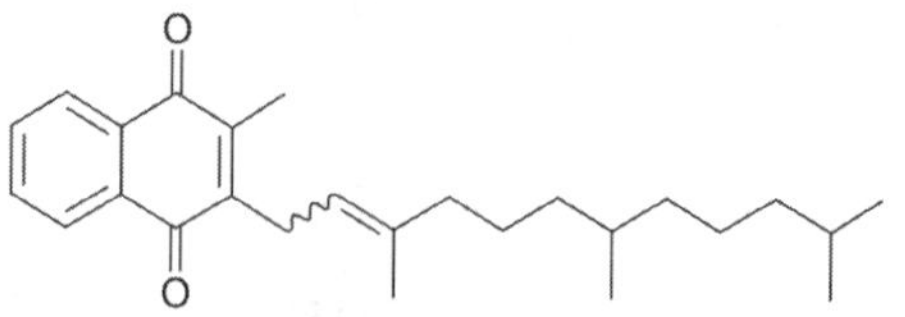

Fig. 4.5: Vitamin K₁

Folic acid: Folic acid, N-[4-[[(2-amino–1,4-dihydro–4-oxo–6-pteridinyl) methyl] amino]benzoyl]-L-glutamic acid, is *de novo* synthesized in microorganisms and plants. These compounds are essential coenzymes for the C1-unit transfer at various oxidation levels.

Carotenoids

Dietary carotenoids are thought to provide health benefits by decreasing the risk of chronic diseases, particularly cancer, cardiovascular disease, and age-related eye diseases. The carotenoids are β-carotene, lycopene, lutein, and zeaxanthin.

Lutein (Fig. 4.6): Lutein is one of the important and widespread natural carotenoids. Lutein can be extracted from natural sources, e.g. from tagetes, or marigold flower petals using various organic solvents.

Zeaxanthin (Fig. 4.7): Zeaxanthin (3R,30R)-dihydroxy-b,β-carotene) is found widespread in nature, e.g. as the yellow colouring in egg yolk and corn. Zeaxanthin reduces the risk of age-related macular degeneration.

Lutein and zeaxanthin are two nutritional carotenoids that are found in a wide variety of fruits and vegetables. Their antioxidant properties, their specific occurrence within the macula at high concentration has led to expectations that the intake of these carotenoids could contribute to reduce the risk for age-related macular degeneration (AMD).

Lycopene (Fig. 4.8): Lycopene (ψ,ψ-carotene) is the red, acyclic carotenoid highly abundant in the tomato. Besides lycopene, tomatoes also contain the carotenoid precursors phytoene and phytofluene, as well as β-carotene and some other minor carotenoids. Other dietary sources are watermelon (23–72 mg/g wet weight), pink guava (~54 mg/g wet weight), pink grapefruit (~33 mg/g wet weight),

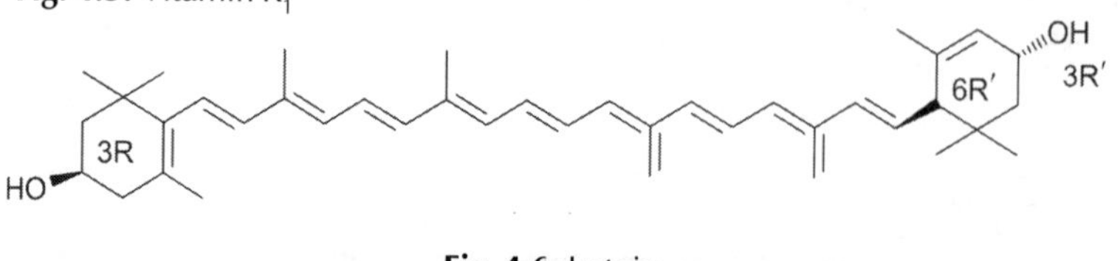

Fig. 4.6: Lutein

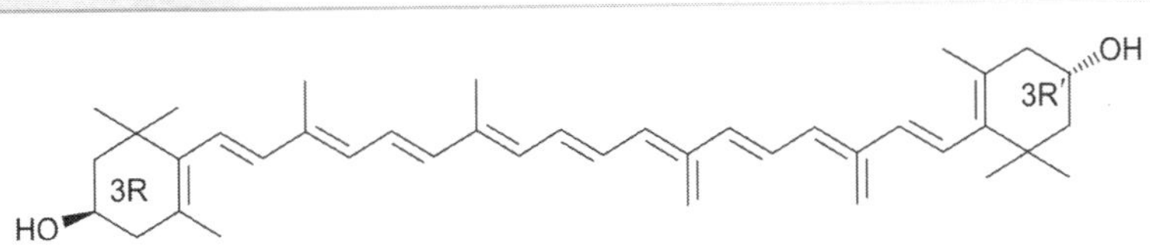

Fig. 4.7: Zeaxanthin

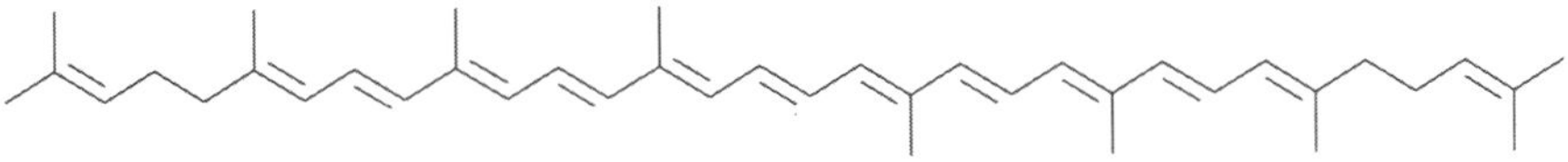

Fig. 4.8: Lycopene (*all-E*)

and papaya (20–53 mg/g wet weight). The high antioxidant properties of lycopene are suggested to be linked with its effect on prevention of cancer and chronic diseases, such as cardiovascular disease. Lycopene might provide protection against oxidative DNA damage suggested to be an early event in carcinogenesis.

Polyunsaturated fatty acids: Polyunsaturated fatty acids (PUFA) are of interest because of their beneficial physiological activities.

ARA (Fig. 4.9): Arachidonic acid (AA), (all-Z)–5,8,11,14-eicosatetraenoic acid, in an essential fatty acid and a precursor in the biosynthesis of prostaglandin, thromboxanes, and leukotriens. AA occurs in liver, brain, glandular organs, and was isolated from liver lipids and beef.

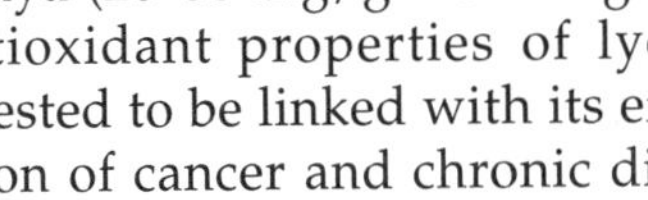

20:4ω6: 20: 4n6; 20Δ5,8,11,14
arachidonic acid, AA

Fig. 4.9: ARA

DHA/EPA (Fig. 4.10): Docosahexaenoic acid (DHA) is an omega-3 PUFA. Fish oils are rich on PUFA, especially eicosopentanoic acid (EPA) docosahexanoic acid (DHA). The content of EPA varies from 5 to 26% and of DHA from

6 to 26% of total fatty acid. PUFA and their ethyl esters are soluble in CO_2, and therefore it is possible to concentrate and separate them using this nonflammable and nontoxic eluent.

CLA: Conjugated linoleic acid (CLA) was identified as a potential mutagen inhibitor. CLA is a term describing several isomers of linoleic acid (LL).

Health effects of PUFA: There are two main classes of PUFA, the omega-6 and the omega-3 that are formed from the two essential fatty acids linoleic and α-linolenic acid, respectively. These fatty acids have a structural role in cell membranes, where they regulate fluidity and affect the function of membrane related proteins. In addition, PUFA are the precursors of eicosanoids, which have a variety of important biological activities and play a role in a number of diseases. The most relevant PUFA in cell membranes are arachidonic acid (AA) and docosahexaenoic acid (DHA), which are important structural and functional components of membranes especially in the central nervous system. Both DHA and AA make up a third of all lipids in the brain's gray matter. These fatty acids must be supplied in sufficient amounts during fetal and infant brain growth. A deficit of omega-3 PUFAs

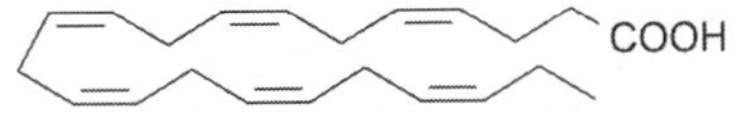

22:6ω3; 22:6n3, 22Δ4,7,10,13,16,19
docosahexaenoic acid, DHA

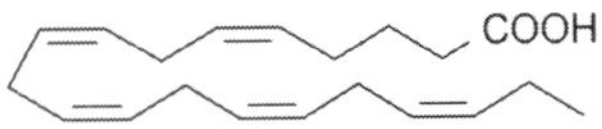

20:5ω3; 20:5n3; 20Δ5,8,11,14,17
eicosapentaenoic acid, EPA

Fig. 4.10: DHA/EPA

during the perinatal brain growth or the retinal development can lead to disorders of the central nervous system and to impairment of vision, which may be irreversible.

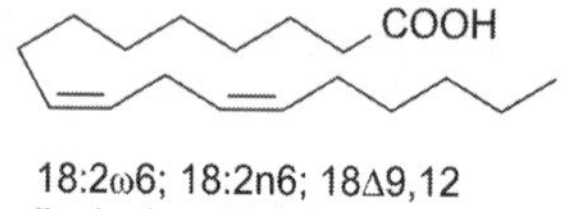

18:2ω6; 18:2n6; 18Δ9,12

Fig. 4.11: Linolenic acid

Polyphenols: Polyphenols have been found to have beneficial health effects.

EGCG: (-)-Epigallocatechin gallate is one of the complex mixtures of polyphenols found in green tea (*Camelia sinensis*). Other catechins found in *Camelia sinensis*, e.g. are epicatechin (EC), and epicatechin gallate (ECG), and epigallocatechin (EGC). EGCG exerts a broad range of activities that include antioxidant, anti-inflammatory, antiangiogenic, antiarthe-rogenic, antithrombotic, and anti-infectious properties. These activities are agreed upon to play an important role in fending off disease.

Flavonoids and isoflavonoids are natural antioxidants and are suggested as agents responsible in the diet for the prevention of coronary diseases, breast cancer, and prostate cancer. Chemically, flavonoids and isoflavo-noids are derivatives of 4H-chromene. Most important are the 4-oxo-chromens, such as flavones and 3-hydroxyflavones. Another important flavone is the plant dye quercetin, 3, 5, 7, 30, 40-penthydroxy-flavone, one of the most important and widely disitributed of the flavonoid family. The following show structures of flavone, 3-hydroxyflavone, and quercetin.

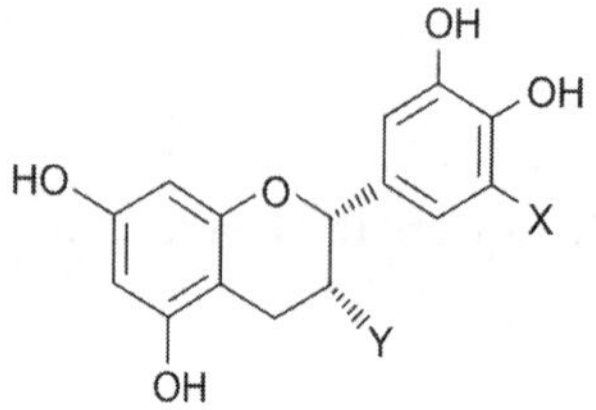

X = H, Y = OH, epicathechin
X = H, Y = C$_7$H$_5$O$_5$, epicatechin gallate
X = OH, Y = OH, epigallocatechin
X = OH, Y = C$_7$H$_5$O$_5$, epicatechin gallate

Fig. 4.12: Structure of polyphenolz

Genistein (Fig. 4.13): Genistein has been associated with reduced incidence of breast and prostate cancer, cardiovascular disease, and osteoporosis.

Phytosterols (Fig. 4.14): Phytosterols are derived from isoprenoid biogenesis and are ubiquitous in higher plants. Usually they are C27–29 substances with a 3-hydroxyl-steran core with C8–10 alkyl and alkenyl side chains at C–17. Various phytosterols such as brassicasterol, stigmasterol, and beta-sitosterol. Phytosterols occur mostly in intracellular organelles, where they appear to play important roles in the stabilization of membranes. They have been found in nearly all plant tissues and organs, including leaves, stems, roots, blossoms, fruits, and seeds. The common dietary phytosterols are most widely established and known for their effects on serum cholesterol. These phytosterols have been shown to competitively inhibit the normally occurring adsorption of endogenous and dietary cholesterol from the intestines. Thus they can lead to lowering of serum cholesterol levels.

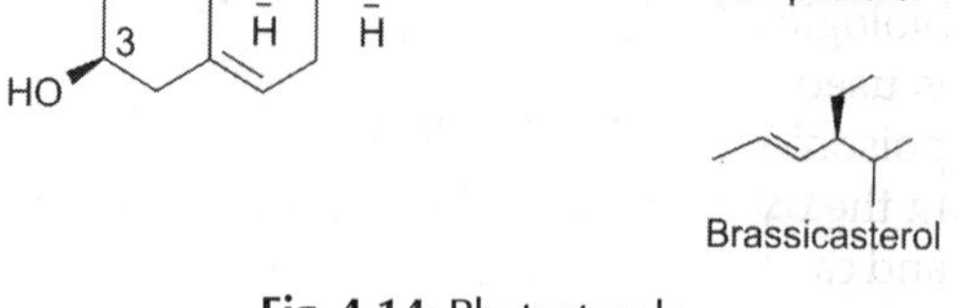

Fig. 4.14: Phytosterols

Others

Creatine (Fig. 4.15): Creatine is a substance that occurs in the human body. The total amount of creatine in a normal healthy person is ~120 g (70 kg) person (256–258). Phosphocre-atine, the phosphorylated creatine and creatine, are important for cellular energy storage, transport, and buffering. In the human organism, creatine is formed from the amino acids argenin,

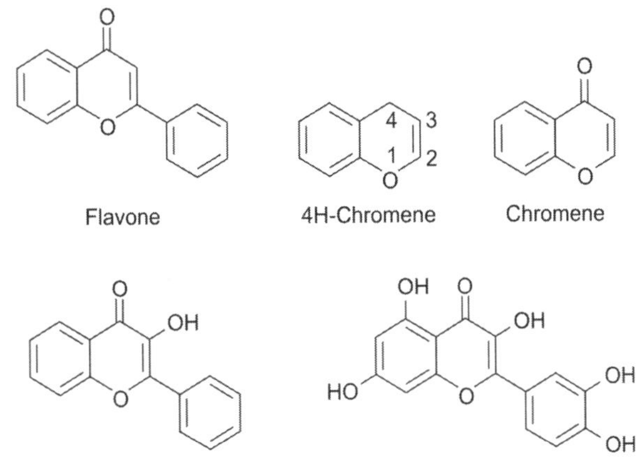

Flavone   4H-Chromene   Chromene

3-hydroxyflavone   quercetin

Fig. 4.13: Genistein

glycin, and methionin. Creatine pyruvate and its salts have several physiological property for treatment of obesity and overweight, and can be used to prevent free radicals and to enhance long-term performance.

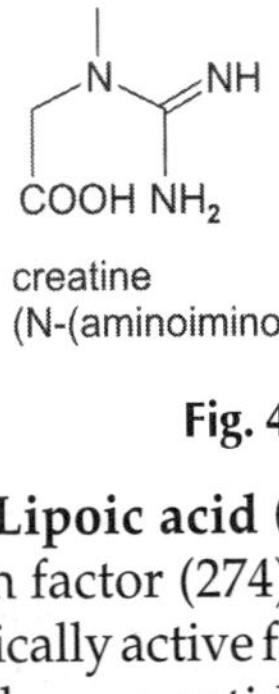

creatine
(N-(aminoiminomethyl)-N-methylglycine)

Fig. 4.15: Creatine

(R)-α-Lipoic acid (Fig. 4.16): Lipoic acid is a growth factor (274). (R)-(α)-Lipoic acid is the biologically active form and racemic lipoic acid is used as an antidote for liver diseases and poisoning. L-Lipoic acid serves as a coenzyme in the oxidative decarboxylation of ketoacids and can be found in every cell of vegetable and animal organisms.

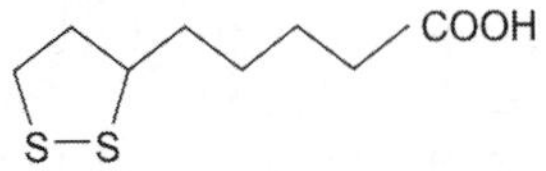

Fig. 4.16: Lipoic acid

Glucosamin (Fig. 4.17): Glucosamin from exogenous sources, e.g., food, is incorporated into the metabolic pathway of glycosaminglycan synthesis. glucosamin increased

the production of proteoglycans and sulfate uptake by articular cartilage.

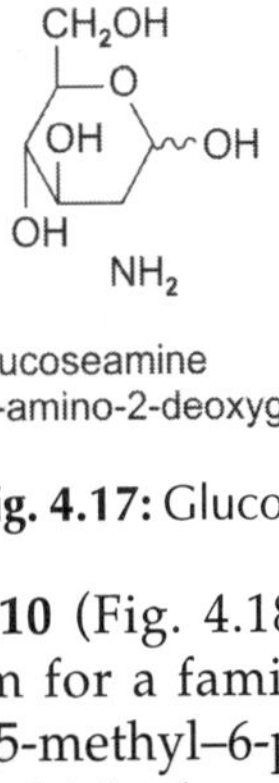

Glucoseamine
(2-amino-2-deoxyglucose)

Fig. 4.17: Glucosamin

Coenzyme Q10 (Fig. 4.18): Ubiquinone is a generic term for a family of quinines (2, 3-dimethoxy–5-methyl–6-polyprenyl-benzoquinone) in which the number of prenyl groups varies from 1 to 10.

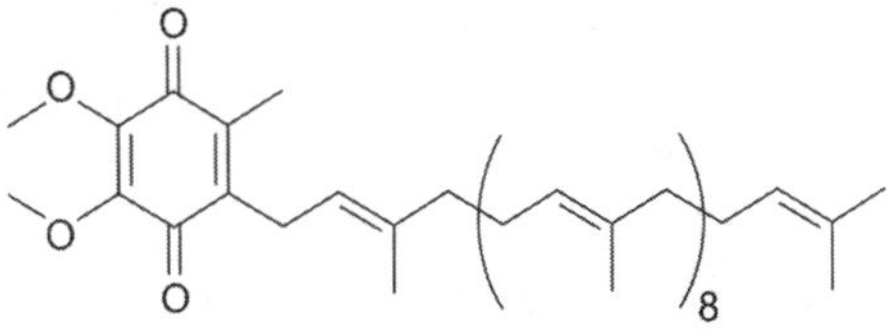

Fig. 4.18: Coenzyme Q10

Economic and Legal Factors

In India, regulatory framework of nutraceuticals needs more attention from the applicable authorities. Worldwide, the regulatory authorities are familiar with changing needs of consumers and proactively protect consumers by amending existing laws to accommo-date changes. But in India old laws such as Prevention of Food Adulteration Act, 1954, which regulates packaged foods, still exist for manufacturers.

Nutraceuticals are grouped under the umbrella of foods by the FSS Act 2006, rules and regulations 2011. Section 22(1) of FSSA, defines 'foods for special dietary uses or functional foods or nutraceutical or health supplements' as:

a. Foods which are specially processed or formulated to satisfy particular dietary requirements which exist because of a particular physical or physiological condition or specific diseases and disorders and which are presented as such, wherein the composition of these foodstuffs must differ significantly from the composition of ordinary foods of comparable nature, if such ordinary foods exist, and may contain one or more of the following ingredients, namely:

   i. Plants or botanicals or their parts in the form of powder, concentrate or extract in water, ethyl alcohol or hydro alcoholic extract, single or in combination;

   ii. Minerals or vitamins or proteins or metals or their compounds or amino acids (in amounts not exceeding the recommended daily allowance for Indians) or enzymes (within permis-sible limits).

   iii. Substances from animal origin;

   iv. A dietary substance for use by human beings to supplement the diet by increasing the total dietary intake;

b. i. A product that is labeled as a 'Food for special dietary uses or functional foods or nutraceuticals or health supplements or similar such foods' which is not represented for use as a conventional food and whereby such products may be formulated in the form of powders, granules, tablets, capsules, liquids, jelly and other dosage forms but not paren-terals, and are meant for oral adminis-tration;

   ii. Such product does not include a drug as defined in clause (b) and Ayurvedic, Siddha and Unani drugs as defined in Clauses (a) and (h) of Section 3 of the Drugs and Cosmetics Act, 1940 (23 of 1940) and rules made thereunder;

   iii. Does not claim to cure or mitigate any specific disease, disorder or condition (except for certain health benefit or such promotion claims) as may be permitted by the regulations made under FSSA.

   iv. Does not include a narcotic drug or a psychotropic substance as defined in the Schedule of the Narcotic Drugs and Psychotropic Substances Act, 1985 and rules made thereunder and substances listed in Schedules E and E(I) of the Drugs and Cosmetics Rules, 1945.

Dietary Supplement Health and Education Act

In 1994 Dietary Supplement Health and Educa-tion Act (DSHEA) passed to govern the human nutraceutical market.

Defines: The law defines as dietary supplement as follows; a dietary supplement is a product that contains one or more of the following dietary ingredients:

   i. Vitamin;

   ii. Mineral;

   iii. Herb or other botanical;

   iv. Amino acid;

   v. A dietary substance for use by humans to supplement the diet by increasing the total dietary intake of that ingredient; and

   vi. A concentrate, metabolite, constituent, extract, or combination of any of the above.

Details of the Act: This Act does not permit FDA to consider a new product a 'drug' or 'food additive' if it falls under the definition of a 'dietary supplement,' which includes among other substances any possible component of the diet as well as concentrates, constituents, extracts or metabolites of these components.

To comply with the regulations, a nutra-ceutical must be labelled as a 'dietary supple-ment' and shall not be represented for use as a conventional food or as a sole item of a meal or diet.

FDA Modernization Act

In 1997, Food and Drug Administration Modernization Act (FDAMA) was passed. Defines:

Additional options for manufacturers of Nutraceuticals are incorporated in this Act by bringing a balance in FDA regulations and by approving therapeutic products so that they can benefit patients and protecting public health with significant changes were also made in the labelling of nutraceuticals.

Indian Regulatory Aspects of Nutraceuticals

There are varieties of laws governing nutraceutical in different names according to the country. In addition, many other cumbersome laws such as:

- Standards of Weights and Measures Act, 1976, and the Standards of Weights and Measures (Packaged commodities) Rules, 1977 (SWMA)
- Infant Milk Substitutes, Feeding Bottles and infant foods (regulation of production, supply and distribution) Act, 1992 with rules, 1993 (IMS)
- Edible Oils Packaging (Regulations) Order, 1998
- Fruit Products Order 1955 (FPO)
- Meat Product Order 1973
- Milk and Milk Products Order 1992
- Vegetable Oils Products (Regulation) Order 1998 (VOP)
- Atomic Energy Act, 1962 and
- Atomic Energy (Control or Irradiation of Food) Rules 1996
- Consumer Protection Act 1986 and the Consumer Protection (Amendment) Act, 2002 and Rules 1987
- Environment Protection Act, 1986 and Rules 1986
- Agricultural Produce (Grading and Marking) Act, 1937 (as amended up to 1986) and 49
- General Grading and Marking Rules 1986 and 1988 (AG Mark)
- Bureau of Indian Standards (BIS) Act 1986

A traditional medicine is not a part of nutraceuticals. A foodstuff (as a fortified food or a dietary supplement) that provides health benefits, if indeed a claim was made that implied medicinal benefit regarding a nutraceutical product, the product would be required to comply with the regulatory requirements for medicinal products, in respect of safety, efficacy, and quality testing and marketing authorization procedures. For decades, FDA regulated dietary supplements as foods to ensure that they were safe and that their labelling was truthful and not misleading.

Food Safety and Standard Act

In 2006, the Indian government passed Food Safety and Standard Act to integrate and streamline the many regulations covering nutraceuticals, foods, and dietary supplements. The Act calls for the creation of the Food Safety and Standard Authority (FSSA).

Food Safety and Standard Authority of India (FSSAI)

Food Safety and Security (FSS) Act was passed by the parliament in 2006. In 2008, FSSAI came into existence.

The FSSA has 12 chapters with 101 sections and two schedules. The FSSA incorporates the salient provisions of the Prevention of Food Adulteration Act 1954, and is based on international legislations, instrumentalities, and the Codex Alimentarius Commission. The aims to establish a single reference point for all matters relating to food safety and standards, by moving from multi-level, multi-departmental control to a single line of command. This unified Act, FSSA, will enable unidirectional compliance and address the need for a single regulatory body.

The FSSA establishes the Food Safety and Standards Authority of India (FSSAI) as an apex regulatory authority, consisting of a Chairperson and 22 members. In their endeavour to carry out the provisions of the FSSA, the FSSAI shall be assisted by a Central Advisory Committee (CAC), Scientific Panels (SPs), and a Scientific Committee (SC); each with specific responsibilities. On September 5,

2008, the GOI notified the establishment of the FSSAI consisting of a chairman and members, who in turn will initiate the rule making process. Nutrition Labeling and Education Act (NLEA): In 1990 (NLEA) defines how food is labeled, including nutrition labeling, in accordance with definitions established by FDA, and providing for the use of claims about the relationship between nutrients and diseases or health-related condition. Benefits of Regulation:

1. Allows greater legal security and more predictable environment.
2. Supports innovation (food and drink products).
3. Prevents unfair competition from manufactures using false or misleading claims.
4. If positive claims cannot be made, the regulation does not oblige anyone to make negative claims about the products.

Scope and Opportunity of Nutraceutical Markets

The nutraceutical market broadly consists of two major segments: Food supplement, vitamins and mineral supplements. The former constituting over 60% of the market and rest 40% comes from the latter. Among vitamins and mineral supplements are continued to be marketed and distributed like prescription drugs in India. Nutraceuticals penetration in urban India is around 22.5% while compartively low in rural India at 6.3%.

Nutraceutical is a new buzzword in Indian healthcare market. This promising term reflects lucrative market opportunities for domestic as well as international pharmaceutical and nutraceutical companies. Nutraceuticals has a spectacular annual growth rate of 25% in Indian healthcare market. Though several scholars have given different definitions for nutraceuticals, essence remains same, and it means 'food as medicine'. Still ambiguity exists in interpreting differences between nutraceuticals and different related terminologies like functional food, dietary supplements, and designer food. Absence of regulatory guidelines for nutraceuticals in India results in mushrooming of nutraceutical manufacturers. In the process of

cut-throat competition, for their survival, they may compromise with the quality of product. Indian scenario: Nutrition is a poorly understood concept in India. The percentage of people who are properly nourished is very small. The imbalances of nourishment patterns give rise to three categories of people: Over-nourished (about 80 million); Under-nourished (about 380 million) and Nourished with calories but not nutrients (about 570 million). The entire population below the poverty line have been considered as undernourished; irrespective of their calorie intake. Similarly, the people who consume less than 175 gm of fruits and vegetables in a day have been considered deficient in micronutrients. Thus the pressing need of the consumer is to supplement food with external nutrients to avert disease conditions. According to current research, global nutraceutical market should reach $285.0 billion by 2021 from $198.7 billion in 2016 at a compound annual growth rate (CAGR) of 7.5%, from 2016 to 2021. The functional beverages market should reach $105.5 billion by 2021 from $71.5 billion in 2016 at a CAGR of 8.1%, from 2016 to 2021. The functional food market should reach $92.5 billion by 2021 from $64.6 billion in 2016 at a CAGR of 7.4%, from 2016 to 2021.

NUTRACEUTICALS AND DISEASES

Nutraceutical Against Alzheimer's Disease (AD) (Fig. 4.19)

Alzheimer's disease (AD), also called senile dementia of the Alzheimer type (SDAT), primary degenerative dementia of the Alzheimer's type (PDDAT), or simply Alzheimer's, is the most common form of dementia.

The various nutraceuticals which are used to cure Alzheimer's disease is as follows (Fig. 4.20).

Antioxidants

Antioxidants are very essential in the treatment of almost all diseases because most chronic diseases carry with them a great pact of oxidative stress. Oxidative stress plays a chief job in neurodegenerative diseases such as

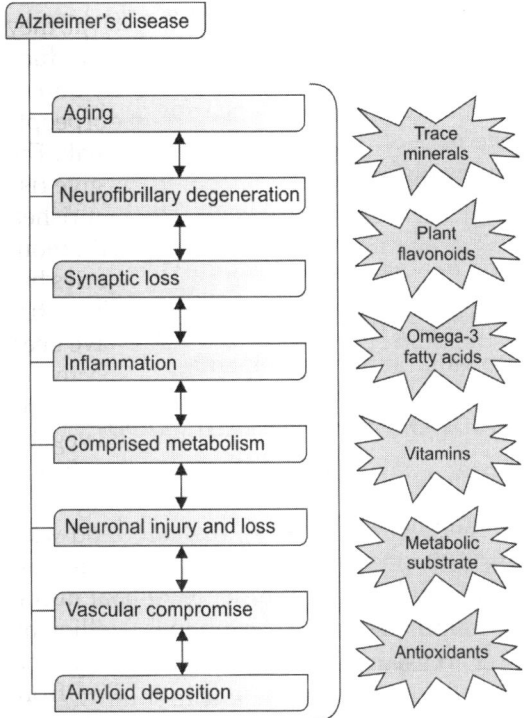

Fig. 4.19: Influences of dietary constituents on neurogeneration in AD

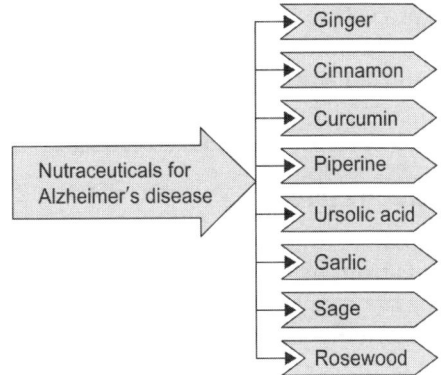

Fig. 4.20: Nutraceuticals for Alzheimer's disease

neurotransmitters: Acetylcholine, norepinephrine, serotonin, and dopamine.

Cardiovascular Diseases Worldwide, the Burdens of Chronic Diseases

Cardiovascular diseases (CVD) is the name for the group of disorders of the heart and blood vessels and include hypertension (high blood pressure), coronary heart disease (heart attack), cerebrovascular disease (stroke), heart failure, peripheral vascular disease, etc. Nutraceuticals in the form of antioxidants, dietary fibers, omega-3 polyunsaturated fatty acids, vitamins, and minerals are recommended together with physical exercise for prevention and treatment of CVD.

The various nutraceuticals which are used to cure cardiovascular diseases are as follows:

Polyphenols present in grapes and in wine alter cellular metabolism and signaling, which is consistent with reducing arterial disease.

Flavonoids in plants available as flavones (containing the flavonoid apigenin found in chamomile); flavanones (hesperidins citrus fruits; silybin milk thistle flavonols (tea: quercetin, kaempferol and rutin grape fruit; rutin buck wheat; ginkgo flavonglycosides ginkgo) play a major role in curing the cardiovascular diseases. Flavonoids block the angiotensin converting enzyme (ACE) that raises blood pressure; by blocking the 'suicide' enzyme cyclooxygenase that breaks down prostaglandins, they prevent platelet stickiness and hence platelet aggregation. Flavonoids

Alzheimer's disease (AD), Parkinson's disease (PD), and Huntington's disease (HD). Oxidative stress is accelerated by the ageing process along with lack of dietary antioxidants. Treatment with antioxidants is a hopeful loom for slowing disease progression.

Alpha Lipoic Acid

Alpha lipoic acid (ALA) also plays a responsibility in brain function. Oxidative stress and energy diminutions are biochemical characteristics and brand of AD. Alpha lipoic acid is potent antioxidant, which also progress glucose metabolism and consumption in the brain.

Phosphatidylserine

Phosphatidylserine is the key phospholipids in the brain and it makes up the basic configuration of the cell membrane. Phosphatidylserine boost cellular metabolism and communication, and oral supplemental outcomes neuronal membranes, cell metabolism and specific

also protect the vascular system and strengthen the tiny capillaries that carry oxygen and essential nutrients to all cells. Flavonoids block the enzymes that produce estrogens, thus reducing the risk of estrogens-induced cancers.

Parkinson's Disease

Parkinson's disease is a brain disorder that results from nerve damage in certain regions of the brain causing muscle rigidity, shaking, and difficult walking. Parkinson's disease (PD) is the second most common aging-related disorder in the world, after Alzheimer's disease. It is characterized by the progressive loss of dopaminergic neurons in the substantia nigra pars compacta and other parts of the brain, leading to motor impairment, cognitive impairment, and dementia. It includes major risk factors including oxidative stress and mitochondrial dysfunction.

These nutraceuticals include vitamins C, D, E, coenzyme Q10, creatine, unsaturated fatty acids, sulphur-containing compounds, polyphenols, stilbenes, and phytoestrogens (Fig. 4.21).

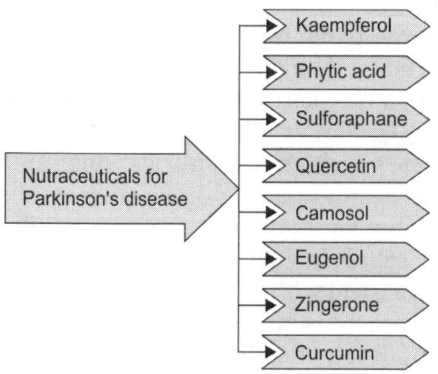

Fig. 4.21: Nutraceuticals for Parkinson's disease

Obesity

Obesity is a complex condition, with serious social and psychological dimensions, affecting virtually all ages and socioeconomic groups. Obesity arises from an energy imbalance whereby energy intake exceeds energy expenditure. Dealing with obesity—by either prevention or treatment—requires modification of

one or both components of energy balance. However, developing functional foods designed for weight management may be a more attractive approach for dealing with the 61% of the population that is currently overweight or obese. There is a very high prevalence of obesity globally; hence nutrition and exercise play key roles in its prevention and treatment. Nutraceuticals like conjugated linoleic acid (CLA), capsaicin, Momordica Charantia (MC), and Psyllium fiber possess potential antiobese properties.

STUDY OF HERBS AS HEALTH FOOD

Alfalfa

Common names: Buffalo grass, chilean clover, lucerne

    Biological source: *Medicago sativa*

    Family: Fabaceae/Leguminosae.

    Part used: Leaves, stems, sprouts

    Habitat: Alfalfa is native to south-western Asia and South-eastern Europe. Also grows in North America and North Africa, Alfalfa is known as the 'Father of all foods' for good reason. It is loaded with important vitamins, minerals, trace minerals and protein.

Chemical Constituents with Mechanism of Action

The leaves and sprouts contain saponins. The saponins appear to decrease serum cholesterol, but not triglycerides, by binding cholesterol and decreasing its absorption. Alfalfa seeds contain the amino acid L-canavanine. L-canavanine is metabolized to produce canaline and urea. Canaline seems to bind pyridoxine phosphate, a cofactor in the metabolism of amino acids, potentially decreasing amino acid enzyme activity. L-canavanine is thought to be responsible for the immunostimulatory effects of alfalfa. Preliminary research suggests the L-canavanine increases immune responses either by decreasing T cell regulation of B cells or by directly binding B cells. Increased activity of B cells can lead to an increase in auto-antibody production and drug induced lupus symptoms.

Uses

➲ Orally, alfalfa is used as a diuretic, for kidney conditions, bladder and prostate conditions, asthma, arthritis, rheumatoid arthritis, diabetes, indigestion, and thrombocytopenic purpura.

➲ It is also used orally as a source of vitamins A, C, E, and K_4; and minerals calcium, potassium, phosphorous, and iron.

➲ This plant also contains chlorophyll, which is good for reducing bad breath and body odour.

➲ This plant is commonly used for arthritis, digestive problems, as a diuretic and for reducing high cholesterol.

➲ It is a very inexpensive source of easily digested nutrients. Alfalfa is high in beta-carotene and builds the immune system.

➲ Sprouted alfalfa seeds contain saponins, which are reported to be toxic to red blood cells *in vitro*.

➲ However, it is harmless to human consumption and has many health beneficial properties like anti-inflammatory, immune-stimulating activity, anti-tumor activity, etc.

➲ Alfalfa sprouts have about 8% saponins content according to commercial sprout growers. When compared with alfalfa seeds sprouting increases the saponin content to 450%. Saponins bind with bile acids. Some large intestinal bacteria converts bile into highly carcinogenic substance where, bile that binds with saponins prevents the formation of toxin.

➲ Presence of saponins in alfalfa sprouts will destroy tumor causing cells particularly in lung and blood cancer it is more effective. It gives more immunity for stomach.

Caution

Pregnant and nursing women should not eat alfalfa seeds due to their content of stachydrine and homostachydrine (may promote menstruation or cause miscarriage). People in general should never eat alfalfa seeds. They contain high levels of the toxic amino acid canavanine. Alfalfa is high in vitamin K and may work as an anti-coagulant so it should not be taken by people taking blood thinning medication.

The cost-effective nutraceutical product containing alfalfa along with other cereals and pulses would serve the humanity to fight undernourishment in an easy and economical way.

Chicory

Biological source: *Cichorium intybus*; Family: Compositae

Part used: Root

Habitat: Chicory has been an esteemed medical plant ever since the Roman physician Galen called it 'the friend of the liver' some 1,800 years ago.

Chemical constituents: The root contains up to 58% inulin and sesquiterpene lactones (lactucine and lactupicrine), sugar, as well as vitamins (B, C, K, P) and minerals. Chicory flowers contain cichoriin, which is 6,7-gluco-hydroxycoumarin. The greens contain chicoric acid (dicaffeoyl tartaric acid), flavonoids, catechol tannins, glycosides, carbohydrates, unsaturated sterols and triterpenoids and tartaric acid.

Medicinal Uses

➲ A syrup of chicory, rhubarb and oats was given to patients with liver ailments. It was also considered valuable for treating a variety of other ailments.

➲ A syrup of the whole plant was prepared with sugar and taken to cure insomnia.

➲ The bruised fresh leaves were applied externally for healing eye inflammations and boiled in broth for strengthening the digestion of the persons with weak stomachs.

➲ An infusion of the leaves was also used to reduce fever in children.

➲ A distilled water of chicory or the juice pressed from it was good for pregnant women and especially to soothe nursing breasts that were swollen from too much milk.

➲ Chicory is an excellent bitter tonic for the liver and digestive tract.

➲ Recommended for loss of appetite and dyspepsia.

➲ The root is therapeutically similar to dandelion root, supporting the action of the stomach and liver and cleansing the urinary tract.

➲ Chicory is also taken for rheumatic conditions and gout, and as milk laxative, one particularly appropriate for children.

➲ An infusion of the leaves and flowers also aids the digestion.

➲ A decoction may alleviate gallstones and kidney stones and aid in the production of bile.

➲ Chicory constituents may be effective in treatment of disorders involving tachycardia, arrhythmias and fibrillation. It also has been found to significantly lower cholesterol and blood sugar levels.

Ginger

Biological source: Ginger is the rhizome of *Zingiber officinale* Rosc., a herbaceous perennial belonging to Zingiberaceae.

Habitat: It is believed to be native of southeastern Asia.

Chemical Constituents

The major constituents in ginger rhizomes are carbohydrates (50–70%), lipids (3–8%), terpenes, and phenolic compounds. Terpene components of ginger include zingiberene, β-bisabolene, β-farnesene, β-sesquiphellandrene, and α-curcumene, while phenolic compounds include gingerol, paradols, and shogaol. These gingerols (23–25%) and shogaol (18–25%) are found in higher quantity than others. Besides these, amino acids, raw fiber, ash, protein, phytosterols, vitamins (e.g., nicotinic acid and vitamin A), and minerals are also present. The aromatic constituents include zingiberene and bisabolene, while the pungent constituents are known as gingerols and shogaols. Other gingerol- or shogaol-related compounds (1–10%), which have been reported in ginger rhizome, include 6-paradol, 1-dehydrogingerdione, 6-gingerdione and 10-gingerdione, 4-gingerdiol, 6-gingerdiol, 8-gingerdiol, and 10-gingerdiol, and diarylheptanoids. The characteristic odour and flavour of ginger are due to a mixture of volatile oils like shogaols and gingerol.

Uses

➲ Ginger and its constituents show antioxidant activity and prevent the damage of macromolecules, caused by the free radicals/oxidative stress.

➲ Ginger and its constituents also show a vital role as anti-inflammatory processes. Earlier studies on *in vitro* investigations of ginger preparations and some isolated gingerol-related compounds showed that anti-inflammatory effects of ginger such as inhibition of COX and inhibition of nuclear factor κB.

➲ Ginger also acts as antitumor via modulation of genetic pathways such as activation tumour suppressor gene, modulation of apoptosis and inhibition of VEGF. Earlier study has shown that terpenoids, constituents of ginger induce apoptosis in endometrial cancer cells through the activation of p53.

➲ Ginger also shows antimicrobial and other biological activities due to gingerol and paradol, shogaols and zingerone.

Fenugreek

Biological source: *Trigonella foenumgraecum; Trigonella foenugraecum.* Family: Fabaceae/Leguminosae.

Habitat: Fenugreek is indigenous to the eastern shores of the Mediterranean sea, but it is grown in India, Morocco, Egypt and England.

Chemical Constituents

Fenugreek seed contains 45–60% carbohydrates, mainly mucilaginous fiber (galactomannans); 20–30% proteins high in lysine and tryptophan; 5–10% fixed oils (lipids); pyridine-type alkaloids, mainly trigonelline (0.2–0.36%), choline (0.5%), gentianine, and carpaine; the flavonoids apigenin, luteolin, orientin, quercetin, vitexin, and isovitexin; free amino acids, such as 4-hydroxyisoleucine

(0.09%); arginine, histidine, and lysine; calcium and iron; saponins (0.6–1.7%); glycosides yielding steroidal sapogenins on hydrolysis (diosgenin, yamogenin, tigogenin, neotigogenin); cholesterol and sitosterol; vitamins A, B$_1$, C, and nicotinic acid; and 0.015% volatile oils (n-alkanes and sesquiterpenes), which are thought to account for many of its presumed therapeutic effects.

Mechanism of Action

The applicable part of fenugreek is the seed. The active constituents include trigonelline, 4-hydroxyisoleucine, and sotolon. Fenugreek seeds have a distinctive bitter taste and odour. Sotolon is frequently used as a flavouring for artificial maple syrup. Soaking fenugreek seeds overnight and washing the seeds in water can decrease some of the taste and odour. Fenugreek seeds contain about 50% dietary fiber and pectin and may affect gastrointestinal transit, slowing glucose absorption. About 80% of the total content of free amino acids in the seeds is present as 4-hydroxyisoleucine, which appears to directly stimulate insulin. This effect is glucose dependent and only occurs in the presence of moderate to high glucose concentrations. Some evidence suggests the seed consumption might decrease calcium oxalate deposition in the kidneys. Fenugreek contains coumarins and other constituents that might affect platelet aggregation, but this might not be significant clinically.

Uses

- Orally, fenugreek is used for lowering blood glucose in people with diabetes, loss of appetite, dyspepsia, gastritis, constipation, atherosclerosis, high serum cholesterol and triglycerides, and for promoting lactation.
- Fenugreek is used orally for kidney ailments, beriberi, hernia, impotence, and other male problems. Fenugreek is also used orally for fever, mouth ulcers, boils, bronchitis, cellulitis, tuberculosis, chronic coughs, chapped lips, baldness, and cancer.
- Topically, fenugreek is used as a poultice for local inflammation, myalgia, lymphadenitis, gout, wounds, leg ulcers, and eczema.

- In foods, fenugreek is included as an ingredient in spice blends. It is also used as a flavouring agent in imitation maple syrup, foods, beverages, and tobacco. In manufacturing, fenugreek extracts are used in soaps and cosmetics.

Garlic

Biological source: Garlic, *Allium sativum* L., is a member of the Alliaceae family, has been widely recognized as a valuable spice and a popular remedy for various ailments and physiological disorders.

Habitat: Cultivated practically throughout the world, garlic appears to have originated in central Asia and then spread to China, the near East, and the Mediterranean region before moving west to Central and Southern Europe, Northern Africa (Egypt) and Mexico.

Chemical Constituents

Garlic contains at least 33 sulphur compounds, several enzymes, 17 amino acids, and minerals such as selenium. It contains a higher concentration of sulphur compounds than any other Allium species. The sulphur compounds are responsible both for garlic's pungent odour and many of its medicinal effects. Dried, powdered garlic contains approximately 1% alliin (S-allyl cysteine sulfoxide). One of the most biologically active compounds, allicin (diallyl thiosulfinate or diallyl disulphide) does not exist in garlic until it is crushed or cut; injury to the garlic bulb activates the enzyme allinase, which metabolizes alliin to allicin. *Sulphur compounds*: alliin, allicin, ajoene, allylpropyl disulphide, diallyl trisulphide, sallylcysteine, vinyldithiines, S-allylmercaptocystein, and others. *Enzymes*: allinase, peroxidases, myrosinase, and others. *Amino acids and their glycosides*: Arginine and others. Selenium, germanium, tellurium and other trace minerals.

Role of Garlic in Various Diseases

- Garlic has demonstrated effects on several risk factors for atherosclerotic disease—hyperlipidemia, hypertension, and platelet aggregation.

➲ Fresh garlic, garlic powder, aged garlic and garlic oil have demonstrated antiplatelet/ anticoagulant effects by interfering with cyclo-oxygenase-mediated thromboxane synthesis. Garlic, *Allium sativum* L., has been used for centuries in many societies against parasitic, fungal, bacterial and viral infections.

➲ Garlic has been proven effective as a hypolipidemic, antimicrobial, antihypertensive, hepatoprotective, and insecticidal agent in various human and animal therapies. The use of garlic extracts reduces serum cholesterol levels and increases blood coagulation time. In aquacultural operations, garlic promotes growth, enhances immunity, stimulates appetite, and strengthens the control of bacterial and fungal pathogens.

➲ Garlic as a natural antibiotic is one of the most effective natural immunostimulants.

➲ Garlic has antioxidant properties and also has beneficial effects on the cardiovascular and immune systems.

➲ Generally, garlic takes effect by facilitates the function of phagocytic cells and increases their bactericidal activities.

➲ Garlic is effective in treating intestinal parasites has been known for a long time. An extract of garlic was effective against a host of protozoa such as *Opalina ranarum, Opalina dimidicita, Balantidium entozoon, Entamoeba histolytica, Trypanosoma, Leishmania, Leptomonas,* and *Crithidia.*

➲ It has been proved that garlic has immunomodulatory properties and is well capable of enhancing protection against pathogens. Hence, it can be concluded that garlic supplemented diets in fish enhance growth rate and improves the immune response in aquaculture. Garlic can also be used as an alternative to antibiotics or chemotherapeutic agents.

Honey

Honey is a sweet food made by bees using nectar from flowers. Honey bees transform nectar into honey by a process of regurgitation and evaporation. They store it as a primary food source in wax honeycombs inside the beehive. Honey gets its sweetness from the monosaccharide's, fructose, and glucose, and has approximately the same relative sweetness as that of granulated sugar.

Habitat: The honey bees are tropical climates and heavily forested areas. Honey bees can thrive in natural or domesticated environments, though they prefer to live in gardens, woodlands, orchards, meadows and other areas.

Chemical Composition

The composition of honey includes sugars such as glucose and fructose and also minerals such as magnesium, potassium, calcium, sodium chlorine, sulphur, iron and phosphate. Depending on the quality of the nectar and pollen, the vitamins contained in honey are B1, B2, C, B6, B5 and B3. The pH of honey is commonly between 3.2 and 4.5. This relatively acidic pH level prevents the growth of many bacteria. Honey is primarily a saturated mixture of two monosaccharides. This mixture has a low water activity.

Uses

➲ It has attractive chemical properties for baking, and a distinctive flavour that leads some people to prefer it over sugar and other sweeteners.

➲ Honey has a long history of human consumption, and is used in various foods and beverages as a sweetener and flavouring.

➲ It also has a role in religion and symbolism. Flavours of honey vary based on the nectar source, and various types and grades of honey are available. It is also used in various medicinal traditions to treat ailments.

➲ Honey have antibacterial effects, attributed to its high osmolarity, low pH, hydrogen peroxide content and content of other, uncharacterized compounds. The low water activity of honey is inhibitory to the growth of the majority of bacteria, many yeasts and moulds.

➲ When applied topically to wounds, osmosis would be expected to draw water from the wound into the honey, helping to dry the infected tissue and reduce bacterial growth. Even when diluted with water absorbed from wounds, honeys would be likely to retain a water activity sufficiently low to inhibit growth of most bacteria.

Amla

Biological source: The fruit, also known as Indian gooseberry (*Emblica officinalis* Gaertn.), is acclaimed for its unique nutritional and rejuvenating properties. It is consumed as a fresh fruit or in the form of food products like preserve.

Amla is a medium-sized deciduous tree with gray bark and reddish wood which success-fully grows in variable agro-climatic and soil conditions. The tree grows to a height of 60 ft (18 m). The leaves are very fine and small, only 1/8 in (3 mm) wide and 1/2 to 3/4 in (1.25–2 cm) long The flowers are small, green-ish-yellow and borne in compact clusters in the axils of the lower leaves. The fruits are round or oval, with smooth textured skin. There are ~6 to 8 pale visible lines, appearing as ridges. unripe fruits are light green turning yellow to red at maturity. The stone is tightly set in the center of the flesh and contains 6 small seeds.

Habitat: Indian gooseberry has been used as a valuable ingredient of various medicines in India and Middle East.

Chemical Composition

It contains tannins, alkaloids and phenols. Fruits have 28% of the total tannins distrib-uted in the whole plant. The fruit contains two hydrolysable tannins: Emblicanin A and B, which have antioxidant properties; one on hydrolysis gives gallic acid, ellagic acid. The fruit also contains phyllemblin, gallic acid, corilagin, furosin and geraniin. Flavonoids like quercetin, alkaloids like phyllantine and phyllantidine are found. Along with these, it primarily contains amino acids and carbo-hydrates its fruit juice contains the highest concentration of vitamin C (478.56 mg/100 ml).

Uses

Amla has been considered the best of the Ayurvedic rejuvenative herbs, because it is tridosaghna. Uniquely, it has a natural balance of tastes (sweet, sour, pungent, bitter and astringent) all in one fruit, it stimulates the brain to rebalance the three main components of all physiological functions, the water, fire, and air elements within the body.

The fresh juice of the round, acidulous fruit is used in combination with that of other Myrobalans-chebulic (*Terminalia chebula*) and Beleric (*Terminalia belerica*) in the form of a decoction known as Triphala (three fruits). It is used as a cooling and refrigerant sherbet, and as an astringent medicine in diarrhoea, haemoptysis (spitting blood), haematemesis (vomiting blood) and other similar conditions.

Ginseng

Ginseng, the root of *Panax species*, is a well-known folk medicine. It has been used as traditional herbal medicine in China, Korea and Japan for thousands of years and today is a popular and worldwide used natural medicine.

Habitat: *Panax ginseng* belongs to the Aralia-ceae family and is found throughout East Asia and Russia. It grows natively in remote forests of Manchuria and North Korea, but has become over-harvested in other parts of Asia. It is culti-vated in Korea, China, and Japan for export and use as a medicinal herb.

Chemical Constituents

The active ingredients of ginseng are ginseno-sides which are also called ginseng saponins. *Panax ginseng* contains triterpene glycosides, or saponins, commonly referred to as ginseno-sides. Many active compounds can be found in all parts of the plant, including amino acids, alkaloids, phenols, proteins, polypeptides, and vitamins B_1 and B_2.

Uses

- Ginseng had been used primarily as a tonic to invigorate week bodies and help the resto-ration of homeostasis.
- It has beneficial effects in a wide range of pathological conditions such as cardiovas-cular diseases, cancer, immune deficiency and hepatotoxicity.

➲ Ginseng products are usually used as general tonic and adaptogen to help the body to resist the adverse influences of a wide range of physical, chemical and biological factors and to restore homeostasis.

➲ These tonic and adaptogenic effects of ginseng are believed to enhance physical performance (including sexual function) and general vitality in healthy individuals, to increase the body's ability to fight stress in stressful circumstances and to support resistance to diseases by strengthening normal body function as well as to reduce the detrimental effects of the aging processes.

Ashwagandha

Ashwagandha (*Withania somnifera*), also known as Indian ginseng, and as Indian Winter Cherry is an important ancient plant, the roots of which have been employed in Indian traditional systems of medicine, Ayurveda and Unani.

Habitat: Cultivated throughout drier parts of India.

Chemical Constituents

It contains constituents like cuseohygrine, anahygrine, tropine, and anaferine, glycosides, Withanolides with starches and amino acid. Withanolides consists of steroidal molecules which is said to fight inflammation. Ashwagandha stimulates the immune system, combats inflammation, increases memory, and helps maintain general health and wellness. Ashwagandha is known to increase the production of bone marrow, semen, and acts anti-aging.

Uses

Ashwgandha has long been considered as an excellent rejuvenator, a general health tonic and a cure for a number of health complaints.

It is a sedative, diuretic, anti-inflammatory and generally respected for increasing energy, endurance, and acts as an-adaptogen that exerts a strong immunostimulatory and an anti-stress agent.

Ashwagandha is taken for treating cold and coughs, ulcers, emaciation, diabetes, conjunctivitis, epilepsy, insomnia, senile dementia, leprosy, Parkinson's disease, nervous disorders, rheumatism, arthritis, intestinal infections, bronchitis, asthma, impotence and a suppressant in HIV/AIDS patients.

Ashwagandha is considered to be one of the best rejuvenating agents in Ayurveda. Its roots, seeds and leaves are used in Ayurvedic and Unani medicines. Ashwagandha root drug finds an important place in treatment of rheumatic pain, inflammation of joints, nervous disorders and epilepsy. Dried roots are used as tonic for hiccup, cold, cough, female disorders, as a sedative, in care of senile debility, ulcers, etc.

Leaves are applied for carbuncles, inflammation and swellings. Leaf juice is useful in conjunctivitis. Bark decoction is taken for asthma and applied locally to bed sores. Ashwagandha and its extracts are used in preparation of herbal tea, powders, tablets and syrups. Ashwagandha has anti-inflammatory, anti-tumour, anti-stress, antioxidant, mind-boosting, immune-enhancing, and rejuvenating properties.

Spirulina

Spirulina, the nutraceutical food, has become widely available as a food ingredient. Spirulina is the most nutritious, concentrated food known to man containing antioxidants, phytonutrients, essential fatty acids, probiotics, and nutraceuticals. Spirulina is the best whole food source of protein, beta carotene, gamma linolenic acid, B-vitamins, minerals, chlorophyll, sulpho-lipids, glyco-lipids, super oxide dismutase, phycocyanin, enzymes.

Spirulina contains its own anti-oxidants like beta-carotene, superoxide dismutase, selenium and vitamin E. Antioxidants helps to protect the body against free radicals formed due to stress, exposure to toxic chemicals, drugs and poor diets. Free radicals can lead to degenerative disease like cancer, aging, age-related macular degeneration, etc. Spirulina is being used as a therapeutic agent because of its antioxidant, anti-cancer properties and its ability to strengthen the immune system.

Spirulina is known to improve malnourishment, and vitamin Spirulina is a good probiotic. Probiotics are good for health as they strengthen the immune system to prevent disease and cancer. Spirulina's probiotic effect helps in maintaining healthy micro flora thus helps in better digestion, absorption and protection from infection. Scientific studies also have indicated that spirulina has got anti-inflammatory, anti-allergic, antimicrobial and anti-stress properties and also helps in the treatment of asthma, arthritis, etc.

Conclusion

At present, nutraceutical represent the fastest growing segment of today's food industry. Although it may be many years before the new designer foods will be stocked on supermarket shelves, the ongoing program will lead to a new generation of foods, which will certainly cause the interface between food and drug to become increasingly permeable. The importance of nutraceuticals to the human organism is that they provide all the essential substances that should be present in a healthy diet. Very often the daily hustle and our diet leads to unhealthy way of life. The right administration of nutraceuticals provides for better quality of life, healthier life, better mood and self-confidence, better working capacity, better social environment. Thus, in the future

we will see the emergency of nutraceutical soups, nutraceutical processed meat, bread and sausage. And many of these foods might be genetically produced. The use of nutraceuticals, as an attempt to accomplish desirable therapeutic outcomes with reduced side effects, as compared with other therapeutic agents has met with great monetary success. 'The movement from treatment to prevention' stimulates demand for nutraceuticals as they offer additional health benefits beyond basic nutrition,' says Ewa Hudson, Head of Health and Wellness Research at Euromonitor. The preference for the discovery and production of nutraceuticals over pharmaceuticals is well seen in pharmaceutical and biotech companies.

The expanding nutraceutical market indicates that end users are seeking minimally processed food with extra nutritional benefits and organoleptic value. Many scientists believe that enzymes represent another exciting frontier in nutraceuticals. For diseases expected to increase in number, but can be prevented by lifestyle change, such as metabolic syndromes, the patients are required to positively change their lifestyles. One of the solutions is to change their diet. Nutraceuticals should contribute to prevent such diseases. The research strategy of the world towards nutraceuticals should be in future for living life healthy and improve quality of life.

5

Herbal-Drug and
Herb-Food Interactions

- General introduction to interaction and classification
- Study of following drugs and their possible side effects and interactions: St John's wort, garlic, kava-kava, black pepper, gingko, ginseng, ephedra and hypercium.
- Other herbs involved in drug interactions
- Minimize herb-drug interactions

INTRODUCTION

Herb-drug interactions are any pharmacological modification caused by an herbal substance(s) to another prescription medication (diagnostic, therapeutic or other action of a drug) in or on the body. It can impact health and the effectiveness of treatments. Adverse effects of herbal-drug interactions are given in Table 5.1

Herbal product is not a single constituent; combination of several components, therefore it may cause certain interactions by reacting with our body constituents.

The chemical makeup and complex nature of herbal product is varied depending on the following factors:

1. Part of the plant used, e.g. bark, stem, leaves, roots, flowers, and rhizomes.
2. Climatic conditions, harvesting and storage conditions, etc.
3. Manufacturing conditions and process.

Some interactions have a beneficial effect on drug therapy, e.g. statin drugs decrease the biosynthesis of endogenous coenzyme Q10, and adverse effects owing to statin therapy may be secondary to decrease in tissue levels of coenzyme Q10. Thus supplementation of coenzyme Q10 by patients on statin therapy may help to prevent adverse effects. Reasons and causes of herbal-drug interactions are stated in Fig. 5.1.

Table 5.1:	Adverse effects of herbal-drug interactions
Herbal-drug interactions and its adverse effects	• Increases the side effect of drug • Increases the toxic profile of drug • Lead to treatment failure • Develops drug resistance • Modify the mechanism of action of drugs • Alter pharmacokinetic and pharmacodynamic profile of drugs • Modify therapeutic effects of drugs • Prolonged treatment duration • Leads to negative metabolism of drug

Mechanisms of Herbal-Drug Interaction (Table 5.2)

Many medical herbs and pharmaceutical drugs are therapeutic at one dose and toxic at another. Interactions between herbs and drugs may increase or decrease the pharmacological or toxicological effects of either component. In essence, interactions between pharmacologically active botanicals and drugs involve the same pharmacokinetic and pharmacodynamic mechanisms as drug–drug interactions.

For example,

1. Herbs such as laxatives can speed up the digestive process, reducing the amount of time a drug is present to be absorbed by the stomach.

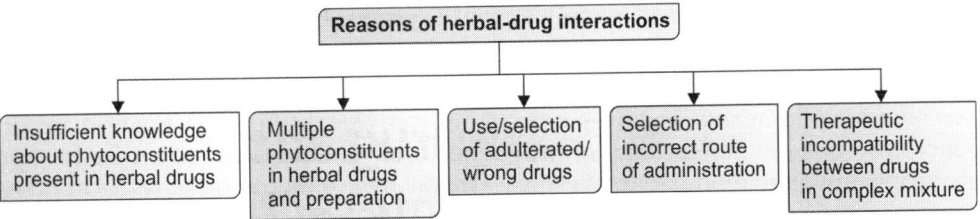

Fig. 5.1: Reasons of herbal-drug interactions

2. Herbs can change the physical environment of the stomach, such as the pH level.
3. Herbs can chemically bind to drugs, causing them to remain in the stomach instead of entering the bloodstream.
4. Herbs such as gums and mucilage (hydrocolloidal carbohydrate) are soluble in water but poorly absorbable; examples include psyllium, rhubarb, flaxseed, marshmallow and aloe bind to other drugs, particularly when consumed in their whole or powdered forms. For example, psyllium (an herb high in mucilage) inhibits the absorption of lithium.
5. Herbs such as rhubarb and aloe reduce the action of drugs that have a narrow therapeutic index (e.g. digoxin, warfarin) and can cause diarrhoea. In order to prevent herbs from binding with drugs should be taken 1 hour before or 2 hours after these herbal products.
6. The use of botanicals containing anthranoid laxatives (e.g. aloe; Aloe spp.) can result in reduction in the extent of drug absorption by increased intestinal transit

Table 5.2: Mechanisms of botanical drug interactions

Mechanisms of botanical drug interactions	Pharmacokinetic interactions	Pharmacokinetic interactions involve alteration in absorption, distribution, metabolism, or excretion of the affected drug or botanical	Drug absorption	• Due to increased intestinal transit time • Due to use of botanicals containing anthranoid laxatives • Due to complex formation between botanical constituents
			Drug distribution	• Due to altered protein binding of highly protein-bound drugs
			Drug metabolism	• Due to drug-metabolizing enzyme inhibition or induction • Due to increased tissue concentration of catalytically active protein involved in drug metabolism.
			Drug excretion	• Botanicals with diuretic effects can increase drug excretion
	Pharmacodynamic interactions	Pharmacodynamic interactions involve alterations in relationship between the drug concentration and the pharmacological response for a drug or botanical	Due to additional, synergistic or antagonistic effect of botanicals	• Mostly based on patient cases or clinicians' experience

time, secondary to or as a result of complex formation between botanical constituents (e.g. polyphenols in green tea).

7. The more significant botanical-drug interaction resulting in altered extent of drug absorption involves modulation of P-glycoprotein within the gastrointestinal tract. However, P-glycoprotein also possesses a physiological protective role by transporting toxic xenobiotics or metabolites out of normal cells.

Types of Herbal-Drug Interaction (Fig. 5.2)

Mechanisms of Herb-Drug Interactions

Pharmacokinetic interactions

Pharmacokinetic interactions involve changes in the way herbs and drugs move through body and can alter the amount, or level, of drug(s) in the body. If the interaction increases the level of a drug, you might experience side effects and/or toxicity. If the interaction decreases the level of a drug, it might not work as well, possibly leading to treatment failure and/or drug resistance.

There are several places in the body where such interactions can happen.

Stomach (gastrointestinal tract): When herbs and drugs are taken orally, they are usually absorbed into the bloodstream through the stomach and intestines. Herbs can affect the way in which drugs are absorbed, leading to changes in the amount of drug that enters the bloodstream. For example, some herbs can change the physical environment of the stomach, such as the pH level, while others might chemically bind to drugs, causing them to remain in the stomach instead of entering the bloodstream. Some herbs, such as laxatives, can speed up the digestive process, reducing the amount of time a drug is present to be absorbed by the stomach.

Liver: Once in the bloodstream, many drugs need to be metabolized (chemically altered) by the liver either in order to become therapeutically active or to be removed from the bloodstream. So the liver plays an important role in controlling the level and effectiveness of drugs in the body. Herbal therapies (and drug therapies too) can change liver metabolism. By inducing or inhibiting liver enzymes, herbs can alter the amount of therapeutically active drug in the blood. A good example of these pharmacokinetic interactions includes the cytochrome P450 system. The interfering drug may act as an inducer, inhibitor and/or substrate of the same CYP P450 enzymes those are responsible for the metabolism of the object drugs. This is the most important mechanism for interactions between herbal therapies and anti-retroviral drugs.

Kidney: Some drugs are eliminated from the bloodstream through the kidney. Herbs that affect the functioning of the kidney can change the level of drug in the blood. If the herb reduces kidney function, the level of drug may increase. If the herb increases kidney functioning, the level of drug may decrease.

Pharmacodynamic interactions

Pharmacodynamic interactions refer to the mutual actions of herbs and drugs inside the body. When taken at the same time, herbs and drugs may work together (synergistically) or in opposition (antagonistically). For example, separately they can have the same toxic effects, so that when taken together, they cause increased side effects. Many herb-drug

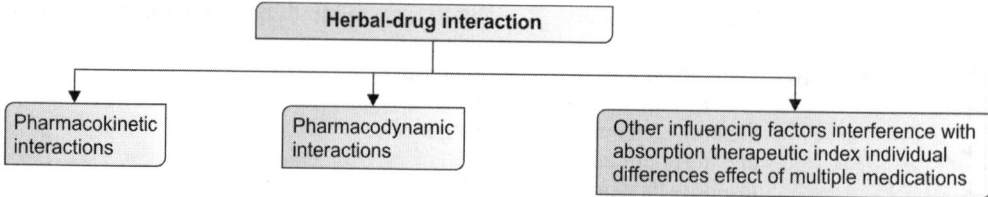

Fig. 5.2: Types of herbal-drug interaction

interactions fall into this category. Pharmaco-dynamic interactions are difficult to predict or prevent than pharmacokinetic interactions. Most of the pharmacodynamic interaction known now is documented through actual cases, as opposed to laboratory experiments. The best way to prevent pharmacodynamic interaction is to follow the patient closely monitor all clinical responses including signs, symptoms and any abnormal reactions.

Pharmacodynamic interactions affect a drug's action in a qualitative way, either through enhancing effects (synergistic or additive actions) or antagonizing effects. Many herb-drug interactions are pharmacodynamic type and are difficult to predict or prevent (Fig. 5.3).

DRUGS AND THEIR POSSIBLE SIDE EFFECTS AND INTERACTIONS: ST JOHN'S WORT, GARLIC, KAVA-KAVA, BLACK PEPPER, GINKO, GINSENG, EPHEDRA AND HYPERCIUM

St John's Wort

St John's wort is obtained from *Hypericum perforatum* L. belonging to family Clusiaceae.

Constituents

The main groups of active constituents of St John's wort are:

- Anthraquinones, including hypericin, isohypericin, pseudohypericin, proto-hypericin, protopseudohypericin and cyclopseudohypericin, and the prenylated phloroglucinols, including hyperforin and adhyperforin.
- Flavonoids, which include kaempferol, quercetin, luteolin, hyperoside, isoquer-citrin, quercitrin and rutin; biflavonoids, which include biapigenin and amentofla-vone, and catechins are also present.
- Other polyphenolic constituents include caffeic and chlorogenic acids,
- Volatile oil containing methyl–2-octane. (Fig. 5.4)

Use and Indications

St John's wort is widely used to treat mild-to-moderate depression, seasonal affective disorder, low mood, anxiety and insomnia, particularly if associated with menopause. It has also been used topically for its astringent properties.

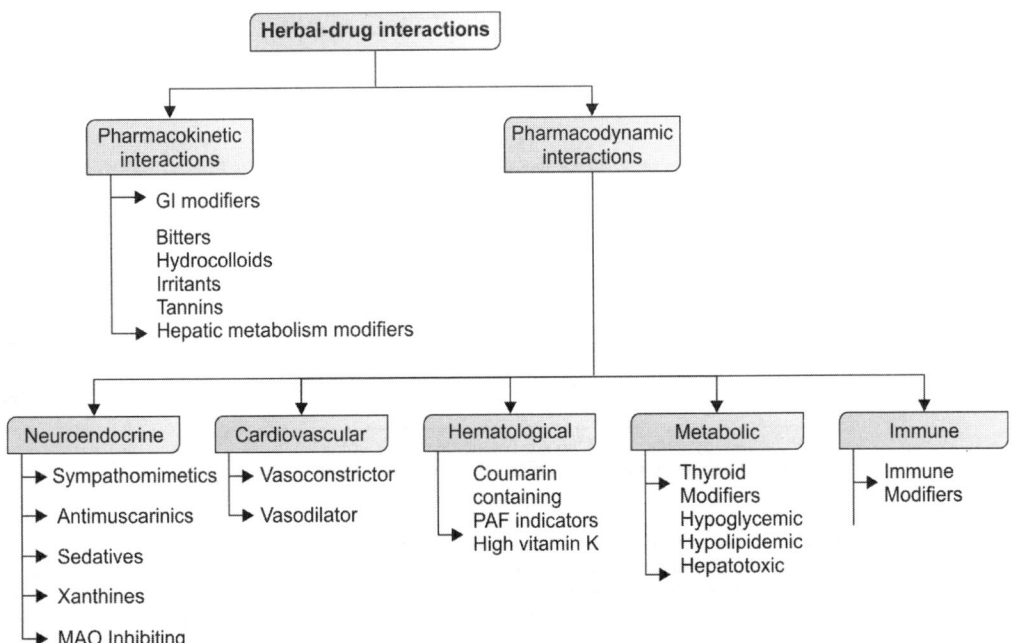

Fig. 5.3: Details of herbal-drug interaction

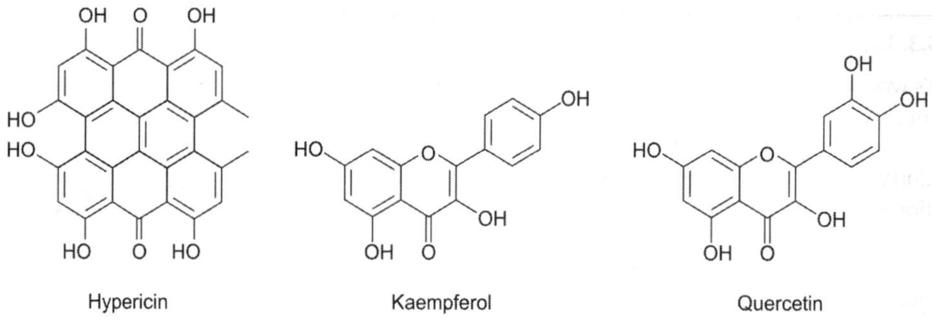

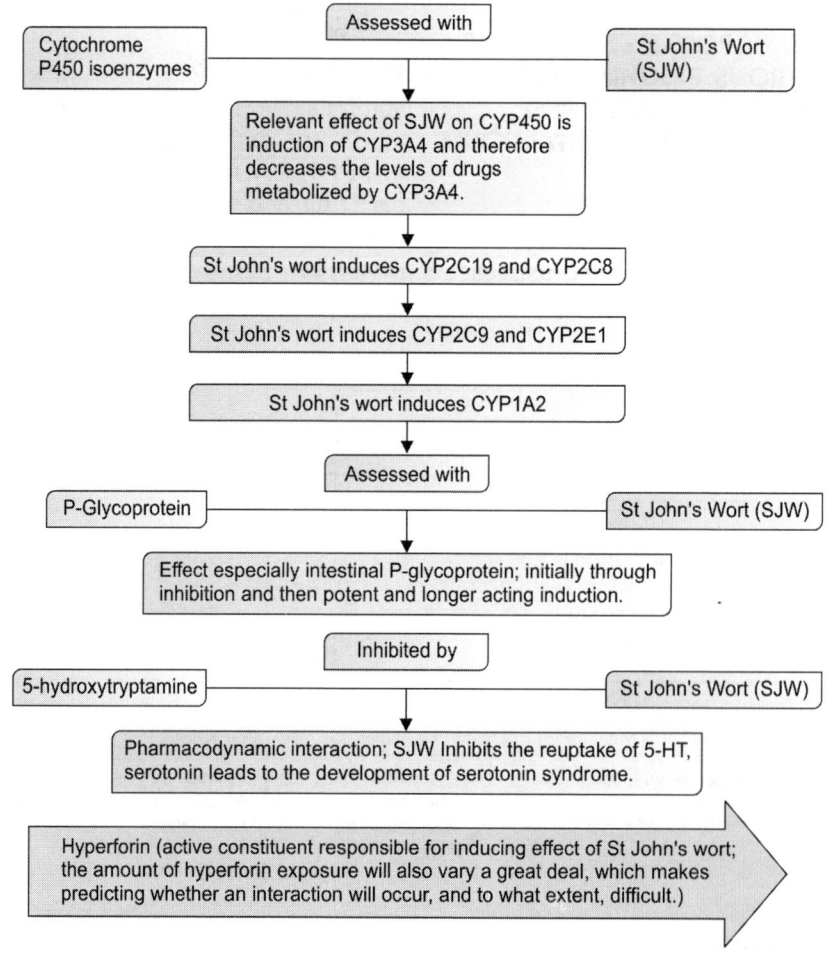

Fig. 5.4: Active constituents of *St John's wort*

Fig. 5.5: Pharmacokinetic drug interactions of herbal drug with *St John's wort*

Table 5.3: Interaction's overview of St John's wort

St John's wort interaction	Effects
Interaction with 5-aminolevulinic acid	Severe phototoxic reaction attributed to a synergistic effect of 5-aminolevulinic acid and St John's wort.
Interaction with general anesthetics	St John's wort may prolong the effects of anesthetics.
Interaction with antidiabetics	St John's wort modestly decreases the AUC of gliclazide and rosiglitazone. Pioglitazone and repaglinide, but it does not affect the metabolism of tolbutamide.
Interaction with antiepileptics	St John's wort modestly increased the clearance of single-dose carbamazepine, but had no effect on multiple-dose carbamazepine pharmacokinetics. Carbamazepine does not appear to significantly affect the pharmacokinetics of hypericin or pseudohypericin (constituents of St John's wort).
Interaction with benzodiazepines	Long-term use of St John's wort decreases the plasma levels of alprazolam, midazolam and quazepam. St John's wort preparations taken as a single dose, or containing low-hyperforin levels, appear to have less of an effect.
Interaction with bupropion	Serotonin syndrome when bupropion was taken with long-term St John's wort.
Interaction with buspirone	Taking buspirone developed marked CNS effects after starting to take herbal medicines including St John's wort.
Interaction with caffeine	Increases the metabolism of caffeine.
Interaction with calcium-channel blockers	It significantly reduces the bioavailability of ifedipine and verapamil. Other calcium-channel blockers are expected to interact similarly.
Interaction with chlorzoxazone	Increases the clearance of chlorzoxazone.
Interaction with ciclosporin	Marked reductions in ciclosporin blood levels and transplant rejection can occur within a few weeks of starting St John's wort.
Interaction with cimetidine	Cimetidine does not significantly alter the metabolism of the constituents of St John's wort, hypericin and pseudohypericin.
Interaction with dextromethorphan	St John's wort does not affect the pharmacokinetics of dextromethorphan or debrisoquine.
Interaction with digoxin	Digoxin toxicity
Interaction with eplerenone	St John's wort slightly decreases the AUC of eplerenone.
Interaction with food; Tyramine-rich	Hypertensive crisis may occur after consuming tyramine-rich food and drink.
Interaction with hormonal contraceptives	St John's wort may affect the pharmacokinetics of desogestrel, ethinylestradiol and norethisterone.
Interaction with imatinib	St John's wort lowers serum imatinib levels.
Interaction with irinotecan	St John's wort increases the metabolism of irinotecan, which may decrease its activity.
Interaction with ivabradine	The metabolism of ivabradine is increased by St John's wort.
Interaction with loperamide	Delirium in a woman taking St John's wort and valerian root who also took loperamide.
Interaction with methylphenidate	St John's wort may decrease the efficacy of methylphenidate in the treatment of attention deficit hyperactivity disorder.
Interaction with warfarin and related drugs	St John's wort can cause a moderate reduction in the anticoagulant effects of phenprocoumon and warfarin.
Interaction with tricyclic antidepressants	The plasma levels of amitriptyline and its active metabolite, nortriptyline, are modestly reduced by St John's wort.

Contd.

Table 5.3: Interaction's overview of St John's wort (*Contd.*)

St John's wort interaction	Effects
Interaction with SSRIs	Sedation, mania and serotonin syndrome
Interaction with proton pump inhibitors	St John's wort induces the metabolism of omeprazole, and this might result in reduced efficacy.
Interaction with protease inhibitors	St John's wort causes a marked reduction in the serum levels of indinavir, which may result in HIV treatment failure. Other protease inhibitors, whether used alone or boosted by ritonavir, are predicted to interact similarly.
Interaction with opioids	St John's wort reduces the plasma concentrations of methadone and withdrawal symptoms may occur.

Pharmacokinetics (Fig. 5.5)

The main constituent found to be responsible for the activity of St John's wort is hyperforin, but other constituents are considered to contribute to its antidepressant activity, such as hypericin and pseudohypericin, the flavonoid quercetin and its glycosides, and rutin. Bioavailability from varying formulations and extracts appears to be low, giving variable steady-state plasma concentrations.

a. Cytochrome P450 Isoenzymes

St John's wort is interacting with wide range of drugs and known to affect several cytochrome P450 isoenzymes, P-glycoprotein and 5 Hydro-xytryptamine. These isoenzymes exert a biphasic effect on, with inhibition occurring in *in vitro* studies with the initial exposure, and induction following long-term use. The interaction overview of *St John's wort* are given in Table 5.3.

Garlic

It is obtained by bulbs (cloves) of *Allium sativum* L. belonging to family Alliaceae.

Constituents

Garlic contains sulphur-containing compounds, alliin, allicin (produced by the action of the enzyme alliinase on alliin) and/or γ-glutamyl-(S)-allyl-L-cysteine. Other sulphur compounds such as allylmethyltrisulphide, allylpropyldisulphide, diallyldisulphide, diallyltrisulphide, ajoene and vinyldithiines, and mercaptan are also present. Garlic also contains various glycosides, monoterpenoids, enzymes, vitamins, minerals and flavonoids based on kaempferol and quercetin (Fig. 5.6).

Use and Indications

Garlic has been used to treat respiratory infections (such as colds, flu, chronic bronchitis, and nasal and throat catarrh) and cardiovascular disorders. It is believed to possess antihypertensive, antithrombotic, fibrinolytic, antimicrobial, anticancer, expectorant, antidiabetic and lipid-lowering properties. It is also used extensively as an ingredient in foods.

Pharmacokinetics (Fig. 5.7)

Allicin is subject to a considerable first-pass effect and passes through the liver

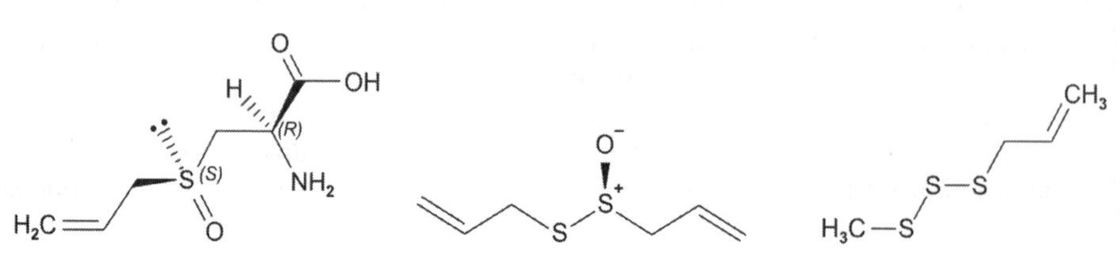

Fig. 5.6: Active constituents of garlic

unmetabolised only at high concentrations, but it is a very unstable compound and, as with ajoene, the vinyldithiins and diallylsuphide, it is not found in blood or urine after oral ingestion.

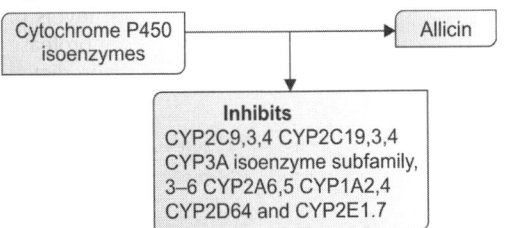

Fig. 5.7: Pharmacokinetic drug interactions of herbal drug with garlic

Garlic causes spontaneous bleeding during and following surgery. Inhibition of platelet aggregation by bio-organic constituents of garlic was demonstrated both *in vitro* and *in vivo*. Garlic may induce hepatic CYP3A4 metabolism of saquinavir resulting in decreased plasma drug levels.

Interactions Overview (Table 5.4)

The garlic may have additive blood pressure-lowering effects with lisinopril, and may cause bleeding in those taking warfarin or fluindione. The antiplatelet effects of garlic may be additive with conventional antiplatelet drugs and NSAIDs, and garlic may reduce isoniazid levels. However, no interaction has been proven with any of these drugs.

In general, garlic seems to have no effect, or have only clinically irrelevant effects when it is given with alcohol, benzodiazepines (such as midazolam), caffeine, chlorzoxazone, dextromethorphan, docetaxel, gentamicin, paracetamol (acetaminophen), rifampicin (rifampin) or ritonavir.

Kava-Kava

It is obtained from rhizomes of *Piper methysticum* belonging to family Piperaceae.

Constituents

The most important constituents are alkaloids 5.5–8.3% kavalactones (kava-pyrones). In traditional medicines, kava root is used to treat extreme states of excitation and exhaustion.

Kavalactones

Use and Indications

Muscle relaxation, analgesic and local anesthetic properties, anti-anxiety and anticonvulsant effects. The kava may directly influence the limbic system, the ancient part of the brain associated with emotions and other brain activities. Kava is a unique anti-anxiety alternative because it does not seem to impair reaction time or alertness when used in proper dosage amounts.

Table 5.4: Interaction's overview of garlic

Garlic interaction	Effects
Interaction with ACE inhibitors	Hypotension vasodilatation and blood pressure reduction
Interaction with antiplatelet drugs	Increase the risk of bleeding with conventional antiplatelet drugs
Interaction with chlorzoxazone	Garlic appears to inhibit the activity of the cytochrome P450 isoenzyme CYP2E1, which metabolises chlorzoxazone to 6-hydroxychlorzoxazone.
Interaction with warfarin and related drugs	Increase in the anticoagulant effects of warfarin, decrease in anticoagulant effects of fluindione. Garlic supplements alone have also rarely been associated with bleeding.
Interaction with protease inhibitors	A garlic supplement reduced the plasma levels of saquinavir
Interaction with herbal medicines; fish oil	Garlic supplements and fish oils may have beneficial effects on blood lipids.

Table 5.5: Interactions overview of kava-kava

Kava interactions	Effects
Interactions with CNS-depressants	Kavalactones potentiate the effects of CNS-depressants like benzodiazepines, barbiturates or alcohol.
Interactions with alcohol	Based on theoretical considerations, that there may be either pharmacokinetic and/or pharmacodynamic interactions between alcohol and kava, resulting perhaps in increased toxicity of either kava or alcohol increased sleeping times in mice when alcohol and a lipid-soluble extract of kava were administered in combination.
Interactions with levodopa	Reduced the effectiveness of levodopa in Parkinson's disease.
Interactions with caffeine	Pharmacodynamic interactions between kava and caffeine are associated with rhabdomyolysis.
Interactions with anti-convulsants	Major kavalactones display anticonvulsive action against maximal electro-shock, strychnine and pentylenetetrazole induced convulsions in mice
Interactions with MAO-inhibitors	Reversible inhibition of platelet MAO-B *in vitro* by kava kava *spissum* extract containing ~ 68% kavalactones avalactones may theoretically display additive effects with MAO-B inhibitors like selegiline used in the treatment of Parkinson disease.
Interactions with anti-platelet medications or anticoagulants	Dose-dependent antithrombotic actions of (±)-kavain on human platelets.

Pharmacokinetic (Fig. 5.8)

Kava is involved in several liver failure cases which led to its ban in many countries and this is matter of discussion on its relative benefits and risks as a social beverage and an herbal remedy.

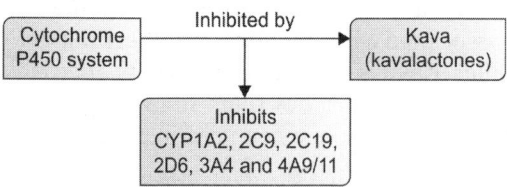

Fig. 5.8: Pharmacokinetic drug interactions of herbal drug with kava

Black Pepper

Black pepper is obtained from unripe fruit of *Piper nigrum* L. belonging to family Piperaceae, when immersed in hot water and dried in the sun, during which the outer pericarp shrinks and darkens into a thin, wrinkled black layer.

White pepper consists of the seed only, prepared by soaking the fully ripe berries, removing the pericarp and drying the naked seed.

Long pepper, *Piper longum* L., is a closely related species where the fruits are smaller and occur embedded in flower 'spikes', which form the seed heads.

Constituents

The major constituents are alkaloids and alkylamides, piperine, with piperanine, piperettine, piperlongumine, pipernonaline, lignans and minor constituents are piperoleins. It also contains a volatile oil composed of bisabolene, sabinene. The pungent taste of pepper is principally due to piperine, which acts at the vanilloid receptor.

Piperine

Use and Indications

It is used as a stimulant and carminative, and is reputed to have anti-asthmatic, antioxidant, antimicrobial, hepatoprotective and hypocholesterolaemic effects. Most of the pharmacological effects reported to date are attributed to piperine. A black pepper extract containing 95% piperine is used in a number of herbal supplements. Both long pepper and black pepper are important ingredients of many Ayurvedic herbal medicines where they are intended to enhance absorption of other medicines.

Pharmacokinetics

1. It has been shown that piperine when administered to mice delay gastrointestinal transit time in a dose-dependent manner.
2. Piperine inhibits the cytochrome P450 isoenzyme CYP3A4 *in vitro*.
3. Methanolic and ethanolic extracts of *Piper nigrum* fruit inhibited CYP3A4 and CYP2D6 *in vitro*.
4. Piperine did not alter CYP2C. *In vitro* studies suggest that piperine may inhibit P-glycoprotein, and ciclosporin.
5. Piperine may inhibit glucuronidation via the UDP glucuronyltransferase enzyme system, which is involved in the metabolism of a number of drugs.

Interactions Overview (Table 5.6)

Piperine, the active alkaloidal constituent of pepper, markedly increased the AUC of a single dose of nevirapine and of theophylline when given at a dose that might easily be achieved with piperine-containing supplements. Some caution might be appropriate with these combinations. The AUC of a single dose of propranolol was similarly increased, but this is less likely to be clinically important. Increases in phenytoin levels have also been demonstrated, and high dose piperine also increased the AUC of rifampicin. Various animal studies have shown increased levels of amoxicillin, barbiturates, NSAIDs and oxytetracycline with piperine, but a little effect on cefadroxil. Piperine also had an antithyroid effect in animals.

Table 5.6: Interaction overview of pepper

Pepper interaction	Effects
Interaction with Coenzyme Q10	Piperine modestly increased the AUC of one dose of coenzyme Q10
Interaction with herbal medicines: Rhodiola	Piperine might reduce the anti-depressant activity of rhodiola
Interaction with turmeric	Piperine increased the bio-availability of curcumin
Interaction with nevirapine	Piperine markedly increases the AUC of a single dose of nevirapine
Interaction with phenytoin	Piperine appears to increase the maximum levels and AUC of phenytoin, although the effect may be less in patients receiving long-term phenytoin.
Interaction with propranolol	Piperine pretreatment increased the AUC of a single dose of propranolol by twofold in a study in healthy subjects.
Interaction with rifampicin (rifampin)	Piperine increased the AUC of rifampicin, but a small dose of Trikatu had no effect.
Interaction with theophylline	Piperine almost doubled the AUC of a single dose of theophylline.

Ginkgo

It is obtained from leaves of *Ginkgo biloba* L. belonging to family Ginkgoaceae.

Synonym(s) and related species: Fossil tree, Kew tree, Maidenhair tree. Salisburia adiantifolia Sm., Salisburia biloba Hoffmanns.

Ginkgetin

Herbal Drug Technology

Isoginkgetin

	R¹	R²	R³
ginkgolide A	OH	H	H
ginkgolide B	OH	OH	H
ginkgolide C	OH	OH	OH

Ginkgolide

Constituents

Ginkgo leaves contain numerous flavonoids including the biflavone glycosides such as ginkgetin, isoginkgetin, bilobetin, sciadopitysin, and also some quercetin and kaempferol derivatives. Terpene lactones are the other major component, and these include ginkgolides A, B and C, and bilobalide, ginkgo extracts may be standardised to contain between 22 and 27% flavonoids (flavone glycosides) and between 5 and 12% terpene lactones, both on the dried basis. The leaves contain only minor amounts of ginkgolic acids, and some pharmacopoeias specify a limit for these. The seeds contain ginkgotoxin (4-O-methylpyridoxine) and ginkgolic acids.

Use and Indications

Ginkgo is often used to improve cognitive function in cases of dementia and memory loss, and it has been investigated for use in the treatment of Alzheimer's disease. The ginkgolides are thought to possess antiplatelet and anti-inflammatory properties and it has been used

Table 5.7: Interaction overview of ginkgo

Interaction with ginkgo	Effects
Interaction with antiepileptics	It may cause seizures taking valproate, or valproate and phenytoin.
Interaction with antiplatelet drugs	Ginkgo biloba has been associated with platelet, bleeding and clotting disorders, and there are isolated reports of serious adverse reactions after its concurrent use with antiplatelet drugs such as aspirin, clopidogrel and ticlopidine.
Interaction with benzodiazepines	Ginkgo does not significantly affect the pharmacokinetics of alprazolam.
Interaction with calcium-channel blockers; Nifedipine	Ginkgo may increase the levels and some of the effects of nifedipine.
Interaction with haloperidol	Ginkgo may increase extrapyramidal effects in response to haloperidol.
Interaction with NSAIDs	Fatal intracerebral bleeding in a patient taking ginkgo with ibuprofen, and another case describes prolonged bleeding and subdural haematomas in another patient taking gingko and rofecoxib.
Interaction with risperidone	An isolated case describes priapism in a patient taking risperidone and ginkgo.
Interaction with proton pump inhibitors	Ginkgo induces the metabolism of omeprazole. Most other proton pump inhibitors are likely to be similarly affected.
Interaction with warfarin and related drugs	Intracerebral haemorrhage associated with the use of ginkgo and warfarin, and there are a few reports of bleeding associated with the use of ginkgo alone.
Interaction with trazodone	Coma developed in an elderly patient with Alzheimer's disease after she took trazodone and ginkgo.

for cerebrovascular and peripheral vascular disorders, tinnitus, asthma and to relieve the symptoms of altitude sickness. Ginkgo seeds contain some toxic constituents; nevertheless, they are used in China and Japan, including as a food.

Pharmacokinetics

The two main active components of ginkgo are flavonoid and terpene lactones. It appears that the flavonoid fraction of ginkgo has more of an effect on the cytochrome P450 isoenzymes than the terpene lactones. *In vitro* ginkgo may have some modest effects on CYP1A2.

Similarly, *in vitro* ginkgo affects CYP2C9, CYP2D6 and CYP1E2, but clinical studies using the specific probe substrates tolbutamide, for CYP2C9, dextromethorphan, for CYP2D6, and chlorzoxazone, for CYP1E2 have found no clinically relevant effect. In contrast, *in vitro* findings suggesting that ginkgo may affect CYP3A4 and induce CYP2C9 are supported by clinical studies with midazolam, and omeprazole, respectively. Ginkgo may affect CYP2B6 and CYP2C8, but the clinical relevance of this needs investigation.

Interactions Overview (Table 5.7)

Ginkgo appears to decrease the levels of omeprazole; it seems likely that most other proton pump inhibitors will be similarly affected. Some evidence suggests that diltiazem and nifedipine levels may be raised by ginkgo, whereas nicardipine levels may be reduced. Isolated cases of bleeding have been seen when ginkgo has been taken with conventional antiplatelet drugs, anticoagulants and NSAIDs, and some cases have occurred with ginkgo alone, although a clinically relevant antiplatelet effect for ginkgo alone is not established. Isolated case reports also suggest that ginkgo may cause seizures in patients taking phenytoin and/or valproate and one case had decreased phenytoin and valproate levels. Phenobarbital levels do not appear to be significantly affected, although this is based on experimental data only. Ginkgo does not appear to affect the pharmacokinetics/ metabolism of alprazolam, caffeine, chlorzoxazone, dextromethorphan, diclofenac, digoxin, donepezil, fexofenadine, flurbiprofen, lopinavir/ritonavir, midazolam, propranolol, theophylline, or tolbutamide to a clinically relevant extent.

Ginseng

Panax ginseng (Araliaceae)

Synonym(s) and related species: *Panax ginseng* is also known as Asian ginseng, Chinese ginseng, Korean ginseng, Oriental ginseng, Renshen. *Panax quinquefolius* L. is also known as American ginseng. Other species used include: *Panax notoginseng* known as Sanchi ginseng, Tienchi ginseng and Panax pseudo-ginseng Wall. also known as Himalayan ginseng.

Ginsenosides

Constituents

The main constituents are the saponin glycosides such as the ginsenosides or the panaxosides in Panax species, or the eleutherosides in *Eleutherococcus senticosus*, which are chemically different. Also present are volatile oils containing mainly sesquiterpenes.

Use and Indications

Ginseng is used to enhance the body's resistance to stress and to improve mental and physical performance. It has also been used for diabetes, insomnia, sexual inadequacy, for degenerative conditions associated with ageing, to improve healing and as a stimulant.

Pharmacokinetics

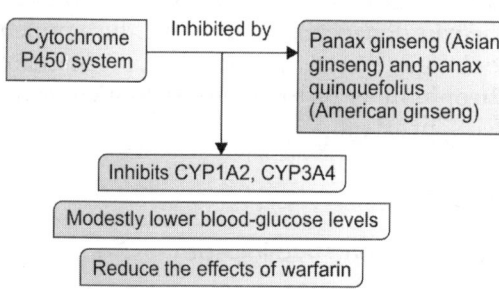

Fig. 5.9: Pharmacokinetic drug interactions of herbal drug with ginseng

Ephedra

Ephedra sinica Stapf, *Ephedra gerardiana* Wall, *Ephedra equisetina* Bunge (Ephedraceae)

Synonym(s) and related species: Ma huang.

Constituents

The main active components of ephedra are the amines (sometimes referred to as alkaloids, or more properly pseudoalkaloids) ephedrine, pseudoephedrine, norephedrine, norpseudoephedrine, N-methylephedrine, ephedroxane, maokonine, a series of ephedradines and others. Other constituents include the diterpenes ephedrannin A and mahuannin, catechins, and a trace of volatile oil containing terpinen-4-ol, α-terpineol, linalool and other monoterpenes.

Ephedrine

Use and Indications

Ephedra is used traditionally for asthma, bronchitis, hayfever and colds, but recently the herb has become liable to abuse as a stimulant and slimming aid. Its main active constituents are ephedrine and pseudoephedrine; however, ephedra herb is claimed to have many more effects than those ascribed to ephedrine and its derivatives. It is these compounds that also give rise to the toxic effects of ephedra.

Interactions Overview (Table 5.8)

Ephedra herb contains ephedrine and pseudo-ephedrine, and therefore has the potential to interact in the same manner as conventional medicines containing these substances. The most notable of these interactions is the potential for hypertensive crises with MAOIs; it would therefore seem unwise to take ephedra during, or for 2 weeks after, the use of an MAOI.

Ephedra + Caffeine

Ephedrine can raise blood pressure and in some cases this may be further increased by caffeine. Combined use has resulted in hypertensive

Table 5.8: Interactions overview of ginseng

Interaction with ginseng	Effects
Interaction with alcohol	Panax ginseng (Asian ginseng) increases the clearance of alcohol and lowers blood-alcohol levels.
Interaction with antidiabetics	Taking various oral antidiabetics, Panax quinquefolius and Panax ginseng have both shown modest reductions in postprandial glucose levels after a glucose tolerance test, but Panax ginseng did not result in any improvement in diabetes control when given for 12 weeks.
Interaction with caffeine	Ginseng and caffeine have stimulant effects.
Interaction with herbal medicines: Guarana	The stimulant effects of guarana, a caffeine-containing herb, appear to be additive to those of Panax ginseng (Asian ginseng).
Ginseng + Laboratory tests	Panax ginseng (Asian ginseng), Panax quinquefolius (American ginseng) and *Eleutherococcus senticosus* (Siberian ginseng) may interfere with the results of digoxin assays.
Interaction with MAOIs	Case reports describe headache, insomnia and tremulousness, which was attributed to the concurrent use of ginseng and phenelzine.

Contd.

Table 5.8: Interaction overview of ginseng (*Contd.*)

Interaction with ginseng	Effects
Interaction with tamoxifen and other oestrogen antagonists	Ginseng may contain oestrogenic compounds that might directly stimulate breast cancer growth and oppose the actions of compe-titive oestrogen receptor antagonists such as tamoxifen. However, there is some evidence that ginseng use before diagnosis might not adversely affect breast cancer survival.
Interaction with tolbutamide	It might increase or decrease the rate of absorption of tolbutamide in animal studies.
Interaction with warfarin and related drugs	Panax quinquefolius (American ginseng) modestly decreased the effect of warfarin, whereas another study found that Panax ginseng (Asian ginseng) did not alter the effect of warfarin.

crises in a few individuals. Isolated reports describe the development of acute psychosis when caffeine was given with ephedra.

Mechanism

Ephedrine and caffeine may cause catechol-amine release and an increase in intracellular calcium release which leads to vasoconstriction. Myocardial ischaemia may occur as a result of this vasoconstriction (in the coronary artery), and this may result in myocardial necrosis and cell death.

Other Herbs Involved In Drug Interactions (Table 5.9)

Chamomile

Chamomile consists of fresh or dried flower heads of *Matricaria recutita* (Fam Asteraceae), is used both externally (for skin and mucous membrane inflammations) and internally (for the treatment of gastrointestinal spasms and inflammatory disease of the gastrointestinal tract). It was believed, but not proven, that the coumarin constituents of chamomile may have worked synergistically or additively with warfarin, resulting in over anticoagulation.

Cranberry

Cranberry is the American name of the fruit of *Vaccinium macrocarpon* (Fam. Ericaceae); it has been used for decades to prevent urinary tract infections, generally in the form of an encap-suled standardized extract, a dilute juice or a dried-juice capsule. Cranberry juice increased the area under the INR-time curve of warfarin by 30%.

Echinacea (Echinacea spp.)

Echinacea preparations derive from under-ground as well as aerial parts of several species of *Echinacea* (Fam Asteraceae), e.g. *E. angustifolia*, *E. pallida* and *E. purpurea*. Due to its immunostimulant properties, echinacea is widely used for the prevention and treatment of common infections, such as respiratory tract infections.

Echinacea seems to pose no serious risk for drug interactions in humans. Echinacea affects caffeine (CYP1A2 probe) and midazolam (CYP3A4 probe) pharmacokinetics.

Eleuthero (Eleutherococcus senticosus)

Eleuthero, also named 'Siberian ginseng', belongs to the same family (Araliaceae) as Asian ginseng (*Panax ginseng*). Like Asian ginseng, eleuthero is promoted as a 'tonic for invigoration and fortification in times of fatigue and debility or declining capacity for work and concentration; also during convales-cence. Eleuthero, generally recommended at

Table 5.9: Interactions overview of ephedra

Interaction with ephedra	Effects
Interaction with Caffeine	Ephedrine can raise blood pressure and in some cases this may be further increased by caffeine. Combined use has resulted in hypertensive crises in a few individuals.

over-the-counter doses, is unlikely to alter the disposition of co-administered medications primarily metabolized by CYP2D6 or CYP3A4.

Green Tea (Camellia sinensis)

Green tea (*Camellia sinensis* leaves, Fam Theaceae) is used both as a beverage and as a herbal drug. Possibly due to its vitamin K content, green tea might reduce the anticoagulant effect of warfarin. Furthermore, green tea has been shown to reduce acid folic and the plasma level of statins through a mechanism that remains to be clarified.

Milk Thistle (Silybum marianum)

Phytotherapeutic milk thistle preparations are obtained from *Silybum marianum* (Fam. Asteraceae) and are used to treat liver diseases. *S. marianum* extracts seem to have minor effects on the pharmacokinetics of drugs metabolized by CYP enzymes or transported by P-glycoprotein. With the exception of one study, several clinical trials have reliably shown that *S. marianum* extracts did not affect the pharmacokinetics of a number of drugs metabolized by various CYP isoforms (e.g. CYP1A2, CYP2D6, CYP2E1 and CYP3A4) and/or transported by P-glycoprotein. Overall, milk thistle seems to pose no risk for drug interactions in humans.

Peppermint (Mentha piperita)

Peppermint leaf and oil from *Mentha piperita* (Fam Labiateae) have a long history of use in digestive disorders. Recent evidence suggests that enteric-coated peppermint oil may be effective in relieving some of the symptoms of irritable bowel syndrome. Some clinical data suggest that peppermint might increase the levels of drugs metabolized by CYP3A4, such as felodipine.

Valerian (Valeriana officinalis)

Valerian (*Valeriana officinalis*, Fam. Valeraniaceae) root preparations are widely available in a variety of commercial preparations as a sleep aid. Clinical evidence supports the notion that valerian is a safe herb associated with only rare adverse events CYP2D6, CYP2E1, CYP1A2.

Valerian might theoretically potentiate the effect of CNS depressants. Hand tremor, dizziness, throbbing and muscular fatigue have been reported in a patient self-medicated with valerian and passion flower (*Passiflora incarnata*) while on lorazepam treatment. Also, a brief episode of acute delirium has been reported in a patient taking the antidiarrhoeal drug loperamide in combination with St. John's wort and valerian.

Other herbal products that have been implicated in drug interactions include betel nut (*Areca catechu*, used for the preparation of a relaxing/refreshing beverage) chlorella (*Chlorella pyrenoidosa*), a unicellular fresh water green alga used mainly as a potential source of food and energy and also believed to have some therapeutic benefits, boldo (*Peumus boldus*) used as a choleretic/cholagogue drug fenugreek (*Trigonella foenum-graecum*), mostly used for the treatment of hypercholesterolaemia and diabetes mellitus evening primrose oil (*Oenothera biennis*), mostly used in dermatology as well as for the treatment of rheumatoid arthritis (*Grifolia frondosa*), an edible mushroom with potential anticancer benefits, mistletoe (*Viscum album*) used as a palliative therapy for malignant tumors, prickly pear cactus (*Opuntia polyacantha*), traditionally used in Mexico for the treatment of diabetes, goji (*Lycium barbarum*), used in traditional Chinese medicine in cases of loss of energy, diabetes and liver disorders and hibiscus (*Hybiscus sabdariffa*), used in folk medicine for the treatment of hypertension.

Gums, mucilages, pectins or fibers contained in several medicinal plants have the ability to bind, trap and form viscous matrices with concurrently administered drugs. Hence, they may reduce their absorption. For example, a decrease in the absorption of lovastatin (associated to increased LDL levels) was observed in patients who took the statin concomitantly with pectin or oat bran. Clinical data have shown that plant products, such as gum guar (from *Cyamopsis tetragonolobus*), acacia gum (from *Acacia senegal*), or guggulipid (a standardized neutral fraction extract of gum guggul, an oleoresin obtained from *Commiphora mukul*) may reduce the absorption of drugs, such as metformin amoxicillin propranolol , and digoxin.

MINIMIZE HERB-DRUG INTERACTIONS

1. Herbs should be administer at least 1½ hours apart from taking drugs, e.g. tetracycline can bind with minerals in the herbs inhibiting their absorption resulting in low drug levels.
2. Preferably taking the drugs first, is so that drug metabolism is already underway by the time the herbs can inhibit enzyme systems, e.g. grapefruit juice and herbs such as angelica, that inhibit the CYP enzyme system, can result in much higher levels of drugs in the bloodstream and longer persistence of the drugs. Saponins in herbs may improve absorption and elimination of drugs, altering the blood levels and rate of change of drug levels.
3. Pectin's resins and fibers in herbs may bind several drugs inhibiting their absorption resulting in low drug levels.
4. Herbs can modify drug absorption and/or elimination, e.g. saponins may improve absorption and elimination of drugs, altering the blood levels and rate of change of drug levels.
5. Avoid using herbs with strong laxative or diuretic action while using cardiac drugs. To compensate for mild diuretic or laxative treatments, consume high-potassium foods.
6. When the drug therapy is already addressing a particular therapeutic goal; avoid adding a potent herbal therapy with the same goal. Intensify monitoring of blood conditions affected by the drugs.
7. One should be aware of drug reactions and take reasonable steps to avoid problematic herbs. For example, MAO inhibitors can cause hypertension when an ordinary food component, tyramine is ingested.
8. One should be aware of herb-drug interactions and avoid using the combinations, if necessary, e.g. avoid mixing herbs or supplements and drugs that have similar actions. For example, gingko has blood thinning properties and may heighten the effects of anticoagulant drugs.
9. Avoid mixing herbs or supplements and drugs that have opposite actions, e.g. ephedra can exacerbate high blood pressure and may cancel out the effects of antihypertensive drugs.

Patient Counselling about Herb-Drug Interactions

Use of herbal and dietary supplements is extremely common. Patients may not be forthcoming about the use of herbal medicine even if it causes severe adverse effects because they fear censure. Clinicians must ask patients about their use of herbs in a non-judgmental, relaxed way. A disapproving manner will ensure only that a patient will conceal further use. The patient should be treated as a partner in watching out for adverse reactions or interactions and should be told about the lack of information on interactions and the need for open communication about the use of herbal remedies. Formulation, brand, dose and reason for use of herbs should be documented on the patient's charts and updated regularly. Patients with clotting disorders, those awaiting surgery or those on anticoagulant therapy should be warned against the concurrent use of ginkgo, danshen, dong quai, papaya or garlic. Although the combined use of anticoagulants with these herbs should be discouraged, patients who insist on the combination should have their bleeding times monitored (most of these herbs interfere with platelet function, not the coagulation cascade and thus will not affect prothrombin time, partial thromboplastin time, or international normalized ratio [INR]). Many other herbs also contain anticoagulant substances; as a precaution, patients on warfarin should have an INR measurement within a week of starting any herbal treatment. Patients on serotonin-reuptake inhibitors, cyclosporin, digoxin, phenprocoumon or any critical chronic medication should avoid St John's wort; those on phenelzine should avoid ginseng and those on tricyclic antidepressants should avoid yohimbine. Patients taking phenytoin should avoid Ayurvedic herbal mixtures for seizures. Liquorice (a very common ingredient in Chinese herb mixtures) may potentiate the action of corticosteroids, and betel nuts have pronounced cholinergic effects. There are doubtless many as yet undiscovered interactions.

Role of Pharmacist in Preventing Herb-Drug Interaction

Pharmacist can play a vital role in preventing drug-herb interaction to occur by appropriately dispensing medicine and taking due care of patient's history and medication profile. In order to ensure that the drugs that he is dispensing to the patient are safe and will not cause any interaction, he should ask the following questions:

➲ Are you taking an herbal product, herbal supplement or other 'natural remedy?'
➲ If so, are you taking any prescription or nonprescription medication for the same purpose as the herbal product?
➲ Have you used this herbal product before?
➲ Are you allergic to any plant products?
➲ Are you pregnant or breast-feeding?

Make sure your pharmacist and your doctor(s) know about every drug you are taking, including prescription and nonprescription drugs, herbal products, and any dietary supplements, including vitamins and minerals; Only take medication that has been specifically prescribed for you by your physician; Medication must be taken properly to ensure its safety and effectiveness; Unless otherwise instructed, take medicine on an empty stomach to achieve a faster onset of action; When taking medicine with food or around a meal time is not recommended, take medicine one hour before meal/food or two hours after meals or eating food; Take your medicine with a full glass (1 cupful or 8 oz.) of water; Avoid concurrent use of alcohol with medicine; Avoid consuming excessive quantities of chocolate and beverages containing caffeine coffee, tea, colas; and if you have any questions or concerns about your medicine or you believe you are having an adverse drug reaction or drug interaction, consult your pharmacist or physician immediately. If there is a problem, your pharmacist can contact your physician, who can prescribe other medication to avoid the risk of drug- related problems. Hence patients prescribed with certain 'known herbs' which are likely to produce interaction with conventional drugs should be periodically monitored. Interactions reported earlier can help to avoid their concurrent use.

Herbal Preparation and Formulation with its Origin

☞ Herbal Cosmetics

☞ Herbal Excipients

☞ Herbal Formulations

6

Herbal Cosmetics

INTRODUCTION

The word cosmetic was derived from the Greek word *kosm tikos* meaning having the power, arrange, skill in decorating.

The term Cosmeceuticals was first used by Raymond Reed founding member of US Society of Cosmetics Chemist in 1961. He actually used the word to brief the active and science-based cosmetics. The above term was further used by Dr Albert Kligman in the year 1984 to refer the substances that have both cosmetic and therapeutic benefits.

Cosmetic is defined as an article intended to be rubbed, poured, sprinkled, or sprayed on, introduced into, or otherwise applied to the human body or any part thereof for cleansing, beautifying, promoting attractiveness, or altering the appearance without affecting structure or function. For example, skin moisturizers, perfumes, lipsticks, fingernail polishes, eye, and facial makeup preparations, shampoos, permanent waves, hair colours, toothpastes, and deodorants, as well as any material intended for use as a component of a cosmetic product. These cosmeceuticals, serving as a bridge between personal care products and pharmaceuticals, have been developed specifically for their medicinal and cosmetic benefits.

Cosmeceuticals are topical cosmetic pharmaceutical hybrids intended to enhance the beauty through ingredients that provide additional health-related function or benefit. The term cosmeceuticals refers to products generally designed for topical application and which contain active ingredients with benefits for improved skin health.

They are applied topically as cosmetics, but contain ingredients that influence the skin's biological function. The variety of ingredients which have been incorporated in cosmeceuticals includes vitamins, antioxidants, minerals, herbs, hormones, anti-inflammatory, mood influencing fragrances (aromatherapy), and even such exotica as placenta, amniotic fluid.

From historical times natural extracts, obtained from animal, botanical, or mineral origin, have been used as 'active ingredients' of drugs or cosmetics. The use of natural ingredients in cosmetic products has a very long history. From ancient Egypt oils, butter, honey, beeswax, lead, and lemon juice were common ingredients of the beauty recipes. A nutritional cosmetic, as nutricosmetics, encompasses the concept that orally ingestible dietary products may support healthier and thus more beautiful skin. The origin of cosmetics forms a continuous narrative throughout the history of man as they developed. The man in prehistoric times 3000 BC used colours for decoration to attract the animals that he wished to hunt and also the man survived attack from the enemy by colouring his skin and adorned his body for protection to provoke fear in an enemy (whether man or animal). The origin of cosmetics was associated with hunting, fighting, religion and superstition and later associated with medicine. The knowledge finally dissociated from medicine and finally to pharmacy. The man from ancient time had the magic tip towards impressing others with their looks; at the time there were no fairness creams or any cosmetics surgeries to modify the appearance. The skin and hair beauty of individuals depends on the health, habits, routine job, climatic conditions and maintenance. The skin due to excessive exposure to heat will dehydrate during summer and causes wrinkle, freckles, blemishes, pigmentation and sunburns. The extreme winter cause damages to the skin in the form of cracks, cuts, maceration and infections. The skin diseases are common among all age groups and can be due to exposure towards microbes, chemical agents, biological toxin present in the environment, and also to some extend due to malnutrition. The only factor they had to rely on was the knowledge of nature compiled in the ayurveda. The science of ayurveda had utilized many herbs and floras to make cosmetics for beautification and protection from external affects. The natural content in the botanicals does not cause any side effects on the human body; instead enrich the body with nutrients and other useful minerals.

Cosmeceuticals could be characterized as follows:

- The product has pharmaceutical activity and can be used on normal or near-normal skin.
- The product should have a defined benefit for minor skin disorders (cosmetic indication).

- As the skin disorder is mild the product should have a very low-risk profile

The cosmeceuticals consist of bioactive such as natural antioxidants, natural preservatives, natural colouring agents, antimicrobiological active compounds, and others. During processing and storing, food, cosmetics, and pharmaceutical products are exposed to environmental factors such as atmospheric composition, light, and temperature. These factors promote their spoilage. The following changes caused by oxidation may occur during cosmetic formulation storage: Fragrance profile change, vitamin and active ingredient decomposition, colour change, and development of rancidity. A major cause of this quality deterioration is the autoxidation of unsaturated lipids initiated by free radicals. Antioxidants are crucial additives in cosmetic preparations for increasing their shelf life. Additionally, they can also be useful bioactive cosmetic ingredients to protect the skin against free radical formation induced by UV radiation and chemical environmental stress. Natural extracts with antioxidant properties recently have gained popularity because many studies show that natural ingredients are better and safer than synthetic ones. The combination of cosmeceuticals and nutraceuticals leads to formation of cosmenutraceuticals (Flowchart 6.1).

THE STRUCTURE OF THE SKIN

Macroscopic Characteristics (Fig. 6.1)

The skin is the largest, most extensive organ of our body. In fact, the average adult has about 170–200 cm² of skin with a weight that varies between 15 kg and 17 kg (obviously varying

Flowchart 6.1: Cosmeceuticals versus nutraceuticals

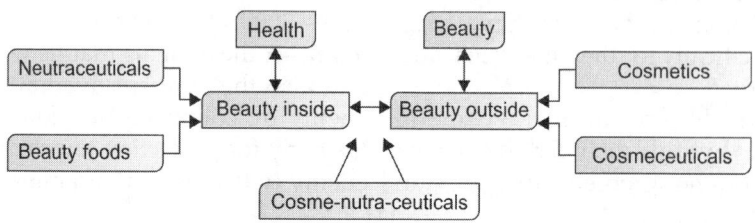

according to the subject's height and dimensions). The thickness of the epidermis, the outermost layer of the skin, can be from 0.5 mm in the thinnest areas (the eyelids, for example) to 4–6 mm at its thickest points (as on the palm of the hand and the sole of the foot). This thickness parameter becomes especially important when a substance is applied to the skin, be it a pharmaceutical or cosmetic product. In fact, once in contact with the skin any substance can penetrate the cutaneous barrier in a way directly proportional to the skin's thickness at that point. The skin tissue houses within its structure other important constituents: Hairs, nails, etc. (the skin's annexes). The whole of the skin is covered with hairs. In some areas the hairs are more developed and more coloured, as on the scalp, in the pubic region, and in the armpit. In other areas they are finer and much paler. These characteristics vary above all according to sex but also with individual biology. Tiny, invisible openings are found over the entire skin surface. These are the outlets of the eccrine sudoriparous glands, which, together with the apocrine sudoriparous glands and the sebaceous glands.

The skin mainly intends to protect human beings against environmental aggressions. It fills this "barrier" part through a complex structure whose external part is made up by the stratum corneum—a horny layer covered with a hydrolipidic protective film.

- ☞ The underlying epidermis also enables to reinforce the skin's defense capacity by ensuring the continuous and functional regeneration of the surface state (keratogenesis) and skin pigmentation (melanogenesis).
- ☞ The dermis also plays this part and appears as a nutritional structure whose function is also particularly important for the maintenance, coherence, elasticity, and thermoregulation of the whole skin.
- ☞ Finally, the hypodermis has a protective and reserve function.

Microscopic Characteristics (Fig. 6.1)

- ☞ **Epidermis**: The most external layer in contact with the environment.
- ☞ **Dermis**: Below the epidermis it is the structural component of the skin and the underlying organs.
- ☞ **Hypodermis**: Immediately below the dermis, composed of a layer of adipose cells and representing a "cushion" of fat between the skin and the organs underneath.

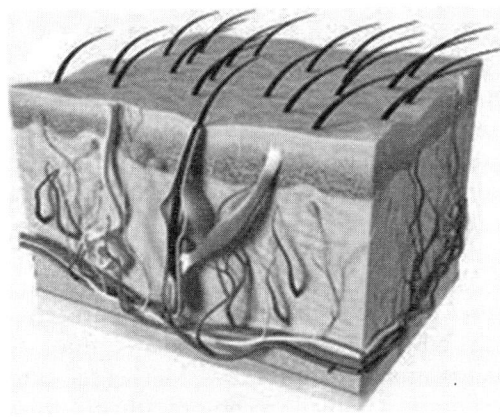

Fig. 6.1: Diagram of a skin section

The Epidermis

The epidermis is composed of different types of cells that overlap, not randomly but in a well-defined manner. There are four different cell types:

1. Keratinocytes
2. Melanocytes
3. Langerhans cells
4. Merkel cells

The Keratinocytes

The "keratinocytes" are the predominant cell type and owe their name to the characteristic protein they produce in the course of their life, "keratin." This protein is responsible for specific, important skin functions.

The Melanocytes

Interposed between the keratinocytes of the basal layer there are "melanocytes" that synthesize "melanin," the pigment responsible for skin colour. The number of melanocytes can vary according to body area and are usually present as a ratio of the number of keratinocytes.

Biochemistry of Melanin: Melanin is the pigment contained in the structures called melanosomes produced by the melanocytes. It is transferred to the surrounding epidermal keratinocytes, which maintain functional contact forming an epidermal melanin unit.

Langerhans Cells

These cells are situated above the basal layer and, like the melanocytes, have a dendritic appearance. The Langerhans cells unite against exogenous antigens and "present" them to both skin and lymph node T lymphocytes. They are also involved in immune surveillance against viral and tumour antigens.

Merkel Cells

These cells are found mainly in certain areas of the body: The fingertips, the oral mucosa, the lips, and the hair follicles. Merkel cells are considered as "tactile receptors," that is, they are the structures responsible for our sense of touch.

The Dermis

The dermis is positioned below the epidermis and is the tissue that supports the skin and its annexes (hair nails, etc). Its thickness varies from area to area, being thinnest on the eyelids and thickest on the back. The dermis tends to become progressively thinner with age. This layer is formed by cells, fibres, and ground substance is richly innervated and vascularized. The most abundant cells are the *fibroblasts*. These cells are the production site of the other dermal components: Both the fibres of the dermis and the ground substance are synthesized within the fibroblasts. In addition to fibroblasts, *mastocytes* (mast cells), *lymphocytes*, and *histiocytes* are present.

The Hypodermis

The hypodermis is situated below the dermis and is composed of "adipocytes" grouped into "lobes" separated by an area of connective tissue. The thickness of the hypodermis varies considerably according to the body site, nutritional state, and sex of the individual. Adipose cells are characterized by the remarkable quantity of lipids they contain. These lipids are grouped into a single globule in the cytoplasm, so large that the nucleus is forced to occupy a peripheral position. In fact, the distribution of subcutaneous fat is a strictly hormone-dependant secondary sexual characteristic. The number of adipose cells changes in the first phases of child development, at first increasing and then remaining stable. During puberty in women there is an increase in subcutaneous fat predominantly in the area of the buttocks, hips, thighs and breasts. In men, on the other hand, the increase in lipid content is in the area of the torso and abdomen.

SKIN CLASSIFICATIONS

Among the numerous skin classifications that are proposed, the one most closely connected with cosmetological requirements distinguishes four different types: Normal, oily, dry, and mixed.

Dry skin would mainly correspond to structural and functional modifications of the components of the epidermis.

Oily skin would result from an excessive seborrheic production, invading skin surface and possibly hair. Resulting from totally independent processes, oily skin and dry skin therefore correspond to two states that must not be opposed to each other, as some skins can be "dry" or "oily" and dehydrated at the same time.

The skin ensures essential functions such as permeation, metabolism, and thermoregulation and actively contributes to the sensorial function. This structural and functional diversity is influenced by intrinsic factors related to subjects, their ethnic group, their age, and their physiological, psychological, and pathological state and by extrinsic factors related to the immediate environment such as the dryness level, sun exposure, temperature, and wind. Numerous skin classifications have been proposed; they are all privilege-specific criteria.

Skin forms a remarkable protective barrier against the external environment, helping to regulate temperature and fluid balance, keeping out harmful microbes and chemicals and offering some protection against sunlight. Skin is a living organ that consists of epidermis, dermis and subcutaneous layers. Natural remedies have been used for centuries for treating skin conditions and a wide variety of dermatological disorders, including inflammation, phototoxicity, psoriasis, atopic dermatitis and alopecia areata. Although they are currently widely accepted by patients, their scientific respect among dermatologists in particular is limited. The alternative medications seem promising, although their true effects are unknown, so further investigations must be performed to assess clinical benefit. Herbal drugs for topical application also deserve consideration because of their widespread use and ill-defined benefit/risk ratio. Human skin manifests conditions ranging from simple dryness to severe erythema and scaling. These indications are sometimes accompanied by pruritis, inflammation and also may exhibit an associated oedema that further increases discomfort. Herbal materials to alleviate these symptoms have presumably been selected by a process of 'trial and error'. However, scientific study shows that plants possess a vast and complex arsenal of phytochemicals that not only calm, restore and heal the skin, but also stand up to the scrutiny of clinical trial and pharmacological testing. A cosmetic formulation, including active principles of strictly natural origin, is designed to protect the skin against exogenous or endogenous harmful agents, as well as to balance again the dermal homeostasis lipids altered by dermatosis and ageing. It is characterized by a lipid composition which is close to human sebum. Thus, treatment of the outermost layers of the epidermis with a relatively high amount of phospholipids, consists of a thin monomolecular layer applied to the skin, permitting natural hydration. The chemical composition of the phospholipids provides antioxidant protection, natural sun-blocking effects, anti-inflammatory and anti-free-radical molecules which are capable, for example, of preventing histidine from being decarboxylated to form histamine. Emollient natural remedies are often found to contain mucilage, consisting of polysaccharides, complex sugars and starch derivatives that relieve dryness and provide a soothing membrane that covers the skin. Protection of the skin hydration, and producing softening effects to skin and hair preparations is achieved using seed oils rich in fatty acids and triglycerides that reduce transepidermal water loss. Those plants with anti-inflammatory properties often have a high level of flavonoids; those that are used to firm and tone the skin are rich in tannins which have an astringent effect; and for skin healing in the case of infections the use of plants with a number of antimicrobial and antifungal biocides are beneficial.

THE HAIR SYSTEM

The entire surface of the skin is supplied with hairs, but on the head the hairs are longer and more pigmented. There are three types of hair:
1. Vellus hair
2. Terminal hair
3. Lanugo hair

Anatomy and Histology of Hair (Fig. 6.2)

Hairs develop from the hair follicles, which are true organs formed by the invagination of the epidermis during the foetal development. These organs are divided into three main parts:

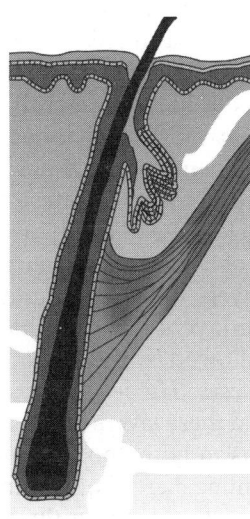

Fig. 6.2: Diagram of a hair follicle

1. The infundibulum is the portion from the opening on the skin surface to the mouth of the sebaceous gland duct.
2. The isthmus is the section between the sebaceous gland duct and the point of intersection with the hair erector muscle.
3. The inferior portion extends from the erector muscle to the bulb of the hair follicle.

The *hair root* is a generic term that includes the entire inferior portion and the isthmus. The *bulb* is the enlarged terminal part of the hair follicle in the root .The root produces the hair *shaft*, which is defined as the hair structure visible above the skin surface. Below the bulb the dermis re-enters the hair follicle, producing the *dermal papillae*, as the hair follicle is formed by introtlexions of the epidermis; this re-establishes the junction with the dermis. In this way the hair follicle is surrounded by the basal membrane. In this region it is particularly thick and assumes the name *vitreous membrane*, because together with the basal membrane it forms a kind of connective sheath that surrounds the whole follicle. The part on the hair follicle between the bulb and the isthmus is known as the *keratogenous zone.* The maturation of the cells that produce the hair shaft occurs in this area.

The most important part of the hair follicle is the bulb. In the basal layer, immediately above the papillae, cells continuously divide and begin their ascent. Slowly as this process proceeds the cells subdivide in the layers that make up the follicle. In fact, if a hair is cut perpendicularly to the follicle one can easily see how, independently of the zones and structure described earlier, each of these is formed by the union of layers and from inwards towards the outside of the follicle we can recognize the following layers: the *medulla, cortex,* and *cuticle.* These three layers form the hair shaft. The cuticle is followed by the *cuticle of the internal epithelial sheath, Huxley's layer,* and *Henle's layer.* Beyond these layers the *external epithelial sheath* begins and this, too, is composed of cell layers becoming increasingly thinner from the epidermal surface to the bulb. **In** the germinative layer, or *hair matrix,* the keratinocytes

are in contact with melanocytes, which are present only in this region. Here the melanocytes produce the pigment that will give rise to our hair colouring. The connective sheath also envelops the sebaceous gland and the hair erector muscle. The latter structure, important in furry animals in controlling the angle of the hair and so regulating heat exchange, is all but useless in man, nevertheless, this thin muscle is able to raise the hair. The follicles are set obliquely to the skin's surface and the erector muscle, by contracting and nipping both the follicle and the epidermis, are able to raise the hair. This is the phenomenon of *horripilation,* commonly called goose flesh, which occurs during shivering due to cold or fear.

HERBAL COSMETICS

Appropriate skin care contributes to successful management of acne. Skin care needs to be rational, flexible, and adaptive. The objective is to keep the skin and hair (scalp) clean, to control oiliness and prevent excessive dryness, to understand the changing needs of the skin on a daily basis brought about by variations in environmental conditions, physical activities, and the effects of topical and systemic treatments, and to compensate for such changes so as to maintain the skin in a near-ideal state. This is possible to achieve by balancing cleansing, moisturizing, and judicious use of supplemental skin care products.

Herbal cosmetics are formulated, using different cosmetic ingredients to form the base in which one or more herbal ingredients are used to cure various skin ailments. Herbal Cosmetics, referred to as Products, are formulated, using various permissible cosmetic ingredients to form the base in which one or more herbal ingredients are used to provide defined cosmetic benefits only, shall be called as "Herbal Cosmetics". Herbs do not produce instant cures. They offer a way to put the body in proper tune with nature.

The demand of herbal medicines is increasing rapidly due to their skin friendliness and lack of side effects. The best thing of the herbal cosmetics is that it is purely made by the herbs and shrubs and thus is side-effects free. The natural content in the herbs does not have any side effects on the human body; instead provide the body with nutrients and other useful minerals. Cosmeceuticals are cosmetic-pharmaceutical hybrids intended to enhance health and beauty through ingredients that influence the skin's biological texture and function.

The cosmetic does not come under the preview of drug license. The herbal cosmetics are the preparations containing phytochemical from a variety of botanical sources, which influence the functions of skin and provide nutrients necessary for the healthy skin or hair. The natural herbs and their products when used for their aromatic value in cosmetic preparation are termed herbal cosmetics.

The increased demand for the natural product has created new avenues in cosmeceuticals market. The Drug and Cosmetics Act specifies that herbs and essential oils used in cosmetics must not claim to penetrate beyond the surface layers of the skin nor should have any therapeutic effect. The legal requirement and the regulatory procedures for herbal cosmetics are same as that for other chemical ingredients used in cosmetic formulations. The use of cosmetic was time back in Pre-Christian Hellenistic period from where the historians had mentioned the use of herbals in cosmetics and aromatic products. Queen Cleopatra, a symbol for the last word in cosmetics and beautification, used aloe vera gel as a skin care product. The Pliny the Elder (A.D. 23-79) has written an interesting section on perfumes and aromatic materials in his Encyclopedia 'Natural History'. The Cornelius Celsus, a Roman physician (B.C. 7–A.D. 53.), discussed about the conditions of the skin cleanser during the 16th century. The Queen Elizabeth encouraged women to cultivate gardens and helped them in preparation of powders, sachets and scented washes (a floral essence with other aromatic substance). The use of ground orris as an ingredient in face powder, red ocher or vermilion as rouge was common during the reign of Elizabeth. The extracts of sandal or Brazil wood were considered a very new and smart cosmetic. The pimples were cured by covering for an hour with powdered sulphur and turpentine and later anointed with fresh butter. The golden-red hair, reddish and yellowish hair became a fashion and was affected by soaking the hair first in a warm solution of alum and then added to a decoction of rhubarb, turmeric and bark of burberry.

Examples:

1. Indian women have long used herbs such as sandalwood and turmeric for skin care and henna to colour the hair.

2. The materials used in cosmetics are aloes, costus, frankincense, lac, myrrh, camphor, musk, saffron.

3. Rose water as attar and sandalwood were common in early period.

4. The herbal ingredients used as perfumes are cassia and nutmeg.

5. The saffron, alkanet, agar, chlorophyll green from nettle plants and indigo were used in body decorations.

6. The use of betel leaves for darkening the lips, vermilion and other colours with waxes for their facial designation of caste.

7. Almond paste for the entire body instead of soap and use of perfumes and aromatics in all religious and social occasions are very common from ancient times.

8. The cracked lips which spoil the beauty of the face can be healed by applying paste made from the rind of *Aegle marmelos* in breast milk.

9. The skin fairness can be attained by preparing a paste with *Sessamum indicum, Pongamia pinnata, Berberis aristata, Saussura lappa.*

10. The dandruff was removed by applying *Papaver somniferum* in milk.

11. The face pack consisting of *Lens culinaris* mixed with honey were used to make the face soft.

12. The pimples were removed from face by applying plaster composed of *Coriandrum sativum, Acorus calamus* and *Saussurea lappa.*

13. The deodorant powder consisting of powder prepared from *Mangifera indica,*

Punica granatum and fragrant shell for removing the bad odour.

14. The presence of hair on arms, legs, face and public area can be removed by applying a mixture consisting of *Emblica officinalis, Piper longum, Euphorbia nivulia* to the desired place and the hair will fall off from the place.

15. The juice of *Eclipta alba, iron oxide, Terminalia chebula, Terminalia bellerica, Phyllanthus emblica* cooked in oil can be used to darken the hair and get relief from dandruff.

16. To make the breast increase the bustline and make it firm and shapely, powder mixture consisting of *Withania somnifera, Scidapsus officinalis, Saussurea lappa and Acorus calamus* added to the butter made from buffalo's milk and massage to the breast.

17. The herbs used were chandana, nagkeshara, padmak, khus, yashtimadhu, manjistha, sariva, payasya, seta (sweta durva) and lata (shyama durva).

18. These ayurvedic herbs are used to purify blood and eliminate vitiated doshas like (vata, pitta, kapha) from the body as they are mainly responsible for skin disorders and other diseases.

Regulatory Status of Cosmeceuticals

The legal difference between a cosmetic and a drug is determined by a product's intended use. Under present concept, the boundary at which a cosmetic product becomes drug is not well-defined and different laws and regulations apply to each type of product. The Drugs and Cosmetic Act 1940 defines a drug and a cosmetic as: Drug—"All medicines for internal or external use of human beings or animals and all substances intended to be used for ; or in the diagnosis, treatment, mitigation or prevention of any disease or disorder in humans or animals". Cosmetic—"Any article intended to be rubbed, poured, sprinkled or sprayed on or introduced into or applied to any part of the human body for cleansing, beautifying, promoting attractiveness or altering the appearance and includes any article intended for use as a component of cosmetic". Cosmetic and drug also categorized as some products meet the definitions of both cosmetics and drugs. This may happen when a product has more than one intended uses. For example, a shampoo is a cosmetic because its intended use is to clean the hair. An antidandruff shampoo is a drug because its intended use is to treat dandruff. Among the cosmetic/drug combinations are toothpastes that contain fluoride, deodorants that are antiperspirants and moisturizers with sun-protection claims. The claims made about drugs are subject to detailed analysis by the Food and Drug Administration (FDA) review and approval process, but cosmetics are not subject to mandatory FDA review. Although there is no legal category called cosmeceuticals, the term has found application to designate the products at the borderline between cosmetics and pharmaceuticals. Federal Food, Drug and Cosmetic Act do not recognize the term itself. It is also often difficult for consumers to determine whether 'claims' about the actions or efficiency of cosmeceuticals are valid unless the product has been approved by the FDA or equivalent agency. Some countries have the classes of products that fall between the two categories of cosmetics and drugs: For example, Japan has 'Quasi-drugs'; Thailand has 'controlled cosmetics' and Hong Kong has 'cosmetic-type drugs'. The regulations of cosmeceuticals have not been harmonized between the USA, European, Asian and other countries.

Advantages of Herbal Cosmetics over Synthetic

Herbal cosmetics are the modern trend in the field of beauty and fashion. These agents are gaining popularity as nowadays over chemicals for their personal care to enhance the beauty as these products supply the body with nutrients and enhance health and provide satisfaction as these are free from synthetic chemicals and have relatively less side-effects compared to the synthetic cosmetics.

Following are some of the advantages of using natural cosmetics which make them a better choice over the synthetic ones.

Natural Products

The herbal cosmetics are natural and free from all the harmful synthetic chemicals which otherwise may prove to be toxic to the skin. Instead of traditional synthetic products different plant parts and plant extracts are used in these products, e.g. aloe-vera gel and coconut oil. They also consist of natural nutrients like vitamin E that keeps skin healthy, glowing and beautiful. For example, aloevera is an herbal plant species belonging to liliaceae family and is naturally and easily available. There are a rising number of consumers concerned about ingredients such as synthetic chemicals, mineral oils who demand more natural products with traceable and more natural ingredients, free from harmful chemicals and with an emphasis on the properties of botanicals.

Safe Usage

Natural cosmetics are safe and harmless in nature. As per dermatologist cosmetics are tested and proven to be hypoallergenic. These cosmetics are made of natural ingredients, henceforth free of all kinds of rashes and skin itchiness. Examples of synthetic antioxidants, e.g. BHA (butylated hydroxyanisole) and BHT (butylated hydroxytoluene) are used as preservatives in lipsticks and moisturizers, can induce allergic reactions in the skin. The International Agency for Research on Cancer classifies BHA as compatible with all skin types.

All types of skin are compatible. Skin tone of dark or fair, it does not matter natural cosmetics like foundation, eye shadow, and lipstick which are appropriate are available as per requirements. Natural cosmetics can be applied on oily or sensitive skin never without degrading their skin condition. Natural colors obtained from herbs are safe to use in cosmetics. Colors derived from coal tar are used extensively in cosmetics but predictable as a human carcinogen which can cause cancer.

Natural cosmetics are suitable for all skin types. No matter if you are dark or fair, you will find natural cosmetics like foundation, eye shadow, and lipstick which are appropriate irrespective of your skin tone. Women with oily or sensitive skin can also use them and never have to worry about degrading their skin condition. Coal tar-derived colours are used extensively in cosmetics, coal tar is recognized as a human carcinogen and the main concern with individual coal tar a colour (whether produced from coal tar or synthetically) which can cause cancer. But natural colours that are obtained from herbs are safer.

Wide Availability

Natural cosmetics may still be a new type in the beauty industry but they already offer a variety of beauty products for all make up crazy people out there to choose from. One will find a variety of foundation, eye shadow, lipstick, blush, mascara, concealer and many more which are all naturally formulated. Furthermore, one will find locally made natural cosmetics or those made by famous designers worldwide. There exist a large variety of herbal extracts, to name a few *Andrographis Paniculata* (Kalmegh), *Asparagus racemosus* (Shatawari), *Boswellia serrata* (Salai Guggal), Asphalt (Shilajit), etc.

Economic

Natural cosmetics are not that expensive. In fact, some of these products are more affordable than synthetic ones. They are offered at discounted prices and are sold for a cheap price during sales. An estimate of WHO demonstrates about 80% of world population depends on natural products for their health care, because of side effects inflicted and rising cost of modern medicine. World Health Organization currently recommends and encourages traditional herbal cures in natural health care programs as these drugs are easily available at low cost and are comparatively safe.

No Need of Animal Studies

Some cosmetics are initially tested on animals to ensure that they are safe and effective to use for human. However, natural cosmetics need not be tested on animals. These natural formulations are tested by experts in laboratories using state-of-the-art equipment with no animals involved.

No Side Effects

The synthetic beauty products can irritate your skin, and cause pimples. They might block your pores and make your skin dry or oily. With natural cosmetics, one need not worry about these. The natural ingredients used assure no side effects; one can apply them anytime, anywhere. For example, herbal cosmetics are free from parabens that are the most widely used preservative in cosmetics and can penetrate the skin.

HERBS USED FOR SKIN (TABLE 6.1)

Coconut oil (or butter) is extracted from mature coconuts that have fallen to the ground. It is stable at high temperatures (up to 76.6°C). It is a colourless to pale brownish yellow oil with a melting point ranging from 23 to 26°C. Modified coconut oil containing polyunsaturated fatty acids in the form of mono-, di- and triglycerides, is useful as a constituent of a barrier lipid mixture in cosmetic and pharmaceutical formulations to protect and prevent drying of the skin. In Ayurvedic medicine, coconut oil is said to nourish the body and increases strength while application of coconut oil to the skin is said to help fixation of vitamin D in the body. The cosmetic application of coconut oil in hair and skin oil includes prevention of dandruff and providing emolliency, in shampoos it aids value, it is also used to prepare massage oils and beauty care products.

Sunflower oil: Sunflower seeds from *Helianthus annuus* (Compositae), contain polyunsaturated fats, rich in triglycerides of linoleic acid, an essential fatty acid, needed by the body to maintain good skin condition. Sunflower oil is rich in essential fatty acids, which have important regulatory actions on skin elasticity and moisture.

1. It is highly recommendable to formulate cosmetic products.
2. To protect the integrity of skin (anti-aging products) and hair (colour protection products).
3. To formulate cosmetic products with photo-protective activity,
4. To formulate cosmetic products to treat hair loss, to formulate cosmetic products with hair conditioning activity.
5. To formulate cosmetic products with purifying and antiseptic activity.

Studies indicate that cutaneous application of the sunflower oil increases the linoleic acid levels of the skin, lowers transepidermal water loss, and helps to eliminate scaly lesions common in patients with essential fatty acid deficiency.

Olive oil. *Olea europaea* (Oleaceae) fruit and oil; used to moisturize dry skin, and as a lip balm, shampoo, hand lotion, soap, massage oil and in dandruff treatment. Olive oil contains fatty acids, triglycerides, tocopherols, squalene, carotenoids, sterols, polyphenols, chlorophylls, volatile and flavour compounds. The extracts of mixtures of olive fruits, leaves and stems show anti-inflammatory and active oxygen scavenging effects. The anti-inflammatory effect is exerted by both unsaponifiable and polar compounds, while the free radical-scavenging effect of virgin olive oil is due to the presence of polyphenols. It is applied topically to treat skin damage, such as contact dermatitis (particularly diaper area dermatitis), atopic dermatitis, xerosis, eczema (including severe hand and foot eczema), rosacea, seborrhoea, psoriasis, thermal and radiation burns, other types of skin inflammation and aging.

Turmeric: Turmeric is the rhizome of *Curcuma longa* L. (Zingiberaceae). It is usually boiled, cleaned and dried, yielding a yellow powder. The major component is curcumin, which is responsible for most of the biological activities. Turmeric helps to remove hairs and impart colour and improve complexion of skin. Several Sanskrit synonyms of turmeric indicate its colour-improving property (such as *varna-datri*—one who gives colour, indicates its use as enhancer of body complexion. It is also used for prevention, treatment or control of psoriasis and other skin conditions such as acne, wounds, burns, eczema, sun damage to the skin and premature aging, due to inhibiting the activity of phosphorylase kinase. Turmeric oil is used as aromatherapy and in perfume industry apart from religious, cultural uses.

Pumpkin: Fatty acids isolated from *Cucurbita pepo* (Cucurbitaceae) seed oil. It contains main fatty acid components being palmitic (10.68%), palmitoleic (0.58%), stearic (8.67%) oleic (38.42%) linoleic (39.84%), linolenic (0.68%), gadoleic (1.14%), total saturated fatty acids (19.35%), and total unsaturated fatty acids (80.65%). The people of Central America and India rub the oil extracted from the seeds of pumpkin on herpes lesions, venereal sores, acne vulgaris and stubborn leg ulcers which refuse to heal up.

Pumpkin is a storehouse of vitamins, mineral and other healthy nutrients. Whether it is the pulp or the seed, pumpkin is magnificent for your health and can offer some inconceivable benefits. Pumpkin leaves are also applied as a poultice on sprains and pulled ligaments. The roots are made into an infusion and used on syphilitic sores, herpes lesions, pimples and blackheads.

Onion: The common red onion, *Allium cepa* (Liliaceae), has been used traditionally for its beneficial effects when used externally as a poultice for acne, boils, abscesses and blackheads to draw out the infection, decrease inflammation and speed healing.

Ginseng: Ginseng is an important traditional drug used for more than 2000 years. *Panax ginseng* is a representative medicinal herb belonging to the Araliaceae family, which is seven major species of ginseng distributed throughout East Asia, Central Asia, and North America. Ginseng is reported to activate the skin's metabolism, reduce keratinization, provide moisture and soften, alleviate wrinkling and enhance skin whiteness. The major active components of ginseng, ginsenosides, are known to exhibit antiaging, antioxidant, and anti-inflammatory activities. It also possesses skin protective and improving effects, as well as protection against excessive sun exposure using *in vitro* and *in vivo* models.

Tea: *Camellia sinensis* (Theaceae) yields both black (red) and green tea. It contains more than 500 chemical compounds, including polysaccharides, tannins, flavonoids, amino acids, vitamins and caffeine. The fermentation process of tea leaves results in black tea while to produce green tea, the leaves are steamed immediately after harvest and then dried.

Green tea: A *Cammelia sinensis* leaf contains flavanols, commonly known as catechins, consists of four major polyphenolic catechins. (-) Epigallocatechin-3-Ogallate (EGCG) is the most abundant and biologically active component, having antioxidant effects. In addition, it is used for prophylaxis, treatment and/or care of dry skin conditions, by stimulating the formation of ceramides and sphingolipids in the skin and thus reinforcing the lipid barrier.

The polyphenols have the potential to protect skin when combined with traditional sunscreens as they found to be particularly potent at suppressing the carcinogenic activity of UV radiation and exerting broad protection against other UV-mediated responses such as sunburn, immunosuppression, and photoaging.

Black tea: Black tea extracts contain polyphenols in a lower amount, and show a rather weaker protective effect against free radicals than green tea, but are still considered to be a good antioxidant.

Grape seed: The seeds of *Vitis vinifera* L. (Vitaceae) and its many varieties contain polyphenolic proanthocyanidins, which in turn can bind to each other to form oligomers known as procyanidins. Grapes contain fruit acids, and the unripe fruit contains oxalic acid. Its seeds contain 6–20% oil, phenols, carbohydrates and fruit acids. The procyanidins are strong antioxidants (compared with vitamins C and E), by inhibition of lipid peroxidation. Grape seed extracts are useful in antiaging and skin-lightening cosmetics as it shows tyrosinase-inhibiting activity.

Chamomile. German chamomile (*Matricaria recutita* L.; often referred to as true chamomile), or the Roman chamomile (*Anthemis nobilis* Linn.) are both members of the family Compositae. The both plants share a similar spectrum of chemical components, though not in the same ratios. Extracts of the plant are used in the form of ointments, lotions and inhalations intended for local application. Chamomile extract, essential oil and isolated constituents possess anti-inflammatory effects and are useful for treating inflammation of skin and mucous membranes, eczema and as an antipruritic adjunct in the treatment and prevention of skin disorders.

Fenugreek Fenugreek (*Trigonella foenum-graecum L.*) locally known as "methi" belonging to the family Leguminosae and subfamily Papilionaceae is widely used as spice and condiment to add flavour in various foods. It was also named, *Trigonella*, from Latin language that means "little triangle" due to its yellowish-white triangular flowers. The Fenugreek extracts are used in cosmetic soaps.

Jojoba: Jojoba oil (*Buxus chinensis* or *Simmondsia chinensis* (Link.) C. Schneider, family Buxaceae), contains fatty acids of broad spectrum such as arachidonic, linolenic, linoleic and oleic as well as triglycerides which have good compatibility with the natural sebum in the skin.

The peanut-sized seed is cold-pressed and expressed to yield about 50% of liquid wax known as jojoba oil. It is a rich extract used in cosmetic preparations, not only as humectant, but it also creates a protective film over the skin that keeps in moisture. Jojoba oils and its hydrogenated derivatives are non-greasy lubricant, therefore, may be useful in the formulation of creams, lotions, soaps, lipsticks and other preparations designed to be spread onto the skin or hair.

Licorice root: *Glycyrrhiza glabra* Linn is one of the most extensively used medicinal herbs from the ancient medical history of Ayurveda. It is also used as a flavouring herb. The word *Glycyrrhiza* is derived from the Greek term glykos (meaning sweet) and rhiza (meaning root). *Glycyrrhiza glabra* Linn, commonly known as 'liquorice' and 'sweet wood' belongs to Leguminosae family. As literature suggests that liquorice extract can be used efficiently to formulate cosmetic products for the protection of skin and hair against oxidative damage. It

is responsible for its powerful antioxidant activity by means of significant free radical scavenging, hydrogen-donating, metal ion chelating, anti-lipid peroxidative and reducing abilities. The extract of liquorice is reported to be an effective pigment lightening agent. It is the safest pigment-lightening agent known with least side effects. Due to good tyrosinase inhibition activity, liquorice extract can be used to formulate cosmetic formulations with depigmenting activity. Licorice is also used for skin irritations and in cosmetics for acne and sunburn.

Aloe vera. Aloe (*Aloe barbadensis*) is an important and traditional medicinal plant belonging to the family Liliaceae. Aloe's benefits can be attributed due to proteins, carbohydrates (including mucopolysaccharides), vitamins (including B_1, B_2, B_3, B_6, C, and folic acid) and minerals. These nutrients are beneficial individually as well as synergistically soothe, heal, moisturize and regenerate the skin. Many cosmetic companies add sap or other derivatives from aloe to products such as makeup, tissues, moisturizers, soaps, sunscreens, incense, razors and shampoos.

Its cosmetic applications are to stimulate the production of collagen and elastin that prevents aging of the skin, used in soaps, shampoos, creams and lotions for beauty purposes, in addition, it lightens the dark spots on the face and reduces the intensity of pigmentation, while applying topically, the gel acts as best moisturizer, removes dead skin cells and rejuvenates the skin and also it hastens the skin repair and hydrates your skin resulting in healthy and glowing skin.

Aloes gel can be applied topically as an emollient for burns, sunburn and mild abrasion, and aloe has antibacterial, antifungal, antiviral, antioxidant, antihistamine and anti-inflammatory effects. In the popular literature aloe gel is also described as a cleanser, anaesthetic, antiseptic, antipyretic, antipruritic, nutrient, and moisturizer.

Cucumber or *Cucumis sativa* Linn. (Cucurbitaceae) is cooling, healing and soothing to irritated skin, whether caused by sun, or the effects of a cutaneous eruption. Analysis of the fruit shows that it is low in nutrient value and little vitamin A but it is a good source of iron, calcium, and vitamins B and C. It is used for the treatment of hyperpigmentation in cosmetic preparations. The cucumber extract and lemon extract both are used; surprisingly, two ingredients do not interfere with each other, and instead increase lightening capabilities.

Antiaging

Rhodiola rosea: It is commonly known as golden root, roseroot, king's crown, *lignum rhodium*. It is a plant in the *Crassulaceae* family that habitats in cold regions of the world. It grows mainly in dry sandy ground at high altitudes in the arctic areas of Europe and Asia, *R. rosea* is rich in phenolic compounds, known to have strong antioxidant properties.

Carrot: It is obtained from the plant *Daucus carota* belonging to family Apiaceae. The richness of a valuable herb is due to vitamin A along with other essential vitamins. Carrot seed oil is used as anti-aging, revitalizing and rejuvenating agent. The carrot gets its characteristic and bright orange colour from β-carotene, and lesser amounts of α-carotene and γ-carotene. α and β-carotenes are partly metabolized into vitamin A in humans.

Gingko: *Ginkgo biloba* L. family *Ginkgoaceae* is the most commercialized medicinal plant worldwide, leaves and nuts have been used for thousands of years to treat various medical conditions, including poor blood circulation; hypertension; poor memory, and depression. In addition, it is gaining a similar reputation as an antioxidant and anti-inflammatory agent. *Ginkgo biloba* belongs to family which grows to a huge size. *G. biloba* is chemically characterized in nutritional and bioactive components, namely due to fatty acids, sugars, organic acids, tocopherols, phenolics and flavonoids. Palmitic, α-linolenic and oleic acids were the main fatty acids found; fructose was the most abundant sugar; quinic acid is the most abundant organic acid and α-tocopherol, which is widely used in various cosmetic preparations and formulations.

Neem: Neem or Margosa is a botanical relative of mahogany. It belongs to the family *Meliaceae*. *Azadirachta indica* is derived from the Persian. Azad=Free, dirakht=Tree, i-Hind=of Indian Origin. It contains nimbin, nimbidin and nimbinene. A large number of medicinals, cosmetics, toiletries and pharmaceuticals are now based on neem derivatives because of its unique properties. Neem bark is cool, bitter, astringent, acrid and refrigerant. It is useful in tiredness, cough, fever, loss of appetite, worm infestation. It heals the wounds and is also used in vomiting, skin diseases and excessive thirst.

Antioxidants

Tamarind: Tamarind or *Tamarindus indica* L. of the *Fabaceae*, subfamily *Caesalpinioideae* consists of amino acids, fatty acids and minerals. The sweet acidic taste of tamarind is most distinguished characteristic of tamarind due to tartaric acid. Apart from this, it is rich source of sugars, excellent source of vitamin B and contains minerals. It exhibits high antioxidant capacity that appear to be associated with a high phenolic content. Biological activity assessment of tamarind seed was reported on the radical scavenging, lipid peroxidation reducing and anti-microbial activities including anti-inflammatory potential. In addition, it is also used in skin lightening and control of sebum in cosmetic formulations.

Vitamin C: Vitamin C is necessary for the hydroxylation of proline, procollagen, and lysine. Vitamin C improves the changes caused by photo damage. Vitamin C has been used effectively to stimulate collagen repair, thus removing some of the effects of photo-aging on skin.

Vitamin E: Alpha-tocopherol is the major lipophilic antioxidant in plasma membranes and tissues. The term vitamin E collectively refers to 30 naturally occurring molecules (4 tocopherols and 4 tocotrienols), all of which exhibit vitamin E activity. Its major role is generally considered to be the arrest of chain propagation and lipid peroxidation by scavenging lipid peroxyl radicals, hence protecting the cell membrane from destruction.

HERBS USED FOR HAIR CARE (TABLE 6.2)

Depending on its moisture content, human hair consists of approximately 65–95% keratin proteins, and the remaining constituents are water, lipids (structural and free), pigment, and trace elements. Proteins are made up of long chains of various mixtures of some 20 or 50 amino acids. Each chain takes up a helical or coiled form. Among numerous amino acids in human hair, cystine is one of the most important amino acids. Every cystine unit contains two cysteine amino acids in different chains which lie near to each other and are linked together by two sulphur atoms, forming a very strong bond known as a disulphide linkage. In addition to disulphide bonds, hair is also rich in peptide bonds, and the abundant CO- and NH-groups present give rise to hydrogen bonds between groups of neighboring chain molecules. The distinct cystine content of various cellular structures of human hair results in a significant effect on their physical properties. High cystine content corresponds to rich disulphide cross-links, leading to high mechanical properties. The species responsible for colour in hair is the pigment melanin, which is located in the cortex of the hair in granular form. An average head contains over 100,000 hair follicles, which are the cavities in the skin surface from which hair fibers grow. Each follicle grows about 20 new hairs.

Plant materials can be used as hair growth stimulation, hair colourants and dyes, and in a number of hair and scalp complaints such as dandruff. Recently, various plant extracts have been patented for use in hair-growth or hair-tonic products, and for the prevention of alopecia.

A. barbadensis gel is used traditionally for hair loss, and for improvement in hair growth following alopecia. Aloenin is the major constituent responsible for promoting hair growth without irritating the skin. Aloe vera has been cited as a treatment for brittle hair, but with no evidence to substantiate this claim.

Henna or *Lawsonia alba* L. (Lythraceae) has been cited as a growth accelerator and was used in an ancient Egyptian formula to cure the loss of hair. The incidence of contact dermatitis appears to be extremely rare with the use of henna, since henna leaf extracts have mild anti-inflammatory and antiallergic action and analgesic effects.

Salvia officinalis L. (Labiatae) also called 'common sage', 'true sage' or 'garden sage' is used as a lotion to improve the condition of hair and skin. Claims of its use, alone or with rosemary, to maintain the sheen of dark curly hair, and to strengthen and stimulate hair growth have been made. The major *S. officinalis* constituents responsible for the effect on hair are the tannins, saponins, as well as borneol and camphor.

Rosemary or *Rosmarinus officinalis* Linn. (Labiatae) is an aromatic herb surrounded by tradition and legends but with important culinary, medicinal and cosmetic properties. In folk medicine it is used to stimulate growth of hair as a rinse. The most important constituents of rosemary are thought to be caffeic acid and its derivatives such as rosmarinic acid; these compounds have antioxidant effects.

Dandruff Treatment

Dandruff is a major problem, yet little is known about the underlying mechanism and subsequent biochemical changes that occur in the scalp skin and lead to its manifestation. The characteristic flaking and scaling of the scalp experienced by dandruff sufferers suggests that the desquamation process is impaired. Dandruff is also associated with a dramatic decrease in free lipid levels, with significant decreases in ceramides, fatty acids and cholesterol. Thus the epidermal water barrier is impaired in the scalp of dandruff sufferers, and the perturbed barrier leaves sufferers more prone to the adverse effects of microbial and fungal toxins, and environmental pollutants, thus perpetuating the impaired barrier.

Traditionally sage (*Salvia officinalis* L.) is an old favourite for dandruff, loss of hair and greasy hair and skin. An extract of sage massaged into the scalp can control dandruff, falling hair or loss of hair if the papilla is dormant and not destroyed.

Rosemary is claimed to be a conditioner for greasy hair, a rinse and a tonic that gives body and sheen to hair, and infused fresh or dried rosemary and sage can be used as a daily rinse for dandruff treatment.

Thyme or *Thymus vulgaris* L. (Labiatae) is also claimed to inhibit dandruff, and used in a scalp rub it prevents hair falling out, and rinses containing rosemary and thyme promote natural hair health.

Garlic or *Allium sativum* (L. Liliaceae) lotion can help to control dandruff. It has been used since ancient times as a vegetable with many properties, including antiseptic, tonic, antioxidant, anti-inflammatory, antibacterial and antifungal effects. Garlic should not be placed directly on the skin since it may cause blisters and a burning sensation in some people or contact dermatitis and allergic reactions in others.

English Walnut or *Juglans regia* L. (Juglandaceae), leaves are used in traditional medicine for external applications such as eczema, acne, loss of hair, scalp itching, peeling and dandruff; and as an adjunctive emollient itch-relieving treatment in skin disorders; as a trophic protective agent for cracks, abrasions, frostbite, chaps and insect bites to treat sunburns and for nappy rashes.

Juglans nigra refers to the black walnut, whose bark is used for dandruff and other scalp problems. Hair colouring vegetable dyes can usually be recommended to patients sensitized to oxidative dyes, due to their low allergenic power. The use of natural dyes on the hair has not made great progress and this is due firstly, to the fact that natural dyes are not very stable in solution, and are prone to oxidation, discolouration, pH colour shift and fading. Secondly, a single natural dye may not give the right colour, and only henna or walnut seems to be suitable to colour the hair. However, many shades can be obtained by mixing with the leaves of other plants.

The leaves of *Lawsonia inermis*, known as henna, has been applied since ancient times

for decorating and dyeing hands and feet, to impart shades of dark red, and for the treatment of certain skin disorders. The compound lawsone, a brown powder isolated from the leaves, is responsible for the red colour in henna. It is used as a staining agent, due to the strong binding of lawsone to the hair, probably upon reaction of thiol groups with keratin. If the hair is dyed with henna and then treated with a hot decoction of *Allium cepa* (onion) skin, a coppery colour will be obtained. The incidence of contact dermatitis from using henna appears to be rare but possible.

Curcumin is the pigment of the spice turmeric and will also give a range of colour from yellow to a deep orange. Turmeric contains three major curcuminoids, of which curcumin is the most significant, and these are responsible for the yellow colour of the herb.

Sweet orange (*Citrus sinensis* [L.] Pers.) Oil is composed largely of terpene hydrocarbons which is a source of flavour and fragrance compounds, it has more than 90% limonene and although it is primarily used in flavours, it does find a use in Eaux des Cologne and soap fragrances.

Grapefruit (*Citrus paradisica* Macfad.) Oil is chemically similar to orange oil but it has a distinctive smell which is largely attributed to a ketone called nootkaton. Grapefruit oil does not find very wide use in perfumery (Barel et al., 2001).

Chamomile oil: It has been mentioned before that the ability of chamomile to reduce inflammation is one of its most highly prized features due to the presence of flavonoids. It is safe for skin care, and it is also credited with a gentle analgesic effect. Its effects as anti-inflammatory, antierythema and antipruritic, at the same time as being gentle, soothing and antiseptic, may help in whitening age spots, take the soreness out of a boil, minor wound, burn, or an insect bite, or used for dry skin, windburn, sunburn, or even chronic skin conditions such as acne and psoriasis.

Geranium oil: *Pelargonium graveolens* (L.) L Her. ex Ait (Geraniaceae), obtained through steam or water plus steam distillation of shoot

Table 6.1: Herbal plant for skin care

Latin name	Common name	Part used	Uses
Acorus calamus	Sweet flag	Rhizome	Aromatic, dusting powders, skin lotions
Allium sativum	Garlic	Bulb	Promotes skin healing, antibacterial controls sore, pimples and acne.
Aloe vera	Aloe	Leaf	Moisturizer, sun screen, emollient
Alpinia galanga	Galanga	Rhizome	Aromatic, dusting powders
Avena sativa	Oat	Fruit	Moisturizer, skin tonic
Asparagus racemosus	Shatavari	Roots	Used to wrinkle on the face.
Azadirachta indica	Neem	Leaf	Antiseptic, reduce dark spots, antibacterial
Andropogon muricates	Khas	Root	Cure irrigated skin and allergies.
Adhatoda vasica nees	Vasca	Leaf	Skin affection and control of scabies
Ailanthus excelsa	Maharukh	Leaf	Check skin eruption and useful in skin creams and lotions
Buchanania lanzan	Chironnji	Seed	Skin ointments, rashes, spots
Butea frondosa	Dhak	Leaf, seed	Leaf used for pimples and seed used for fungal infection
Carica papaya	Papaya	Fruit	Skin soft and remove blemishes
Cassia tora	Panwar	Leaf and seed	Skin infection, ringworm and eruption.
Citrus limon	Nimbu	Fruit	Skin nourishment, useful as facial ingredients.
Cocos nucifera	Nariyal	Oil	Skin itches and rashes
Cucumis sativus	Khira	Fruit and seeds	Protect skin from sunburn
Curcuma longa	Haldi	Rhizome	Anti-inflammatory, antioxidant, enhance colour of skin
Curcuma amada	Amhaldi	Dry rhizome	Face pack, acne and blemishes
Cuscuta refexa	Akash bhel	Whole plant	Dermatitis, itching and ringworm
Callicarpa marcophylla	Priyangu	Dry fruits	Treat acne, pimples and allergic skin patches
Echinacea purpurea	Echinacea	Roots, stem, and leaves	Skin regeneration
Centella asiatica	Gotu kola	Plant	Wound healing
Symphytum officinale	Comfrey	leaves	Cell regeneration, stimulates the growth of new cells
Crocus sativus	Kesar	Flowering top	Skin cleansing lotion
Eclipta alba	Bhringraj	Whole plant	Skin diseases and eczema
Euphorbia thymifolia	Choti dhudhi	Whole plant	Ringworm and skin infections
Jasminum grandiflorum	Chameli	Flowers	Skin diseases, protection from sunburn
Juniperus communis	Aaraar	Whole plant	Skin rejuvenation
Lavendula vera	Lavender	Essential oil	Antiacne cream
Leucas aspera	Hul khusa	Leaves	Control scabies, skin psoriases, chronic skin, skin eruption and eczema
Mallotus philippensis	Kamala	Flower	Control scabies, ringworm
Mangifera indica	Mango	Plant	Antioxidant
Matricaria chamomilla	Babuna	Leaves	Anti acne
Mimosa pudica	Lajwanti	Plant	Skin cream and control itching
Ocimum sanctum	Tulsi	leaves	Skin infection and rejuvenation
Phyllanthus emblica	Amla	Fruit	Antioxidant

Contd.

Table 6.1: Herbal plant for skin care (*Contd.*)

Latin name	Common name	Part used	Uses
Prunus amygdalus	Badam	Fruit	Skin beautification
Psoralea corylifolia	Babchi	Seed	Skin diseases
Rosa damascena	Lal gulab	Flowers	Beautification, smoothness and protection from sunburns
Rubia cordifolia	Manjit	Dry roots and stem	Dark spots on face
Santalum album	Chandan	Hardwood	Skin beautification, protection of sunburn, antioxidant properties
Saussurea lappa	Kuth	Root	Treatment of chronic skin diseases
Sesamum indicum	Til	Seed	Skin protection and rejuvenation
Swertia chirayita	Til	Bark	Antioxidant
Withania Somnifera	Aswagandha	Root	Skin cleansing formulations and antioxidant

Table 6.2: Herbal plant for hair care

Latin name	Common name	Part used	Uses
Emblica officinalis	Amla	Dry fruits	Hair care, hair tonic
Acacia concinna	Ritha, shikakai	Pods	Hair growth, prevent hair splitting, hair falling and dandruff
Aloe barbadensis	Aloe	Leaves	Hair falling, dandruff, sunburn
Azadirachta indica	Neems	Whole plant	Hair and scalp care
Callicarpa macrophylla	Priyangu	Fruits	Prevent acne
Eclipta prostrata	Bhringraj	Whole Plant	Keep hairs in their original colour
Lawsonia inermis	Mehandi	Leaves	Colour the hairs
Centella asiatica	Brahmi	Herb	Maintain proper bodily environment that leads to healthy hairs.
Eclipta alba	Bhringraj		Hair tonic
Cocos nucifera	Coconut	fruit	Oil of coconut fruit is used in different hair formulations such as shampoos and hair oil
Eucalyptus globulus	Eucalyptus	Fruit	Prevents dandruff
Lawsonia inermis	Henna	Leaves	Hair colour
Azadirachta indica	Neem	Leaves	Hair tonic and conditioners
Hibiscus rosa sinensis	Gurhal	Petal	Prevent premature graying, hair loss and scalp disorders.
Nardostachys jatamansi	Jatamansi	Rhizomes	Hair tonic and impart blackness to hairs.
Trigonella foenum graecum	Fenugreek	Seeds	Hair grow, preserves natural colour, keeps hair silky and also cures dandruff
Juniperus virginiana	Cedar wood oil	Woods	Hair loss and dandruff.
Rosmarinus officinale	Rosemary	Oil	Promote hair growth and shining
Arnica montana	Arnica	Flower	Tonic and stimulates hair follicles.
Betula pendula	Birch	Leaves	Antidandruff
Calendula officinalis	Marigold	Flowers	Hair cream for smoothing effect
Carthamus tinctorius	Safflower	Whole plant	Hair tonic
Centella asiatica	Mandukaparni	Whole plant	Growth and maintenance of hairs

Contd.

Table 6.2: Herbal plant for hair care (Contd.)

Latin name	Common name	Part used	Uses
Ficus racemosus	Bargad	Root	Checks hair fall
Salvia officinalis	Sage	Whole plant	Hair conditioner
Sapindus mukorossi	Ritha	Fruit	Natural shampoo and hair cleanser
Saussurea lappa	Kuth	Root	Hair dyeing
Terminilia bellirica	Behera	Seed	Hair dyeing preparations
Thymus serphyllum	Banajwain	Whole herb	Preparing hair tonic

biomass, is extensively used in the fragrance industry and in aromatherapy. Geranium oil is a cleansing, toning and sharpening oil and is so helpful with those problems that come with greasy, over-oily skin, acne, congested skin and eczema. Care should be taken since there is the possibility of contact dermatitis in hypersensitive individuals. It is a very important component of high grade perfumes due to its strong rose-like odour.

Lavender oil: Essential oils distilled from members of the genus Lavandula have been used both cosmetically and therapeutically for centuries. It is extensively employed in all types of soaps, lotions and perfumes, with the most commonly used species being *Lavendula angustifolia*, *L. latifolia*, *L. stoechas* and *L. intermedia*. Among the claims made for lavender oil are that it is antibacterial, antifungal and effective for burns and insect bites. This oil in the herbal tradition is said to encourage cell growth and so should be used to help with mending and regeneration in all kinds of skin ailments: Bites, stings, boils, burns, stretch marks, rashes, spots, cold sores, sunburns. Lavender oil inhibits immediate-type allergic reaction in mice and rats. Topical and intradermal lavender oil inhibited the ear swelling response in mice and passive cutaneous anaphylaxis in rats.

Amla: Amla is the name given to the fruit of a small leafy tree (*Emblica Officinalis*), which grows throughout India and yields an characteristics odor. There are mainly four species of roses for oil production. These are *Rosa damascena* Mill., *R. gallica* L., *R. moschata* Herrm. and *R. centifolia* L. Rose oil and rose water have many therapeutic effects. Rose oil helps soothe the mind and heals depression, grief, nervous stress and tension. It also helps to heal wound and skin health.

Eucalyptus oil: There are around 700 different species of Eucalyptus in the world, of which at least 500 produce a type of essential oil. It is produced by steam distillation from the leaves of *Eucalyptus* species (*E. cinerea F. Muell.*, *E. baueriana F. Muell.*, *E. smithii R. T. Baker*, *E. bridgesiana R. T. Baker*, *E. microtheca F. Muell.*, *E. foecunda Schau.*, *E. pulverulenta Sims*, *E. propinqua Deane and Maiden*, *E. erythrocorys F. Muell.*, etc.). They are widely used in the preparation of liniments, inhalants, cough syrups, ointments, toothpaste and also as pharmaceutical flavours. The European Pharmacopoeia monograph for *Eucalyptus* oil sports a chromatographic profile: 1,8-cineole (eucalyptol; not less than70%), limonene (4–12%), α-pinene (2-8%), α- phellandrene (less than1.5%), β-pinene (less than 0.5%), camphor (less than 0.1%).

Ayurveda has numerous natural medications wherein the most common herbs include neem, kapoor (naphthalene), and henna, hirda, behada, and amalaki, magic nut, bringaraj, rosary pea, sweet flag, cashmere tree and mandor.

Henna: Henna comes from the plant *Lawsonia inermis* family Lythraceae, which contain a dye molecule called Lawsone, which when processed produces henna powder. Besides lawsone other constituents present are gallic acid, glucose, mannitol, fats, resin (2%), mucilage and traces of an alkaloid. Leaves yield hennatannic acid and an olive oil green resin, soluble in ether and alcohol. Lawsone edible fruit. It is highly praised both for its high vitamin C content and for the precious oil, which is extracted from its seeds and pulp and used as a treatment for hair and scalp problems. It is used in eye syndromes, hair loss, and children ailments, etc.

Shikakai: *Acacia concinna Linn. (Leguminosae)* is a medicinal plant that grows in tropical rainforests of southern Asia. The fruits of this plant are used for washing hair, for improving hair growth, as an expectorant, emetic, and purgative. The powder of *Acacia concinna Linn* shows the presence of saponins, alkaloid, sugar, tannin, flavanoids, anthraquinone glycosides.

Essential Oils

Rose oil: Roses are widely referred to as the world's favourite flower in part due to their vast diversity in plant habitat and floral from the underground stems of the tropical perennial herb *Curcuma longa* of the family *Zingiberaceae*. Turmeric contains a wide range of phytochemicals including, demethoxycurcumin, bisdemethoxycurcumin, zingiberene, curcumol, curcumenol, eugenol, tetrahydrocurcumin, triethylcurcumin, curcumin, turmerin, turmerones, and turmeronols. Curcumin is the phytochemical that gives a yellow colour to turmeric and is now recognized as being responsible for most of the therapeutic effects. Uses of turmeric include antiseptic, analgesic, anti-inflammatory, antioxidant, antimalarial, insect-repellant, and other activities associated to turmeric.

CONCLUSION

Natural ingredients are everywhere and are continually gaining popularity, and the use of plant extracts in cosmetic formulation is on the rise. A cosmetic formulation including active principles of natural origin can protect the skin against exogenous or endogenous harmful agents, and help to remedy many skin conditions. In addition, natural products can be used in hair care, and as hair colourants or dyes. Aromatic plants and oils have been used for thousands of years, as incense, perfumes, cosmetics, and for their medicinal and culinary applications. Essential oils impart many benefits, such as a pleasant aroma, especially in perfumes and to impart shine or conditioning in a hair care product, and for emolliency or improving the elasticity of the skin. In the future, it is possible that many new plants, extracts and oils of commercial significance will be identified, and many ethnobotanical uses and claims of many widespread herbs will be proven, new isolation and extraction techniques will be shown to give higher quality products. But this requires the multidisciplinary cooperation of botanists, preparative chemists, analytical chemists, toxicologists and biologists to assess cosmetic, rather than just pharmaceutical activity.

7

Herbal Excipients

- Herbal Excipients
- Significance of substances of natural origin as excipients—colourants, sweeteners, binders, diluents, viscosity builders, disintegrants, flavours and perfumes.

HERBAL EXCIPIENTS

Pharmaceutical excipients can be defined as nonactive ingredients that are mixed with therapeutically active compound(s) to form medicines. Excipients are defined as 'the substance used as a medium for giving a medicament'. The ingredient which is not an active compound is regarded as an excipient. Excipients affect the behaviour and effectiveness of the drug product more and more functionality and significantly. The variability of active compounds, excipients and process is obvious components for the product variability.

Natural excipients and derivatives occur ubiquitously throughout the plant and animal kingdoms. Examples of several pharmaceutical excipients of plant origin, like starch, agar, alginates, carrageenan, guar gum, xanthan gum, gelatin, pectin, acacia, tragacanth, and cellulose have applications in the pharmaceutical industry as binding agents, disintegrates, sustaining agents, protectives, colloids, thickening agents, gelling agents, bases in suppositories, stabilizers, and coating materials.

Classification of Excipients

Excipients are commonly classified according to their application and function in the drug products: Binders, diluents, lubricants, glidants, disintegrants, plasticizers, colourings suspending agents, preservatives, antioxidants, polishing film formers and coatings agents flavourings, sweeteners and taste improving agents.

Advantages of Herbal Excipients

There are various advantages of herbal and natural excipients; some of them are described below:

- Biodegradable
- They show no adverse effects on the environment or human being.
- Biocompatible and non-toxic
- Economic and cheaper and their production cost is less than synthetic material.
- Safe and devoid of side effects
- Easy availability

Disadvantages of Herbal Excipients

- Microbial contamination
- Variation
- The uncontrolled rate of hydration
- Slow process
- Heavy metal contamination

COLOURING AGENTS AND COLOURANTS

Natural dyes are dyes or colourants derived from plants, invertebrates, or minerals. The majority of natural dyes are vegetable dyes from plant sources—roots, berries, bark, leaves, and wood—and other organic sources such as fungi and lichens.

Colouring agents and colourants are mainly used to impart distinctive appearance to the pharmaceutical dosage forms. The colourant increases acceptability of the formulation. As it is well known and believed that the brightly coloured tonics, cherry red children's cough mixtures and flesh-tinted powders and ointments are more likely to be used because they are attractive.

Colour Psychology: The Psychological Effects of Colour

- The study of colour is complex, involving variety of systems like aesthetic, psychological, physiological, associative, and symbolic.
- Colour psychology says that the colour of the product may also influence the efficacy of therapy and its effects have universal meaning.
- Colours in the red area of the colour spectrum include red, orange and yellow. These warm colours evoke emotions ranging from feelings of warmth and comfort to feelings of anger and hostility.
- Colours on the blue side of the spectrum are known as "cool colours" and include blue, purple and green. These colours are often described as calm, but can also call to mind feelings of sadness or indifference.
- Colours on the blue side of the spectrum are known as 'cool colours' and include blue, purple and green. These colours are often described as calm, but can also call to mind feelings of sadness or indifference.

Ideal Properties of a Colourant

- Nontoxic, have no physiological activity and free from harmful impurities.
- It is a definite chemical compound because then only its colouring power will be reliable, its assay will be practicable and easier.
- Its tinctorial (colouring) power should be high so that only small quantities are required.
- Unaffected by light, tropical temperatures, hydrolysis and micro-organisms and, therefore, be stable on storage.
- Unaffected by oxidizing or reducing agents and pH changes.

- Compatible with medicaments and not interfere with them.
- Ready solubility in water is desirable in most cases but some oil-soluble and spirit-soluble colours are necessary.
- Does not interferes with the tests and assays to which the preparations containing it are subject. Should not be appreciably adsorbed on to suspended matter.
- Free from objectionable taste and odour.
- Readily available and inexpensive.

The Food, Drug, and Cosmetic Act of 1938 created three categories of coal tar dyes, of which only the first two are applicable to the manufacture of chewable tablets.

- **FD&C colours:** These are colourants that are certifiable for use in foods, drugs, and cosmetics.
- **D&C colours:** These are dyes and pigments considered safe for use in drugs and cosmetics when in contact with mucous membranes or when ingested.
- **External D&C colours:** These colourants, due to their oral toxicity, are not certifiable for use in products intended for ingestion but are considered safe for use in products applied externally.

Categories of Natural Colourants

Table 7.1: Categories of natural colourants

Colours	Chemical classifications	Examples
Yellow and brown	Flavone dyes	Weld, Quercitron, Fustic, Osage, Chamomile, Tesu, Dolu, Marigold, Cutch
Yellow	Iso-quinoline dyes: Polyene colourants: Pyran colourants	Barberry beta-carotene, lycopene only gentisin and gentiain Turmeric rhizome
		(Curcuma domestica) Safflower (Carthamus tinctorius) Carrot (Daucus carota) Big marigold (Tagetes erecta)

Contd.

Table 7.1: Categories of natural colourants (*Contd.*)

Colours	Chemical classifications	Examples
Orange-yellow	Chromene dyes	Kamala
		Sweet peppers, paprika (*Capsicum annuum*) Annato (*Bixa orellana*) Saffron red stigmas (*Crocus sativus*) bloodroot (*Sanguinaria canadensis*)
Brown and purple-grey red	Naphtho-chinone dyes	Henna, walnut, alkanet, Pitti
	Chinone and Anthrachinone dyes; Chromene dyes	Lac, cochineal, Madder (Majithro) Santalin
Purple and black	Benzophy-rone' dyes	Logwood alkanet root (*Alkanna tinctoria*)
blue	Indigoid dyes and indole colourants	Woad *Isatis tinctoria* (Brassicaceae)
		Indigo Indigofera tinctoria (Fabaceae) Cornflower flower *Centaurea cyanus* Bilberry fruits *Vaccinium myrtillus* Fruits of Common Elderberry (*Sambucus nigra*) European ash (*Fraxinus excelsior*)

Plants have been used for the extraction of a majority of natural dyes. Various plant parts including roots, leaves, twigs, stems, heart wood, bark, wood shavings, flowers, fruits, rinds, hulls, husks, and the like serve as natural dye sources. The Categories of natural Colorants with examples are enlisted in Table 7.1

Blue Dyes

This very important dye popularly known as the "king of natural dyes" has been used from ancient times till now for producing blue colour. Indigo leaves *indigofera tinctoria* are the best source of this dye. The colouring matter is present in indigo plant leaves as a light yellow substance called indicant.

Red Dyes

There are several plant sources of red natural dyes. Some of the prominent sources are listed below.

Madder: Madder popularly known as the "queen of natural dyes". It is the red colour producing natural dyes from the plants of various Rubia species. The dye is obtained from the roots of the plant. The main colouring constituent of European madder *Rubia tinctorum* is alizarin.

It is extracted by boiling dried root chips or stem pieces with water but sometimes, these are merely steeped in cold water for a few hours. As it is a mordant dye, it produces brightly coloured insoluble complexes or lakes.

Alum: It is widely used to get pink and red shades. A mixture of alum and iron produces purple shades. Alum can be used as a primary metallic salt in combination with other mordants to develop a range of red shades.

Brazil wood/Sappan wood: A red coloured dye obtained from the wood of small tree *Caesalpina sappan* found in India, Malaysia, and the Philippines also known as Sappan wood or "Patang." The same dye is also present in Brazil wood (*Caesalpinia echinata*), means glowing like fire due to the bright red colour of its wood.

Morinda: Morinda obtained from root and bark of the tree *Morinda citrifolia* growing in India and Sri Lanka is used for getting red shades. Dye is extracted from the chipped material with water after a preliminary wash to remove free acids. Various shades including purple and chocolate can be produced with the use of this dye.

Yellow Dyes

These dyes are available from several plant resources. A few popular sources are listed as follows.

Turmeric: Turmeric is a natural dye extracted from the fresh or dried rhizomes of *Curcuma longa*. It consists of curcumin belonging to the Diaroylmethane class.

Saffron: Saffron is a yellow dye obtained from the dried stigmas of the plant *Crocus sativus* belonging to the family Iridaceae. It is mainly found in the Mediterranean, Iran, and India, and used for cooking as well as medicinal purposes. The dye is extracted from the stigmas of flowers by boiling them in water.

Annatto: Annatto is a yellow orange dye obtained from seeds of *Bixa orellana* belonging to the family Bixaceae. It is used for colouring butter, cheese, and the like. The pulp is rich in tannin.

Barberry: *Berberis aristata* roots, bark, and stems are used to extract the dye. The main constituent of the dye is alkaloid which is berberine. It is a basic dye.

Pomegranate: Rinds of pomegranate (*Punica granatum*) fruits are rich in tannins and are used for mordanting purposes.

Myrobolan: Dried myrobolan (*Terminalia chebula*) fruits have high tannin content and also contain a natural dye that is used for producing bright yellow shades. Myrobolan is a part of the triphala which is famous Ayurvedic preparation and dyed materials are also imparted with medicinal properties such as antimicrobial and antifungal.

Marigold: Marigold (*Tagetus spp.*) is a bright yellow flower-yielding plant. It is commonly used for making garlands and floral decorations. It is available in different colours including yellow, golden yellow, orange, and the like. The main colouring component is quercetagetol, a flavonol along with two of its glycosides and lutein.

Kamala: The dried fruit capsules of kamala (*Mallotus phillipensis*) yield a red-orange powder that can be used for dyeing wool and silk to bright orange-yellow and golden-yellow colours.

Onion: The outer skin of onion (*Allium cepa*) which is generally thrown away as waste can be used to extract yellow colour natural dye.

BINDERS

Binders are agents employed to impart cohesiveness to the granules. This ensures the tablet remains intact after compression. Natural binders like different starches, gums, mucilages dried fruits possess binding capacity as well as some other properties like disintegrant, filler, sustain release, and these natural polymers are much safer and economical than polymers like PVP. Different starches like rice, potato, maize, corn, wheat, tapioca starch and gums like ferula gummosa boiss, gum olibanum, beilschmiedia seed gum, okro gum, aegle marmelod gum, gum cordial, okra gum and cassia roxburghii seeds gum and plant fruit like date palm fruit and orange peel pectin show good potency as a binding agent. Binders are added to tablet formulation to impart plasticity and thus increase the interparticulate bonding strength within the tablet. Binders are agents employed to impart cohesiveness to the granules. This ensures the tablet remains intact after compression as well as improving the flow qualities by the formulation of granules of derived hardness and size. The choice of a suitable binder for a tablet formulation requires extensive knowledge of the relative importance of binder properties for enhancing the strength of the tablet and also of the interactions between the various materials constituting a tablet.

Natural polymers: Starch, pregelatinised starch, gelatin, acacia, tragacanth and gums.

Advantages of Natural Binder

1. Natural polysaccharides are widely used in the pharmaceutical and food industry as excipients and additives due to their low toxicity, biodegradable, availability and low cost.

2. They can also be used to modify the release of drug, thereby influencing the absorption and subsequent bioavailability of the incorporated drug.

3. They act as vehicles which transport the incorporated drug to the site of absorption and are expected to guarantee the stability of the incorporated drug, the precision and

accuracy of the dosage, and also improve the organoleptic properties of the drugs where necessary in order to enhance patient adherence.

4. They should optimize the performances of dosage forms during manufacturing as well as when patients ingest them.

Starch

Starch is a typical multipurpose excipient, which can be applied as filler, disintegrant or binder in many tablet formulations. Pharmaceutical tablets need to be hard enough to avoid physical damage. Therefore, a good binder is needed to improve tablet friability and subsequent loss of active ingredient during processing. The most commonly employed binder historically has been cooked starch or pregelatinised starch, its cold water swelling equivalent. Because of their unique rheological properties starch binders are applied when different ingredients need to be granulated prior to compressing into tablets. Uncooked (native) starch, however, is used as a disintegrant in tablets. Although tablet hardness is required to withstand physical stress, the tablet should also disintegrate quickly when the active is to be released. Native starch granules have the ability to swell slightly in an aqueous environment, resulting in the rupture of the physical tablet structure.

Gelatin

Gelatin is hydrated by soaking in cold water for hours or by keeping it overnight. The soaked gelatin is heated to boil, so as to form gelatin solution. This hot gelatin solution must be used as early as possible to prevent gelling upon cooling Tablets of gelatin are hard to disintegrate. It acts as a media for the growth of bacteria and molds. Hence preservatives are added.

Acacia

Gum acacia is also known as gum arabic; it is natural material made of hardened exudate from *Acacia senegal*. It is complex mixture of polysaccharides and glycoproteins used in food industry as an emulsion stabilizer. Acacia is functional binder used to form strong tablets and granules.

Gum acacia or gum arabic is the dried gummy exudate obtained from the stem and branches of *Acacia senegal (Linne) Willdenow* and other related species of acacia (Family Leguminosae). The gum has been recognized as an acidic polysaccharide containing Dgalactose, L-arabinose, L-rhamnose, and D-glucuronic acid. Acacia is mainly used in oral and topical pharmaceutical formulations as a suspending and emulsifying agent, often in combination with tragacanth. It is also used in the preparation of pastilles and lozenges and as a tablet binder.

Tragacanth

This gum is obtained from the branches of *Astragalus gummifer*, Family Leguminosae. Tragacanth when used as the carrier in the formulation of 1- and 3-layer matrices produced satisfactory release prolongation.

GUMS

Gums possess a complex, branched polymeric structure because of which they exhibit high cohesive and adhesive properties, such properties used in pharmaceutical preparation. Hence gums find diverse application in pharmacy. They are ingredients in dental and other adhesive and as bulk laxative. These polymers are useful as tablets binder, disintegrating agent, emulsifier, suspending agent, thickener, gelling agent, stabilizing agent protective colloids in suspension and sustain agent in tablets. They act as adjuvant in some pharmaceutical formulation. Gums are translucent and amorphous substances produced by the plants. Usually pathological products, gums are produced when the plant is growing under unfavourable conditions or when injured. Gums are plant hydrocolloids and may be anionic or nonionic polysaccharides. On hydrolysis gums yield sugar and salts of uronic acid.

FILLERS AND DILUENTS

Fillers fill out the size of a tablet or capsule, making it practical to produce and convenient for the consumer to use. By increasing the bulk volume, the fillers make it possible for the final product to have the proper volume for patient handling. Good filler must be inert, compatible with the other components of the formulation, non-hygroscopic, relatively cheap, compactible, and preferably tasteless or pleasant tasting.

Diluents are fillers used to make required bulk of tablet when the drug dosage itself is inadequate to produce the bulk. The range of diluents may vary from 5–80%. It also provided better tablet properties such as improve cohesion, permit use of direct compression manufacturing, promote flow as well as adjust weight of tablet as per die capacity.

Other examples of fillers include: Lactose, sucrose, glucose, mannitol, sorbitol, calcium carbonate, and magnesium stearate.

Diluent should be nontoxic, physiologically inert, physically and chemically stable, free from all microbial contamination, should not alter the bioavailability of the drugs, colour compatible. Diluents are classified as

1. **Insoluble tablet fillers** or diluents as starch, powdered cellulose, microcrystalline cellulose and calcium phosphate.
2. **Soluble tablet fillers** or diluents as lactose, sucrose, mannitol and sorbitol.

Lactose

Lactose ($C_{12}H_{22}O_{11}$) is milk sugar. It is a disaccharide composed of one galactose and one glucose molecule. In the pharmaceutical industry, lactose is used to help form tablets because it has excellent compressibility properties. It is also used to form diluent powder for dry-powder inhalations. Lactose may be listed as lactose hydrous, lactose anhydrous, lactose monohydrate, or lactose spray-dried.

Disintegrating Agents

Disintegrating agents is a substance or mixture of substances added to tablets to facilitate its break up or disintegration. The active constituents must be released from the tablet as efficiently as possible to allow its rapid action. Hence the therapeutic action is based on the amount of drug released from the tablet, these disintegrants which allow rapid de-aggregation of solid into solution and followed by which absorption of the drug takes place.

Disintegrants are the agents that are added to tablet and some encapsulated formulations to promote the breakup of the tablet and capsule 'slugs' into smaller fragments in an aqueous environment, thereby increasing the available surface area and promoting a more rapid release of the drug substance. They promote moisture penetration and dispersion of the tablet matrix. Tablet disintegration has received considerable attention as an essential step in obtaining fast drug release. The emphasis on the availability of drug highlights the importance of the relatively rapid disintegration of a tablet as a criterion for ensuring uninhibited drug dissolution behaviour.

The proper choice of disintegrant and its consistency of performance are of critical importance to the formulation development of tablet.

Ideal Properties of Disintegrants

⮞ Poor solubility
⮞ Poor gel formation
⮞ Good hydration capacity
⮞ Good flow properties
⮞ No tendency to form complexes with the drugs

Cross Carmellose Sodium

It is modified cellulose and is a cross-linked polymer of carboxymethylcellulose. The disintegration rate of cross carmellose sodium is higher than that of sodium starch glycolate and the mechanism is also different. The carboxymethyl groups themselves are used to cross link the cellulose chains, process is accomplished by dehydration. Cross-linking makes it insoluble, hydrophilic, highly absorbent material, resulting in excellent swelling properties and its unique fibrous nature gives it excellent water wicking capabilities. It is used in oral pharmaceutical formulations as a superdisintegrant for capsules, tablets and granules. Concentrations of cross carmellose sodium range between 1 and 5% w/w, although normally 1–3% w/w is used in tablets prepared by direct compression and 2–4% w/w in tablets prepared by a wet granulation process.

Sodium Starch Glycolate

It is a cross-linked polymer of carboxymethyl starch. It is possible to synthesize sodium starch glycolate from a wide range of native starches but in practice potato starch is used as it gives the product with the best disintegrating properties. The effect of introduction of the large hydrophilic carboxymethyl groups is to disrupt the hydrogen bonding within the polymer structure. This allows water to penetrate the molecule and the polymer becomes cold water soluble. The effect of the cross-linking is to reduce both the water soluble fraction of the polymer and the viscosity of dispersion in water. The mechanism by which disintegration action takes place is rapid absorption of water and swell leading to an enormous increase in volume of granules which result in rapid and uniform disintegration. The natural predried starches swell in water to the extent of 10–20 percent and the modified starches increase in volume by 200–300 percent in water. The tablets formulated by using these super-disintegrant are disintegrated in less than two minutes.

Cross-Linked Polypyrrolidine

Cross povidones are synthetic, insoluble, cross-linked homopolymers of N-vinyl-2-pyrrolidone. Cross povidones are highly compressible materials as a result of their unique particle morphology. Cross povidone is used as super-disintegrant at low concentration levels (2–5%) in direct compression, wet and dry granulation processes. Cross povidone uses a combination of swelling, wicking and deformation mechanism for rapid disintegration of tablets, swells rapidly in water without forming gel, is highly compressible, unaffected by pH media.

Gums

Gums have been used as disintegrants because of their tendency to swell in water. They can display good binding characteristics (1 to 10 percent of tablet weight). This property can oppose the desired property of assisting disintegration and the amount of gum must be carefully titrated to determine the optimum level for the tablet. Common gums used as disintegrant include agar, locust bean, karaya, pectin and tragacanth.

Guar Gums

It is naturally occurring gum (marketed under the trade name jaguar). It is free flowing, completely soluble, neutral polymer composed of sugar units and is approved for use in food. It is not sensitive to pH, moisture contents or solubility of the tablet matrix. It is not always pure white and sometimes varies in colour from off-white to tan tends to discolour with time in alkaline tablets. It is used as disintegrants in the range of 0.5–5% showed rapid rate disintegration due to swelling of the gum.

Gum Karaya

Karaya has the natural gum exudates from the traces of Sterculia urens belonging to family sterculiacea. The high viscosity nature of gum limits its uses as binder and disintegrant in the development of conventional dosage form.

Gellan Gum

Gellan gum is a linear anionic polysaccharide, biodegradable polymer obtained from *Pseudomonos elodea* consisting of a linear tetra-saccharide repeat structure and use as a food additive.

Alginates

These are hydrophilic colloidal substances extracted naturally from certain species of Kelp or chemically modified from natural sources like alginic acid or salt of alginic acid. They are having higher affinity for water absorption and capable for an excellent disintegrants. They can be successfully used with ascorbic acid, multi-vitamins formulation.

Isapghula Husk

It is a natural substance as disintegrant. It consists of dried seeds of the plant known as plantago ovata. It contains mucilage which is present in the epidermis of the seeds. The mucilage is used as binding agent in the granulation of material for compressed tablets. *Plantago ovata* seeds husk has high swellability and gives uniform and slightly viscous solution, hence it is used as thickening and suspending agent.

SWEETENERS

The overall pleasure and enjoyment of a food or drink is contributed by the taste. The taste plays a crucial role in determining the quality of a food. Sweet taste within the five basic tastes permits the identification of energy rich nutrients. Sweeteners enhance the perception of sweet taste due to their ability to interact with taste buds and evoke characteristic response.

Classification

The potential area for global consumption of herbs as medicine, nutraceuticals, food additives, and cosmeceuticals are natural sweeteners. Sweeteners can be broadly classified into two categories:

- Natural sweeteners are made from saps, syrups and nectars are subdivided into saccharide and non-saccharide.
- Synthetic/artificial sweeteners

On the basis of nutritional property the sweeteners are categorized as nutritive and non-nutritive (Fig. 7.1).

Nutritive sweeteners: It provides calories or energy to the diet at about four calories per gram. Examples include sucrose, honey and syrups such as maple and corn. Nutritive sweeteners provide energy and high intake increases the risk of obesity, diabetes and cardiovascular disease. Some of them are sorbitol, mannitol, xylitol and maltitol.

Non-nutritive sweeteners: They are zero or low calorie alternatives to nutritive sweeteners. The non-nutritive sweeteners are much

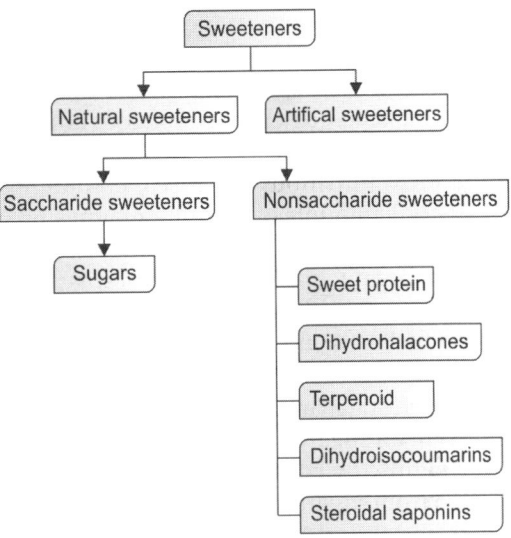

Fig. 7.1: Classification of sweeteners

sweeter than sugar. Examples are aspartame, neotame, sucralose and stevioside.

Natural Sweeteners

Natural sweeteners exist or are produced by nature, without added chemicals or fancy machinery. The only sugars that are optimal to eat are wild, non-hybridized, seeded fruits, and the natural sugars and starches in living vegetables, trees, seeds, nuts, and roots. The following are considered natural sweeteners: Maple syrup, honey, Stevia, molasses, coconut sugar, date sugar, agave nectar and xylitol.

Stevia is wonderful alternative to sources and artificial sweetener for those who are diabetic. One more reason to recommend Stevia for diabetics is its advantage of safe, non-calorie herbal sweetener and also nourishment to the pancreas. It does not lower the blood glucose level in normal subjects. The leaves of the Stevia are sweeter than cane sugar having slight liquorice sensation and a good alternative for the synthetic sweetener. The herb is 300 times sweetener than table sugar. But 100% calorie free. The fresh leaf of Stevia is itself 3–5 times sweetener than table sugar and dried leaf powder is about 30 times sweeter.

Blackstrap molasses, unlike other sugar-cane sweeteners, contains significant amounts of vitamins and minerals. 'First' molasses is left over when sugarcane juice is boiled, cooled, and removed of its crystals. If this product is boiled again, the result is called second molasses. Blackstrap molasses is made from the third boiling of the sugar syrup and is the most nutritious molasses, containing substantial amounts of calcium, magnesium, potassium, and iron. When buying, consider choosing organic blackstrap molasses, as pesticides are more likely to be concentrated due to the production of molasses.

Rapadura is the Portuguese name for unrefined dried sugarcane juice. Probably the least refined of all sugarcane products, rapadura is made simply by cooking juice that has been pressed from sugarcane until it is very concentrated, and then drying and granulating it, or traditionally, pouring it into a mold to dry in brick form, which is then shaved. Because the only thing that has been removed from the original sugarcane juice is the water, rapadura contains all of the vitamins and minerals that are normally found in sugarcane juice, namely iron.

Sucanat stands for sugarcane-natural, and is very similar to rapadura. It is made by mechanically extracting sugarcane juice, which is then heated and cooled until tiny brown (thanks to the molasses content) crystals form. It contains less sucrose than table sugar (88 percent and 99 percent, respectively).

Turbinado sugar is often confused with sucanat, but the two are different. After the sugarcane is pressed to extract the juice, the juice is then boiled, cooled, and allowed to crystallize into granules. Next, these granules are refined to a light tan colour by washing them in a centrifuge to remove impurities and surface molasses. Turbinado is lighter in colour and contains less molasses than both rapadura and sucanat.

Evaporated cane juice is essentially a finer, lighter-coloured version of turbinado sugar. Still less refined than table sugar, it also contains some trace nutrients (that regular sugar does not), including vitamin B_2.

Agave nectar is produced from the juice of the core of the agave, a succulent plant native to Mexico. Far from a whole food, agave juice is extracted, filtered, heated and hydrolyzed into agave syrup. Vegans often use agave as a honey substitute, although it is even sweeter and a little thinner than honey. It contains trace amounts of iron, calcium, potassium and magnesium. Agave nectar syrup is available in the baking aisle at most natural foods stores. The fructose content of agave syrup is much higher than that of high fructose corn syrup, which is of concern since some research has linked high fructose intake to weight gain (especially around the abdominal area), high triglycerides, heart disease and insulin resistance. High fructose corn syrup contains 55% fructose while agave nectar syrup contains 90%. Despite this, it has a low glycemic index because of its low glucose content.

Brown rice syrup is made when cooked rice is cultured with enzymes, which break down the starch in the rice. The resulting liquid is cooked down to a thick syrup, which is about half as sweet as white sugar and has a mild butterscotch flavour. It is composed of about 50% complex carbohydrates, which break down more slowly in the bloodstream than simple carbohydrates, resulting in a less dramatic spike in blood glucose levels. It is worth noting that the name 'brown rice syrup' describes the colour of the syrup, not the rice it is made from, which is white.

Honey, made by bees from the nectar of flowers, is a ready-made sweetener that contains traces of nutrients.

Maple syrup comes from the sap of maple trees, which is collected, filtered, and boiled down to an extremely sweet syrup with a distinctive flavour. It contains fewer calories and a higher concentration of minerals (like manganese and zinc) than honey. 'Maple-flavoured syrups' are imitations of real maple syrup. True maple syrup contains nothing but 'maple syrup.' Imitation syrups are primarily made of high fructose corn syrup, sugar, and/ or artificial sweeteners, and contains 3 percent maple syrup (or less).

Artificial Sweeteners

Artificial sweeteners or synthetic sweeteners are natural occurring synthetic sweeteners/

sugar sweeteners are substances used to replace sugar in foods and beverages. They can be divided into two large groups: Nutritive sweeteners, which add some energy value (calories) to food; and non-nutritive sweeteners, which are also called high-intensity sweeteners because they are used in very small quantities, adding no energy value to food. Examples: Cyclammate, Aspartame, Alitame, Acesulfame potassium and sucralose.

There are five artificial sweeteners that have been tested and approved by the U.S. Food and Drug Administration (FDA): Acesulfame potassium (also called acesulfame K), aspartame, saccharin, sucralose, neotame. These sweeteners are used by food companies to make diet drinks, baked goods, frozen desserts, candy, light yogurt, and chewing gum. You can buy them to use as table top sweeteners. Add them to coffee, tea, or sprinkle them on top of fruit. Some are also available in 'granular' versions which can be used in cooking and baking.

Types of artificial sweeteners

Aspartame: The familiar blue packet in the sugar substitutes bowl usually contains aspartame. With no saccharin-like aftertaste, equal has become one of the most popular sugar substitute brands. There are four calories per packet.

Sucralose: Sucralose is an artificial sweetener. The majority of ingested sucralose is not broken down by the body, so it is noncaloric. In the European Union, it is also known under the E number E955. Sucralose is approximately 600 times as sweet as sucrose (table sugar), twice as sweet as saccharin, and three times as sweet as aspartame. It is stable under heat and over a broad range of pH conditions. Therefore, it can be used in baking or in products that require a longer shelf life. The commercial success of sucralose-based products stems from its favorable comparison to other low-calorie sweeteners in terms of taste, stability, and safety. Common brand names of sucralose-based sweeteners are Splenda, Sukrana, SucraPlus, Candys, Cukren and Nevella.

Saccharin: Saccharin is an artificial sweetener. The basic substance, benzoic sulfilimine, has effectively no food energy and is much sweeter than sucrose, but has a bitter or metallic aftertaste, especially at high concentrations. It is used to sweeten products such as drinks, candies, cookies, medicines, and toothpaste.

Neotame: Neotame is an artificial sweetener made by Nutrasweet that is between 7,000 and 13,000 times as sweet as sucrose (table sugar). In the European Union, it is known by the E number E961. It is moderately heat-stable, extremely potent, rapidly metabolized, completely eliminated and does not appear to accumulate in the body. The product is attractive to food manufacturers, as its use greatly lowers the cost of production compared to using sugar or high fructose corn syrup (due to the lower quantities needed to achieve the same sweetening), while also benefiting the consumer by providing fewer 'empty' sugar calories and a lower impact on blood sugar.

FLAVOURS AND PERFUMES

Fragrances used for external applications such as—spray perfumes, body care, home care, cosmetics, soaps and detergents and incense. These are non-consumables.

Ingredients used by flavourists and perfumers can be broadly placed in 2 categories, viz.:

➲ Natural ingredients
➲ Synthetic/semi-synthetic ingredients

Cinnamon bark oil possesses the delicate aroma of the spice and a sweet and pungent taste. Its major constituent is cinnamaldehyde but other minor components impart the characteristic odour and flavour. It is employed mainly in the flavouring industry where it is used in meat and fast food seasonings, sauces and pickles, baked goods, confectionery, cola-type drinks, tobacco flavours and in dental and pharmaceutical preparations. Perfumery applications are far fewer than in flavours because the oil has some skin-sensitizing properties, but it has limited use in some perfumes.

Cinnamon leaf oil has a warm, spicy, but rather harsh odour, lacking the rich body of the bark oil. Its major constituent is eugenol rather than cinnamaldehyde. It is used as a flavouring agent for seasonings and savory snacks. As a cheap fragrance it is added to soaps and insecticides. The oil's high eugenol content also makes it valuable as a source of this chemical for subsequent conversion into iso-eugenol, another flavouring agent.

Cassia oil is distilled from a mixture of leaves, twigs and fragments of bark. Cinnamaldehyde is the major constituent and it is used mainly for flavouring cola-type drinks, with smaller amounts used in bakery products, sauces, confectionery and liqueurs. Like cinnamon bark oil, its use as a fragrance is limited by its skin sensitizing properties.

Rosewood oil is obtained by steam distilling the comminuted trunkwood. The oil ('bois de rose') possesses a characteristic aroma and is a long-established ingredient in the more expensive perfumes. Rosewood oil is rich in linalool, a chemical which can be transformed into a number of derivatives of value to the flavour and fragrance industries.

Eucalyptus oils are obtained by distillation of the leaves of Eucalyptus and have aromas characteristic of the particular species used. The oils are classified in the trade into three broad types according to their composition and main end-use: Medicinal, perfumery and industrial. It is used as an inhalant or chest rub to ease breathing difficulties, as a mouthwash in water to refresh or ease the throat, and as a skin rub to provide relief from aches and pains. Eucalyptus oil is also used as a general disinfectant, cleaner and deodorizer about the house. Of the two principal perfumery oils, that from *Eucalyptus citriodora* is produced in the greatest volume. It differs from the medicinal oils in containing citrinellal, rather than cineole, as the major constituent. The oil is employed in whole form for fragrance purposes, usually in the lower cost soaps, perfumes and disinfectants, but also as a source of citrinellal for the chemical industry.

Sandalwood oil: Indian sandalwood oil distilled from the heartwood and roots of *Santalum album*. Sandalwood oil has a characteristic sweet, woody odour which is widely employed in the fragrance industry, but more particularly in the higher-priced perfumes. It has excellent blending properties and the presence of a large proportion of high-boiling constituents in the oil (about 90 percent santalols) also makes it valuable as a fixative for other fragrances. In India, where it is produced, it is used in this manner for the manufacture of traditional attars such as rose attar; the delicate floral oils are distilled directly into sandalwood oil.

Cedarwood oils each have characteristic woody odours which may change somewhat in the course of drying out. The crude oils are often yellowish or even darker in colour and some, such as Texas cedarwood oil, are quite viscous and deposit crystals on standing. They find use (sometimes after rectification) in a range of fragrance applications such as soap perfumes, household sprays, floor polishes and insecticides. Small quantities are used in microscope work as a clearing oil.

Regulatory Bodies for Regulations in Excipients

The excipients are the integral component of drugs in synthetic as well as modified dosage form. Therefore, the demand of the excipient in pharmaceutical industry is increasing. The search of its excipient quality and suitability is a burning issue as sometimes excipient content in formulation is more than active pharmaceutical ingredients.

In the scenario of commercialization and globalization, it is necessary to ensure quality, safety and cost effective excipient for which several regulatory organization and notifications play their role.

World Health Organization through its technical report 885:1999, provides guideline, definition of the pharmaceutical excipient in addition to the quality, safety and their required standards.

ICH produces its ICH-Q8 (R2) guideline for excipient and its relevancy in drug development. IPEC (The International Pharmaceutical Excipients Council), an international industry association formed in 1991 by manufacturers, distributors and end-users of excipients.

IPEC Federation formed in 2010 officially having member IPEC-Americas, IPEC-Europe, IPEC-Japan and IPEC-China. IPEC India is now in the process to be a key player and is in the formation stages. IPEC India will work actively to promote excipients safety and harmonization of regulatory standards and pharmacopoeial monographs.

The excipient certification scheme (EXCI-PACT) was launched in May 2008 with EFCG (European Fine Chemical Group) and IPEC Europe, now comprises 5 trade associations:

1. FECC European Association of Chemical Distributors
2. IPEC-Americas (International Pharmaceutical Excipients Council Americas)
3. IPEC-Europe (International Pharmaceutical Excipients Council Europe)
4. PQG-UK (Pharmaceutical Quality Group)
5. EFCG with the aim to more safety (through certified compliance to recognized GMP and GDP standard), cost and time savings (only a single audit is needed to prove GMP/GDP compliance) and worldwide acceptance (building on existing ISO standards, and supported by major industry organizations).

Globalized market of excipient: According to the publication "Excipients market global industry analysis, market size, share, trends, analysis, growth and forecast, 2012–2018" the global excipients market, which was valued at US$5, 260.0 million in 2011, is expected to be worth US$7,586.6 million by the end of 2018. Driven by factors such as the expansion of the pharmaceuticals market, the global excipients market is poised to grow at a 5.4% CAGR between 2012 and 2018. The pharmaceutical excipients market is expected to reach around $8,439.0 million by 2019 at a CAGR of 6.7% during the forecast period from 2015 to 2019.

CONCLUSION

Excipients, a partner of the API in a dosage form meanwhile have major share in a formulation sometimes and showing their unique pharmacokinetics and pharmacodynamics apart from active pharmaceutical ingredients to complete the motive of medicine. The natural excipients used in pharmaceutics may play a major role as advance nurture for medicament as well as modern medicaments to fulfil the requirement of time demanding dosage form with quality, safety and efficacy along with cost effectiveness and serve the creation of nature by its natural nurture and medicament.

8

Herbal Formulations

- Introduction
- Recent patents on novel herbal formulations

- Conventional herbal formulations like syrups, powders and tablets and novel dosage forms like phytosomes

INTRODUCTION

Herbal drug formulations define as dosage form consisting of one or more herbs or processed herb(s), herbal preparations in specified quantities to provide specific nutritional, cosmetic benefits, and/or other benefits meant for use to diagnose treat, mitigate diseases of human beings or animals and/or to alter the structure or physiology of human beings or animals. Herbal drug formulations are the means by which plant drug or preparation or isolate are delivered to sites of action within the body through topical, parental, nasal, and ophthalmic route of administration.

Herbal formulations are obtained by subjecting herbal substances to treatments such as extraction, distillation, expression, fraction-ation, purification, concentration or fermentation include comminuted or powdered. Whole, fragmented or cut plants, plants parts, algae, fungi, lichen in an unprocessed, usually dried

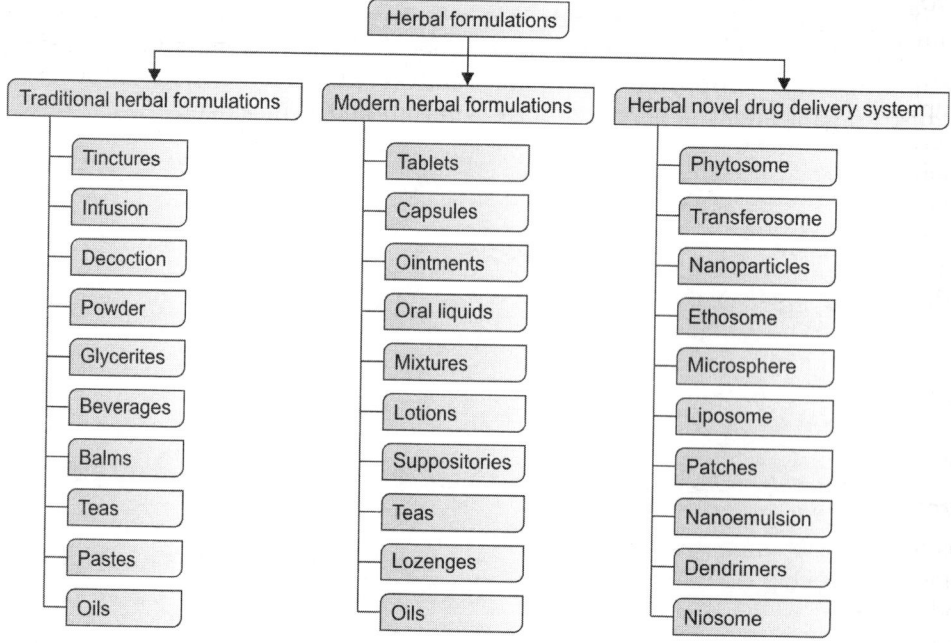

Fig. 8.1: Classification of herbal formulations

form but sometimes fresh were used in the preparations of herbal formulations. Herbal substances are precisely defined by the plant part used and the botanical name according to the binomial system (genus, species, variety and author). Different herbal formulations are tinctures, extracts, essential oils, expressed juices and processed exudates (Fig. 8.1).

CONVENTIONAL HERBAL FORMULATIONS

Syrup

Syrups are viscous oral liquids that may contain one or more plant drug or plant preparations in solution. The vehicle usually contains large amounts of sucrose or other sugars to which certain polyhydric alcohols may be added to inhibit crystallisation or to modify solubilisation, taste and other vehicle properties. Sugarless syrups may contain sweetening agents and thickening agents. Syrups may contain ethanol (95%) as a preservative or as a solvent to incorporate flavouring agents. Antimicrobial agents may also be added to syrups.

Advantages of Syrup

- Ability to disguise the bad taste of medications.
- Syrups are thicker than aqueous solutions, therefore only a portion of the medication dissolved in the syrup comes in contact with the taste buds. The remainder of the medication is held above the tongue by the thick syrup so it is not tasted as it is swallowed.
- The high sugar content of syrups gives them a sweet taste that helps conceal the bad taste of the medicine. This is why syrups are commonly used for pediatric medications.
- The thick character of syrups also has a soothing effect on irritated tissues.

Preparation of Syrups

Syrups should be carefully prepared in clean equipment to prevent contamination. Three methods may be used to prepare syrups:
- Solution with heat
- Agitation without heat
- Percolation

Although the hot method is quickest, it is not applicable to syrups of thermolabile or volatile ingredients. When using heat, temperature must be carefully controlled to avoid decomposing and darkening the syrup (caramelization).

Syrups may be prepared from sugars other than sucrose (glucose, fructose), non-sugar polyols (sorbitol, glycerin, propylene glycol, mannitol), or other non-nutritive artificial sweeteners (aspartame, saccharin) when a reduction in calories or glucogenic properties is desired, as with the diabetic patient. The non- nutritive sweeteners do not impart the characteristic viscosity of syrups and require the addition of viscosity adjusters, such as methylcellulose. The polyols, though less sweet than sucrose, have the advantage of providing favourable viscosity, reducing cap-locking (which occurs when sucrose crystallizes), and in some cases acting as cosolvents and preservatives. A 70% sorbitol solution is commercially available for use as a vehicle.

Quality Control Tests for Syrups

1. Visual inspection/physical appearance.
2. Light transmission matter/colour.
3. pH measurement.
4. Physical stability in syrups.
5. Sucrose concentration.
6. Weight per ml.
7. Viscosity.
8. Optical rotation.
9. Solubility.
10. Assay of active ingredients

Powders

Powders are finely divided powders that contain one or more plant drugs or dried extracts with or without auxilliary substances including, where specified, flavouring and colouring agents. They are simple to prepare, less perishable than decoctions, rapidly absorbed, and fast acting. They are intended to be taken internally with or without the aid of water or any other suitable liquid. Patient compliance is better with powders than with decoctions because they are easier and faster to prepare. Powders contain the whole herb; therefore, patients rely on good digestion to break down the herbal matter to release the active constituents. Poor digestion can be circumvented, somewhat by boiling and then straining the drugs before drinking. This is known as a draft. Powders require a smaller dose, generally, than is prescribed for most decoctions. This is due to the type of conditions, typically functional, treated with powders, and because more of the active ingredients are released due to the increased surface area of powders compared to bulk herbs. Also, there is less binding of constituents and less damage to heat sensitive compounds as happens with the prolonged boiling of decoctions.

Powders may be single dose or multiple dose preparations. For single dose powders, each dose is enclosed in a separate container, e.g. a sachet, a paper packet or a vial. With multiple dose powders it may be necessary to provide a measuring device capable of delivering the quantity prescribed.

Advantages of Powder

- ➲ Powders are one of the oldest dosage forms and are used both internally and externally.
- ➲ Powders are more stable than liquid dosage form
- ➲ The changes of incompatibility are less as compared to liquid dosage form.
- ➲ Powders are easier to transport than the liquid dosage form.
- ➲ The onset of action of powdered drug is rapid as compared to other solid dosage form, e.g. tablets, capsules.

Preparation of Powder

In the manufacture of powders, means are taken to ensure a suitable particle size with regard to the intended use of the product. Plant materials or extracts are dried and pulverized into uniform particle size separately and mixed appropriately as per prescribed formula. During manufacture, packaging, storage and distribution of oral powders, suitable means shall be taken to ensure their microbial quality. Store in containers protected from moisture.

Quality Control Tests For Powder

1. Particle size and shape determination
2. Surface area
3. *Density:* Bulk density, true density and granular density
4. Granule strength and friability
5. *Flow properties:* Angle of repose, percentage compressibility and Hausner's ratio
6. Moisture content
7. Percentage fine
8. Uniformity of content
9. Uniformity of weight

Tablets

Tablets are solid dosage forms each containing a unit dose of one or more medicaments. They are intended for oral administration. Some tablets are swallowed whole or after being chewed, some are dissolved or dispersed in water before administration and some are retained in the mouth where the active ingredient is liberated.

Herbal tablets are a convenient dosage form and no problems with taste or alcohol are associated with their use. However, tablets contain fixed formulations which cannot be exactly adapted to the needs of the individual patient. Therefore, it is critical that the herbs contained in a tablet are carefully chosen for the disorder they are intended to treat. Even then, the degree of treatment flexibility is limited.

A major potential problem with tablets is the degree of processing required. Processing is minimal for tablets containing the powdered herb, but the amount of herb which can be incorporated into such tablets is limited (without making them excessively large). Tablets are, therefore, usually made from extracts, which are more concentrated than the original dried herb. In order to achieve this, the herb is first extracted with a solvent. Often water is used to keep costs down. The resultant liquid is then dried to either a soft or a powdered concentrate using processes such as vacuum concentration or spray drying. Heat-sensitive or volatile components can be damaged or lost by this process. Heat is also sometimes used in the tablet-making process via a granulation step: The tablet mixture may be wetted and then dried in an oven before the final pressing. These risk further damage active components. Hence, when manufacturing tablets, quality may be sacrificed for the sake of quantity.

Because of their composition, method of manufacture or intended use, tablets present a variety of characteristics and consequently there are several categories of tablets.

Unless otherwise stated in the individual monograph, tablets are uncoated. Where coating is permitted, the monograph states: "The tablets may be coated". Where the monograph directs coating the statement reads: "The tablets are coated". Unless otherwise directed, tablets may be coated in one of different ways.

Tablets are usually solid, right circular cylinders, the end surfaces of which are flat or convex and the edges of which may be bevelled. They may exist in other shapes like triangular, rectangular, etc also. They may have lines or break-marks and may bear a symbol or other markings. They are sufficiently hard to withstand handling without crumbling or breaking.

Advantages of Tablet

1. Unit dosage forms with dose precision
2. Least content variability
3. Administration of accurate amounts of minute doses of a drug is possible
4. Economical of all oral dosage forms as its production does not require additional processing steps
5. Easy transportation
6. Sustain release of a drug can be achieved through enteric coating
7. Medicaments with bitter taste can be masked with coating technique (sugar coating)
8. Tablet dosage form is stable when compared to all oral dosage forms.

Production

Tablets are obtained by compression of uniform volumes of powders or granules by applying high pressures and using punches and dies.

The particles to be compressed consist of one or more medicaments, with or without auxiliary substances such as diluents, binders, disintegrating agents, lubricants, glidants, permitted colours and substances capable of modifying the behaviour of the medicaments in the digestive tract. Such substances must be innocuous and therapeutically inert in the quantities present.

In the production of tablets, measures are taken to ensure that they have sufficient strength to avoid crumbling or breaking on handling or subsequent handling. Chewing tablets are manufactured to ensure that they are easily crushed by chewing.

During manufacture, packaging, storage and distribution of tablets, suitable means shall be taken to ensure their microbial quality.

Quality Control Tests For Tablet

1. *General appearance:* Size, shape, odour, taste, texture, legibility, identifying marks
2. Content of active ingredients
3. Uniformity of weight
4. Dissolution
5. Disintegration

Herbal Novel Drug Delivery System (Fig 8.4)

Herbal medicines have gained worldwide appreciation due to their therapeutic potency and fewer adverse effects as compared to the synthetic ones. Novel drug delivery technologies have gained importance to achieve modified delivery of herbal drugs, thereby increasing the therapeutic value as well as reducing toxicity. Novel herbal drug carriers cure particular disease by targeting exactly the affected zone inside a patient's body and transporting the drug to that area. Novel drug delivery system is advantageous in delivering the herbal drug at predetermined rate and delivery of drug at the site of action which minimizes the toxic effects with the increase in bioavailability of the drugs.

NDD technologies: Used to achieve modified delivery of herbal drugs, increasing its therapeutic value as well as reducing toxicity.

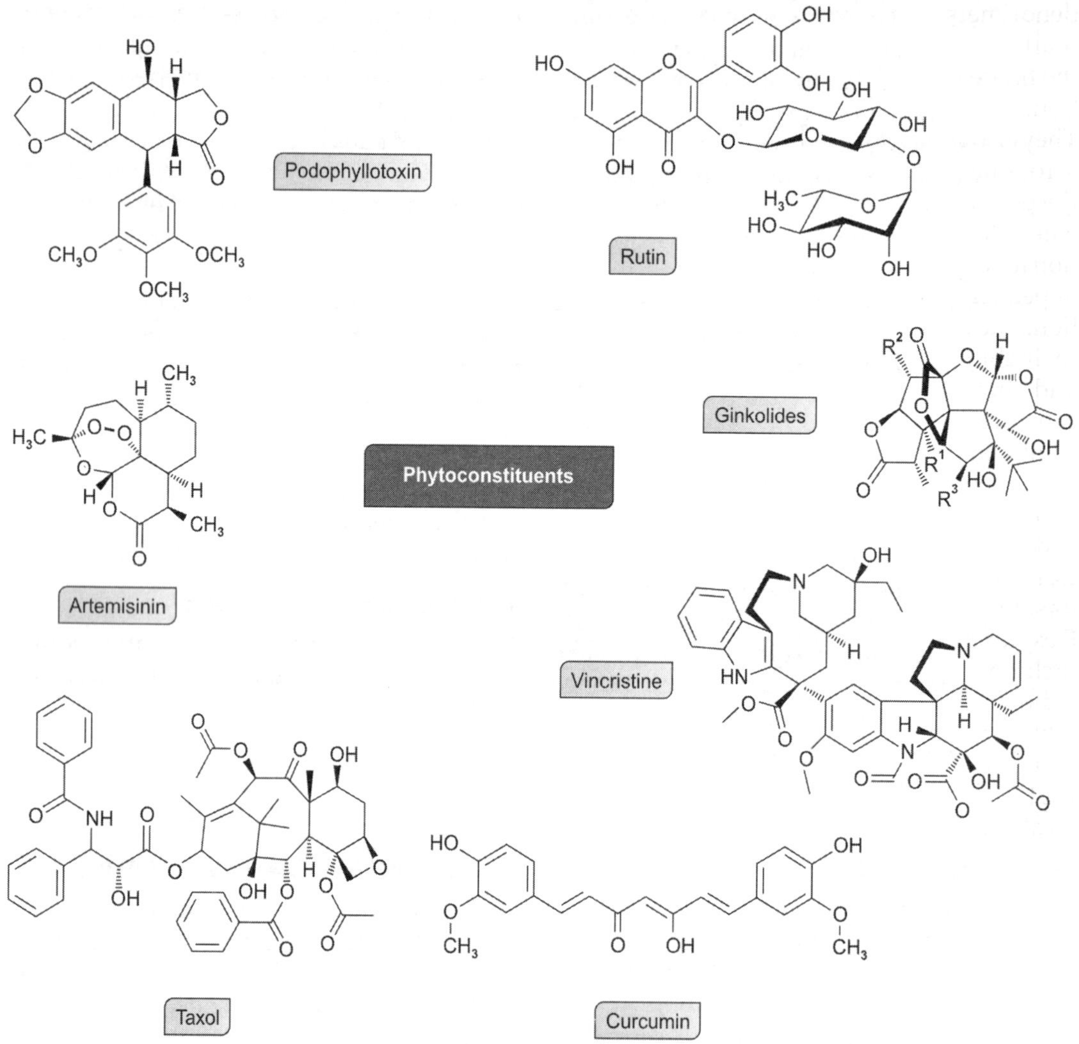

Fig. 8.2: Phytoconstituents delivered through NDDS

Novel herbal drug carriers: Cure disease by targeting the affected zone inside a patient's body and transporting the drug to that area. Few examples of phytoconstituents delivered through NDDS are cited in Fig. 8.2.

NDDS: Advantageous in delivering the herbal drug at predetermined rate and delivery of drug at the site of action. Reduce toxic effects and the increase in bioavailability.

Phytochemical Bioavailability and Efficacy in Preventing Chronic Diseases

Since ancient times, plant-derived compounds have been a great source of materials used in beneficial medical treatments. The several other factors could also play a role in limiting bioavailability, such as solubility of the compound, stability due to gastric and colonic pH, metabolism by gut microflora, absorption across the intestinal wall, active efflux mechanism and first-pass metabolic effects. Examples of compounds that are only sparingly water-soluble include ellagic acid, curcumin and resveratrol. A promising approach to overcome low bioavailability and systemic toxicity is the application of drug-loaded nanosized drug carriers, such as polymeric nanoparticles (NPs), liposomes, dendrimers and micelles. NPs may enhance the oral bioavailability of poorly soluble drugs and the tissue uptake after parenteral administration, through adherence to the capillary wall. They also enhance the delivery of certain drugs across membranes. Being small in size, NP have the potential to leave the vascular system and enter sites of inflammation. The NP size limitation for crossing different biological barriers is dependent on the tissue, target site and circulation. The distinct advantages of liposomes are their ability to encapsulate various materials and their structural versatility. Liposomes can encapsulate drugs with widely varying solubility or lipophilicity, either entrapped in the aqueous core of the phospholipid bilayer or at the bilayer interface. Liposomes are able to deliver drugs into cells by fusion or endocytosis, and practically any drug, irrespective of its solubility, can be entrapped into liposomes. Despite the many advantages of liposomes, including safety and biocompatibility, their main drawback as nanocarriers is their instability in plasma. The polymeric micelle system, owing to its solubilization, selective targeting, P-glycoprotein inhibition and subcellular localization properties, has received growing

scientific attention as an effective drug carrier. Niosomes are a promising vehicle for drug delivery, and since they are non-ionic, they are less toxic and improve the therapeutic index of drugs by restricting their action to target cells. The characteristics of the vesicle formulation are variable and controllable. Niosomes are osmotically active, stable and increase the stability of the entrapped drug. They improve oral bioavailability of poorly absorbed drugs and enhance skin penetration. Niosomal dispersion in an aqueous phase can be emulsified in a non-aqueous phase to regulate the delivery rate of drug and administer normal vesicle in an external non-aqueous phase.

Cyclodextrins (CDs) enhance bioavailability of insoluble drugs by increasing drug solubility and dissolution. They also increase the permeability of insoluble, hydrophobic drugs by making the drug available at the surface of the biological barrier (e.g. skin and mucosa) from whence it partitions into the membrane without disrupting the lipid layers of the barrier. CDs enhance the bioavailability of insoluble drugs by molecular dispersion, protection from degradation, and delivery to the surface of the intestinal wall.

Implants of drug-loaded polymers, either as millirods, pellets or microspheres, are able to deliver drugs for prolonged periods. The benefits of this subcutaneous implantation include greater assurance of patient compliance, which then leads to better therapeutic outcome, particularly for chronic medication. Site of bioavailability of herbal drugs is given in Fig. 8.3.

Phytochemicals With Low Bioavailability

- ⮕ Most of the biologically active polyphenolic phytoconstituents are associated with the problem of either
- ⮕ Poor absorption
- ⮕ Poor permeation
- ⮕ Poor availability

Flavonoids

Problem: Good water solubility, but they are poorly absorbed.

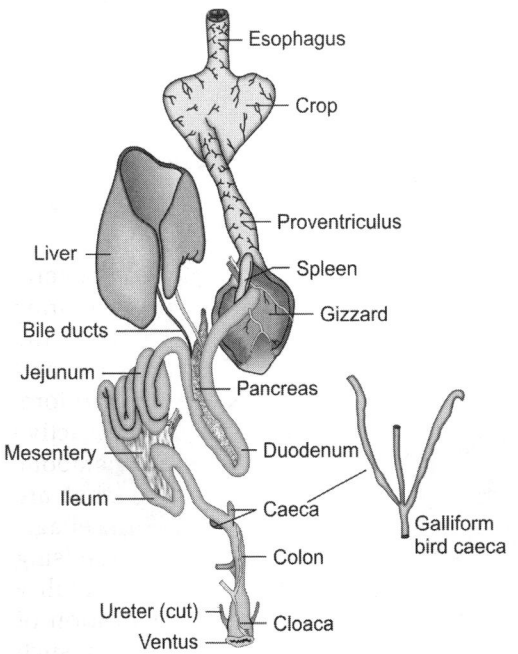

Esophagus
Crop
Proventriculus
Liver
Spleen
Gizzard
Bile ducts
Jejunum
Pancreas
Mesentery
Duodenum
Ileum
Caeca
Galliform bird caeca
Colon
Ureter (cut)
Cloaca
Ventus

Fig. 8.3: Site of bioavailability of herbal drug

Curcumin

Problem: Insoluble in water, highly unstable undergoing rapid hydrolytic degradation.

Andrographolides

Problem: High lipophilicity and low aqueous solubility and poor bioavailability.

Rutin

Problem: Poor bioavailability and is not significantly absorbed before 2 hours, peak plasma concentrations—6 hours.

Paclitaxel (for Malignancies)

Problem: Limited aqueous solubility

Formulated with mixture of Cremophor EL (formulation vehicle used for poorly water soluable drugs) and ethanol.

Thus, patients receive Cremophor EL, resulting in plasma levels of Cremophor EL.

Cremophor EL causes (severe) hypersensitivity.

Artemisinin

Problem: Low bioavailability after oral administration probably due to incomplete absorption, t_{max}—2 to 3 hours postdose; elimination is rapid.

Ginsenoside

Problem: Pre-systemic elimination (degradation in acidic condition), low solubility and low bioavailability.

Etoposide (Anticancers)

Problem: Bioavailability limitation, because of poor water solubility.

Incorporation of drugs in the novel delivery systems helps in
- Increased solubility
- Enhanced stability

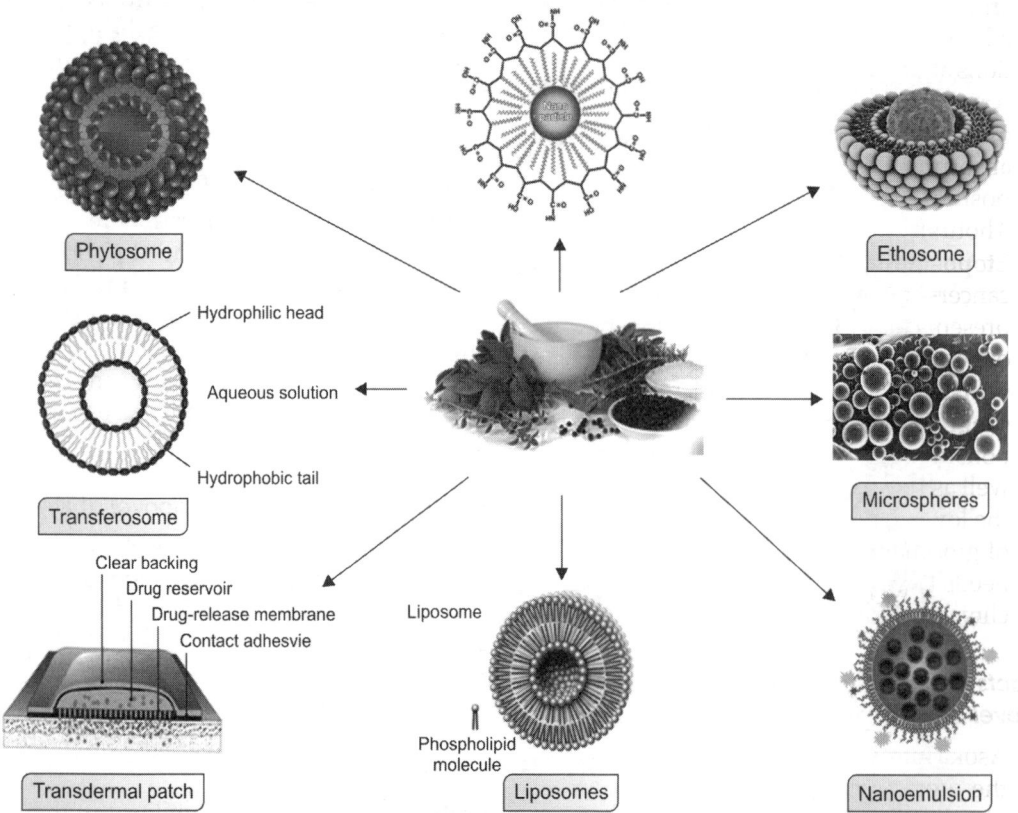

Fig. 8.4: Novel carriers for drug delivery

- Protection from toxicity
- Enhanced pharmacological activity
- Improved tissue macrophage distribution
- Sustained delivery
- Targeted delivery
- Enhanced bioavailability
- Protection from physical and chemical degradation.

Some Phytochemicals With Low Bioavailability

- **Curcumin,** a naturally occurring polyphenolic phytoconstituent, is highly unstable undergoing rapid hydrolytic degradation in neutral or alkaline conditions to feruloyl methane and ferulic acid. It is reported to be stable below pH 6.0.
- **Andrographolides** have poor bioavailability due to high lipophilicity and low aqueous solubility.
- **Rutin** has the lowest relative bioavailability and is not significantly absorbed before 2 hours, showing peak plasma concentrations at 6 hours after intake.
- **Artemisinin** has low bioavailability after oral administration due to incomplete absorption, t_{max} occurs approx. 2 to 3 hours postdose; elimination is rapid ($t_1/2\beta$: 2 to 3 hours).
- **Etoposide** is active in the treatment of many cancers and is widely used in the therapy, it presents bioavailability limitation, because of poor water solubility.
- **Ginsenoside** pre-systemic elimination (degradation in acidic condition; metabolism in intestine tissue and contents), as well as low solubility largely accounted for the low bioavailability. Low bioavailability of ginsenoside is one of the major hurdles needs to be overcome to advance its use in clinical settings.

Facts About Herbal Drugs in Novel Delivery Systems

- Asoka Life Science Limited launched Res-Q, the world's first poly-herbal fast mouth dissolving tablet, effective for lung problems and other respiratory ailments like asthma.

In Ayurvedic medicine segment, this was the first attempt to make medicines more effective in managing chronic ailments.

- This unique mouth dissolving drug delivery system ensures that the drug reaches the blood directly and the first pass metabolism is by passed. It dissolves in mouth by mixing with the saliva and gets absorbed, thereby providing relief from respiratory distress within fifteen minutes. This way, this drug resembles the efficacy of Sorbitrate, a revolutionary mouth dissolving drug used in cardiac distress.
- An investigation aimed to formulate transdermal films incorporating herbal drug components such as Boswellic acid (Boswellia serrata) and curcumin (Curcuma longa) is one of the first few attempts to utilize ayurvedic drugs through transdermal drug delivery system (TDDS), which utilizes skin as a site for continuous drug administration into the systemic circulation.
- This avoids the first pass metabolism of the drug without the pain associated with injection; moreover, the system provides a sustained drug delivery with infrequent dosing via zero-order kinetics and the therapy can be easily terminated at any time.
- Use of turmeric in TDDS for the local action of the drug at the site of administration can also be considered as a new version of ayurvedic turmeric poultice or lepa.
- A patent describes a herbal-based oral composition for periodic retention within the buccal cavity, comprising of Radix polygoni, *Rhizoma drynariae, Rhizoma ligustici Calculus bovis, Indigo naturalis, Herba ecliptae, Pericarpium trichosanthis, Radix sophorae, Spina gleditsiae, Radix angelicae,* and *Fructus mori.*
- The herbal ingredients were selected and prepared to provide a composition effective in causing human scalp and facial hair to darken, to reduce loss of scalp hair and to promote hair growth after a period of repeated usage.
- ArthriBlend-SR is a marketed formulation containing glucosamine sulfate, boswellin

(*Boswellia serrata* extract) and Curcumin (*Curcuma longa*) to support healthy joints and connective tissues in the body.

➲ It is a proprietary clinically validated blend of natural actives for joint care applications. The composition has the added advantage of sustained release technology, which benefits the continuous management of symptoms of arthritis. Novel sustained release implant of herb extract using chitosan has proved to be very useful.

➲ The extract of Danshen (*Radix salvia*), a medicinal herbal, was developed with chitosan—gelatin as an implant for the promotion of healing on muscles and tissues at the organic incision site in abdominal cavities.

➲ Nanoparticles of TCH (traditional Chinese herbs) are helpful to improve their absorption and distribution in body, and therefore enhance their efficacies.

➲ Traditional Chinese herbs, including peach seed, safflower, angelica root, Szechwan lovage rhizome, Rehmannia root, red peony root, leech, gadfly, earthworm and ground beetle, were mixed and prepared through drying, mincing, extracting, crushing into liquid particles with ultrasonic wave, filtering and nanometerizing into nanoparticles with nanometer collider.

➲ These showed significant thrombolytic effects, resulting in quick recovery from arterial embolism and diminution of thrombi.

Phytosomes (Fig. 8.5)

Phytosomes are advanced forms of herbal products that are better absorbed, utilized, and as a result produce better results than conventional herbal extracts. Phytosomes are produced via a patented process whereby the individual components of an herbal extract are bound to phosphatidylcholine—an emulsifying compound derived from soy. Phosphatidylcholine is also one of the chief components of the membranes in our cells. Most of the bioactive constituents of phytomedicines are flavonoids (e.g. anthocyanidins from bilberry, catechins from green tea, silymarin from milk thistle). However, many flavonoids are poorly

absorbed. The poor absorption of flavonoid nutrients is likely due to two factors. First, they are multiple-ring molecules too large to be absorbed by simple diffusion, while they are not absorbed actively, as occurs with some vitamins and minerals. Second, flavonoid molecules typically have poor miscibility with oils and other lipids, severely limiting their ability to pass across the lipid-rich outer membranes of the enterocytes of the small intestine. Water-soluble flavonoid molecules can be converted into lipid-compatible molecular complexes, aptly called phytosomes. Phytosomes are better able to transition from a hydrophilic environment into the lipid-friendly environment of the enterocyte cell membrane and from there into the cell, finally reaching the blood. The lipid-phase substances employed to make flavonoids lipid-compatible are phospholipids from soy, mainly phosphatidylcholine (PC). PC, the principal molecular building block of cell membranes, is miscible both in water and in oil/lipid environments, and is well absorbed when taken by mouth. Precise chemical analysis indicates a phytosome is usually a flavonoid molecule linked with at least one PC molecule. A bond is formed between the two molecules, creating a hybrid molecule. This highly lipid-miscible hybrid bond is better suited to merge into the lipid phase of the enterocyte's outer cell membrane. Phosphatidylcholine is not merely a passive "carrier" for the bioactive flavonoids of the phytosomes, but is itself a bioactive nutrient with documented clinical efficacy for liver disease, including alcoholic hepatic steatosis, drug-induced liver damage, and hepatitis. The intakes of phytosome preparations sufficient to provide reliable clinical benefit often also provide substantial PC intakes. Phytosomes are not liposomes; structurally, the two are distinctly different. The phytosome is a unit of several molecules bonded together, while the liposome is an aggregate of many phospholipid molecules that can enclose active phytomolecules, but without specifically bonding to them. Few examples of phytosomal herbal products are enlisted in Table 8.1.

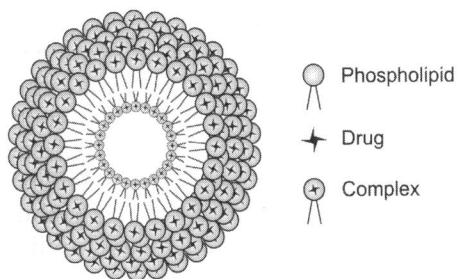

Phospholipid

Drug

Complex

Fig. 8.5: Phytosomes

Table 8.1: Phytosomal herbal products

Phytosomes	Source	Use
Silybin	Silybin flavonoids from *Silybium marianum*	Hepato-protective, antioxidant for liver
Ginseng	Ginsenosides from Panax ginseng	Nutraceutical and immuno-modulator
Green tea	Epigallocatechin from *Thea sinensis*	Anti-cancer, nutraceutical
Grape seed	Procyanidins from *Vitis vinifera*	Nutraceutical, systemic antioxidant, cardioprotective

Properties of Phytosomes

Phytosome is a complex between a natural product and natural phospholipids, like soy phospholipids. Such a complex is obtained by reaction of stoichiometric amounts of phospholipid and the substrate in an appropriate solvent. On the basis of spectroscopic data it has been shown that the main phospholipid-substrate interaction is due to the formation of hydrogen bonds between the polar head of phospholipids (i.e. phosphate and ammonium groups) and the polar functionalities of the substrate.

When treated with water, phytosome assumes a micellar shape forming liposomal-like structures, but while in liposomes the active principle is dissolved in the internal pocket or it is floating in the layer membrane, in phytosome the active principle is anchored to the polar head of phospholipids, becoming an integral part of the membrane. In the case of the catechin distearoyl phosphatidyl choline complex, for example, there is the formation of H-bonds between the phenolic hydroxyls of the flavone moiety and the phosphate ion on the phosphatidylcholine side. This can be deduced from the comparison of the NMR of the complex with those of the pure precursors.

The signals of the fatty chain are almost unchanged. Such evidences inferred that the two long aliphatic chains are wrapped around the active principle, producing a lipophilic envelope which shields the polar head of the phospholipids and the catechins. Additional evidences of the phytosome structure are obtained applying the solid state NMR technique. Proton relaxation studies, by means of spin diffusion process, show that the phytosomes are not mechanical mixture but a complex due to dipolar interactions between the two constituents. This can be confirmed by IR spectroscopy, comparing the spectrum of the complex to the one of the individual components and their mechanical mixture. The particular structure of phytosome elicits peculiar properties and advantages in cosmetic application. Phytosome retain the solubility in fats and in lipophylic media of the precursor phospholipid. Furthermore they act as a carrier of the active principle through lipophilic membranes.

Their low solubility in aqueous media allows the formation of stable emulsions or creams.

The increased bioavailability of the phytosome over the noncomplexed botanical derivatives has been demonstrated by pharmacokinetics studies or by pharmacodynamic tests in experimental animals and in human subjects. The similar things have been studied in some marketed products.

Leucoselect® is composed of oligomeric polyphenols (grape procyanidins) complexed with soy phospholipids. This results in a markedly improved oral bioavailability of procyanidins, which are widely recognized to exert a protective activity on the cardiovascular system through an integrated network of specific mechanisms of action including a unique antioxidant effect. It is composed of oligomeric polyphenols (grape procyanidins) of varying molecular size, complexed with phospholipids. The markedly improved oral bioavailability of these procyanidins flavonoids offers marked protection for the cardiovascular system and other organs through a network of mechanisms that extend beyond their great antioxidant potency.

Ginkgoselect® is an easy absorbable form of the standardized extract of *Ginkgo biloba* leaves. Its major indications are cerebral insufficiency and peripheral vascular disorders, and it is an appropriate aid in situations of reduced cerebral performance. Its better oral bioavailability and the good tolerability make it the ideal product even for long-term treatments. It is a more fully absorbable form of the standardized extract of Ginkgo biloba leaves. Its major indications are cerebral insufficiency and peripheral vascular disorders, and it can also ameliorate reduced cerebral circulation. Its improved oral bioavailability and good tolerability makes it the ideal Ginkgo product even for long-term treatment.

Greenselect® contains a totally standardized polyphenolic fraction (not less than 66.5%) obtained from green tea leaves and mainly characterized by the presence of epigallocatechin and its derivatives. These compounds are demostrated to be strong *in vitro* modulators of several biochemical processes mainly involved in the pathogenesis of major chronic-degenerative diseases such as cancer and atherosclerosis. The complexation of green tea polyphenols with phospholipids strongly improves their low and erratic oral bioavailability. It contains a totally standardized polyphenolic fraction (not less than 66.5 percent) obtained from green tea leaves and mainly characterized by the presence of epigallocatechin and its derivatives. These compounds are potent modulators of several biochemical processes linked to the breakdown of homeostasis in major chronic-degenerative diseases such as cancer and atherosclerosis. The complexation of green tea polyphenols with phospholipids strongly improves their poor oral bioavailability.

Siliphos® prevents liver damage of different etiology. Siliphos® is the most absorbable form of silybin known up to now, as it allows silybin to reach the target organ, the liver, in concentrations which are reported to be effective as antihepatotoxic.

Mirtoselect® contains an extract of bilberry which provides anthocyanosides. These improve capillary tone, reduce abnormal blood vessel permeability, and are potent antioxidants. They hold great potential for the management of retinal blood vessel problems and venous insufficiency.

Sabalselect®18 includes an extract prepared from saw palmetto berries through supercritical CO_2 (carbon dioxide) extraction. It delivers fatty acids, alcohols and sterols that benefit prostate health. In particular this extract may benefit non-cancerous prostate enlargement.

Lymphaselect™ includes a standardized extract from *Melilotus officinalis*. This preparation is particularly indicated for venous disorders, including chronic venous insufficiency of the lower limbs.

Oleaselect™ is a newer preparation from olive oil polyphenols. These are potent free radical scavengers (antioxidants), inhibit harmful oxidation of LDL cholesterol, and also have anti-inflammatory activity.

Polinacea™ is an immunomodulating preparation made from *Echinacea angustifolia*. It includes echinacosides and a unique high-molecular weight polysaccharide. This preparation especially enhances immune function in response to a toxic challenge. For all these breakthrough phytomedicines, the phytosome technology enables cost-effective delivery and synergistic benefits from the phospholipid nutraceuticals intrinsic to life.

HERBAL CONSTITUENTS USED IN PHYTOSOMAL DRUG DELIVERY

Flavonoids

Plants are endowed with myriad health giving substances, prominent among these being the flavonoids. First recognized for their antioxidant properties, flavonoids are widely distributed in food and medicinal plants. To date, more than 4,000 naturally occurring flavonoids have been identified, each with its own distinctive molecular structure and 3-D shape. Flavonoids are part of a broader class of dietary antioxidants called polyphenols (literally, having more than one phenolic ring). The flavonoids are distinctive for their triple ring structures. Subclasses of the flavonoids exist, classified mostly on the degree of oxidation of the oxygen heterocycle or C-ring. Molecular 3-D shape or "configuration" is an important aspect of flavonoid biology. Individual flavonoids have been found to specifically protect vulnerable molecular sites on cells, to stimulate or inhibit the active sites.

Among foodstuffs, the flavonoids are most abundant in berries and other fruits, a few vegetables, and in cocoa and tea beverages. As a rule, the flavonoids are poorly absorbed from foods—for greater than 10% of the administered dose to reach the blood is the rare exception. Epidemiological evidence suggests that the lower intakes of flavonoids are associated with heightened risk of cardiovascular disease, but is not yet conclusive. A very active area of current research is focused on flavonoids that downregulate receptors for prostaglandins, cytokines, or hormones on cancerous or other abnormal cells. Molecular configuration may prove to be just as important as antioxidant action in the diverse anti-inflammatory, anti-allergic, antiviral, anticancer, and immune-stimulant applications of flavonoids. Then by taking flavonoid preparations with the greatest health giving potential and making them into phytosomal preparations, Indena scientists achieved a breakthrough in phytomedicine.

Terpenoids: Natural products and related compounds formally derived from isoprene units. They contain oxygen in various functional groups. This class is subdivided according to the number of carbon atoms in the same manner as are *terpenes*. The skeleton of terpenoid may differ from strict additivity of isoprene units by the loss or shift of a fragment, generally a methyl group.

Carotenoids: Carotenoids are a large class of lipid-soluble isoprenoid compounds located in plant plastids and belong to two chemical classes: The oxygen-free carotenes (orange and red pigments) and the oxygen-containing xanthophylls (yellow pigments).

Isoprenoids: Compounds formally derived from isoprene (2-methylbuta-1,3-diene), the skeleton of which can generally be discerned in repeated occurrence in the molecule. The skeleton of isoprenoids may differ from strict additivity of isoprene units by loss or shift of a fragment, commonly a methyl group. The class includes both *hydrocarbon* and oxygenated derivatives.

Terpenes: Hydrocarbons of biological origin having carbon skeletons formally derived from isoprene [$CH_2=C(CH_3)CH=CH_2$]. This class is subdivided into the C5 hemiterpenes, C_{10} monoterpenes, C_{15} sesquiterpenes, C_{20} diterpenes, C_{25} sesterterpenes, C_{30} triterpenes, C_{40} tetraterpenes (carotenoids), and C_{5n} polyterpenes.

The lipid-phase substances that successfully employed to make flavonoids lipid compatible are phospholipids from soy, mainly phosphatidylcholine (PC). PC is miscible both in the water phase and in oil/lipid phases, and is excellently absorbed when taken by mouth. PC is the principal molecular building block for cell membranes, and the molecular properties that suit PC for this role also render it close to ideal for its Phytosome® role. Precise chemical analysis indicates the unit phytosome is usually a flavonoid molecule linked with at least one PC molecule. A bond is formed between the two molecules to create a hybrid molecule; this hybrid is highly lipid—miscible, better suited to merge into the lipid phase of the enterocyte's outer cell membrane.

Advantages and Applications

1. **Better bioavailability (Silybin Phytosomes):** There is a growing body of scientific studies showing improved absorption, utilization, and results with the phytosome process. Siliphost (silybin phytosome) is the well-studied. Silybin is the chief component of silymarin, the flavonoid

complex from milk thistle valued for its ability to protect and restore the liver. Silybin is the most potent of these active substances. Siliphost contains one part silybin to one part phosphatidylcholine while milk thistle phytosome is a less potent version as it contains all three flavonoids of silymarin and the ratio of phosphatidylcholine to silymarin is 2:1. The research has shown in both human and animal studies is that Siliphost is better absorbed compared to an equal amount of silybin in conventional milk thistle extracts.

2. Antitumor activity of the silybin-phosphatidylcholine complex, IdB 1016, against human ovarian cancer was studied. This study aimed to assess, in an *in vivo* experimental model, the growth inhibitory effects of IdB 1016 (silipide, a complex of silybin/phosphatidylcholine) when used as a single agent against human ovarian cancer.

3. **New effects and applications of silybin and silymarin:** The polyphenolic fraction from the seeds of *silybum marianum* and its main component silybin. Silymarin and silybin were studied as hepatoprotectants shown to have other interesting activities, e.g. anticancer and canceroprotective. These activities were demonstrated in a large variety of illnesses of different organs as, e.g. prostate, lungs, CNS, kidneys, pancreas and others. Besides the cytoprotective activity of silybin mediated by its antioxidative and radical-scavenging properties, also new activities based on the specific receptor interaction were discovered, e.g. inhibition and modulation of drug transporters, P-glycoproteins, estrogenic receptors, nuclear receptors and some others. New derivatives of silybin open new ways to its therapeutic applications. Pharmacology dealing with optically pure silybin diastereomers may suggest new mechanisms of its action.

4. **Vessel maturation effects on tumor growth:** In an experiment, validation of a computer model in implanted human ovarian carcinoma spheroids. Measurements of tumor growth, neovascular maturation and function in human epithelial ovarian carcinoma xenografts were performed. Results suggest that vascular maturation and mature and immature vessel regression occur continuously during tumor neovascularisation. Moreover, in these spheroids, a high tumor growth-rate is associated with monotonic changes in vessel density (VD) and with large proportions of mature blood vessels, whereas a lower tumor growth-rate is associated with fluctuating VD and lower proportions of mature vessels. These results corroborated a mathematical model for tumor dynamics, including vascular maturation and immature and mature vessel regression.

5. Peritoneal dissemination of ovarian cancer and tumor angiogenesis was studied in Pyrrolo[2,1-c][1,4]benzodiazepine dimer SJG-136 (NSC 694501) selectively cross-links guanine residues located on opposite strands of DNA, and found to exhibit potent *in vitro* cytotoxicity. In addition, SJG-136 was highly active *in vivo* in hollow fiber assays.

Herbal drugs/plant actives possess a lot of therapeutic potential that should be explored via application of novel drug delivery technology. Large molecular size, lipid solubility, degradation in acidic stomach are certain problems which limit the therapeutic activity of these extracts *in vivo* though these possess excellent bioactivity *in vitro*. Application of novel drug delivery systems led to enhanced bioavailability of plant actives by increasing the permeability and solubility as well as reduction in side effects. A number of plant constituents like flavanoids, tannins, terpenoids, etc. showed enhanced therapeutic effect at similar or less dose when incorporated into novel drug delivery vehicles as compared to conventional plant extracts. Hence there is great potential in development of NDDS for valuable herbal drugs as it provides efficient and economical drug delivery and the trends of incorporating NDDS for herbal drugs have also been adopted at industrial scale.

Liposomes

Liposomes are biodegradeable, colloidal and spherical vesicles (0.05–5.0 μm in diameter) composed of a bilayer membrane entrapping an aqueous core. Liposomal-based drug delivery is advantageous specifically in enhancing the therapeutic index, either by increasing the drug concentration in the tumour cells and by decreasing the exposure to normal cells. Liposomes have been used to change the pharmacokinetic profile of various drugs, herbs, enzymes, etc. (Fig. 8.6). The liposomal herbal formulations are enlisted in Table 8.2.

Microspheres (Fig. 8.7)

Microspheres are spherical particles consisting of size ideally 1–300 μm. Each particle is matrix of the drug dispersed in the polymer and drug is released as a first order process. The polymers used for the fabrication of the microspheres are biodegradable or non-bio-degradable. Various polymers have been used for fabrication of these microparticulate carriers such as albumin, gelatin, modified starch, polypropylene, dextran, polylactic acid and polylactide co-glycolide, etc. Microsphere herbal formulations are enlisted in Table 8.3.

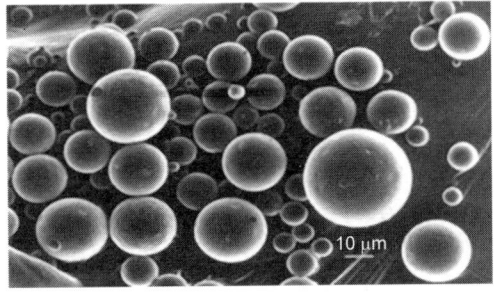

Fig. 8.7: Microsphere

Table 8.2: Liposomal herbal formulations	
Name of bioactive component/plant	Application
Essential oil from *Atractylodes macrocephala Koidz*	Increase in solubility and bioavailability
Essential oil of *Origanum dictamnus*	Increase in activity
Quercetin	Increase in bioavailability and reduction in side effects
Silymarin extract	Increase in hepato-protective activity
Capsaicin	Increase in permeation as prolongation of action
Taxanes	Decrease in toxicity

Table 8.3: Microsphere herbal formulations	
Name of bioactive component/plant	Application
Silymarin	Sustained release
Zedoary turmeric oil (Microencapsulation techniques)	Increase in bioavailability as well as sustained release occurs
Rutin	Specific delivery to cardiovascular and cerebrovascular region
Camptothecin (Spray dry process)	Significant decrease in dose by enhancing the solubility

Nanoparticles (Fig. 8.8)

Nanoparticles are the submicron size particles having size range 10 to 1000 nm. The main advantages of the nanoparticles is their stability and long-term storage. The particle size and surface characteristics of nanoparticles can be easily modified for controlled and targeted drug delivery. Nanosizing leads to increased solubility of components and reduction in the dose via improved absorption of active ingredient. Nanoparticles are efficient delivery systems for the delivery of both hydrophilic and hydrophobic drugs. Examples

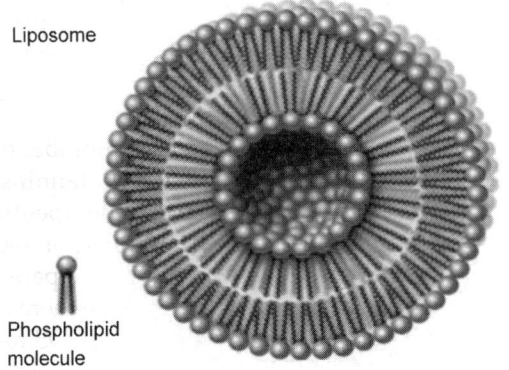

Liposome

Phospholipid molecule

Fig. 8.6: Liposomes

of nanoparticle containing herbal drug with application are enlisted in Table 8.4.

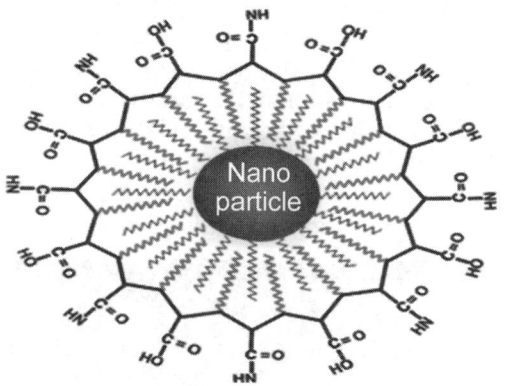

Fig. 8.8: Nanoparticles

Table 8.4: Nanoparticle containing herbal drugs

Name of bioactive component/plant	Application
Paclitaxel (contro-lled nanosystem)	Reduction in side effects
Curcumin (poor aqueous solubility)	Increase in solubility/ potential carrier for the treatment of cancer
Triptolide	Increase in solubility
Quercetin	Increased drug release and antioxidant effect (Approx 74 times)
Taxol (emulsion solvent evaporation technique)	Sustained release/enhanced bioavailability
Paclitaxel and Doxorubicin (using Brij 78 surfactant, P-glycoprotein mediated drug)	Inhibition of resistance and thus increases anticancer activity
Cuscata chinensis (Flavonoid/Lignan)	Nanosuspension reduced the dose 5 times compared to alcoholic extract

Transferosomes (Fig. 8.9)

Transferosomes are phospholipid vesicles which act as potential carriers for the transdermal delivery of the drug. They overcome the difficulty of penetration through the *stratum corneum* and can easily penetrate through the intracellular pores of the skin due to their flexibility. Transferosomes are fabricated by using

phospholipids (act as vesicle forming material), surfactant (providing flexibility), alcohol (solvent) and buffering agent (as hydrating medium). Examples of herbal transferosomes with their applications are given in Table 8.5.

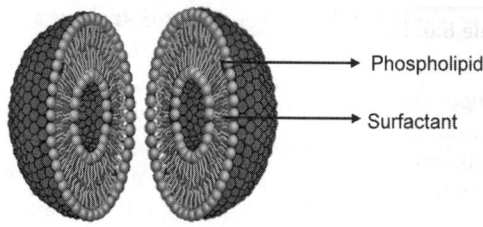

Fig. 8.9: Herbal transferosomes

Table 8.5: Herbal transferosomes

Name of bioactive component/plant	Application
Capsaicin transferosomes	Increased skin penetration
Curcumin transferosomes	Increased skin pene-tration (potent anti-inflammatory)
Vincristine sulphate trans-ferosomes (prepared with lecithin and sodium deoxy cholate)	Increase in permeability
Colchicine transferosomes (by Shaking method)	Reduction in GIT side effects

Ethosomes (Fig. 8.10)

Ethosomes are vesicles composed of phospholipids and high concentration of ethanol. High concentration of ethanol in the vesicles leads to enhancement in their permeability through the skin by fluidizing the lipid domain of the skin. Ethosomes have been reported for transdermal delivery of the hydrophilic and impermeable drugs such as minoxidil, testosterone,

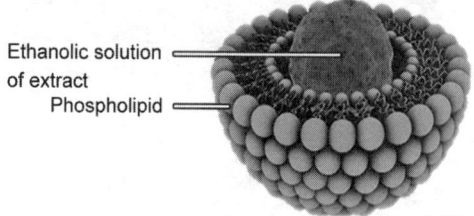

Fig. 8.10: Herbal ethosomes

bacitracin and cannabidol. It is efficient carrier for topical/ transdermal route. It is also used for both hydrophillic and hydrophobic drug. Herbal Ethosomes with their applications are given in Table 8.6.

Table 8.6: Herbal ethosomes

Name of bioactive component/plant	Application
Ethosomal suspension of ammonium Glycyrrhizinate	Increased drug permeation through dermis for inflammatory disorders
Triptolide	Increase in bioavailability
Sophora alopencerides (ethosomes prepared by using isolated alkaloids)	Increase in permeability and useful for topical delivery of alkaloids

Nanoemulsions/Microemulsions (Fig. 8.11)

Nanoemulsions and microemulsions are the emulsions of O/W type having the size range of several microns. They are prepared by using the surfactants which are considered safe for the human use and approved by the FDA. These types of emulsions have higher surface area and hence can easily penetrate through the skin. They are also nontoxic and nonirritant in nature and can be used in the animals and veterinary purpose.

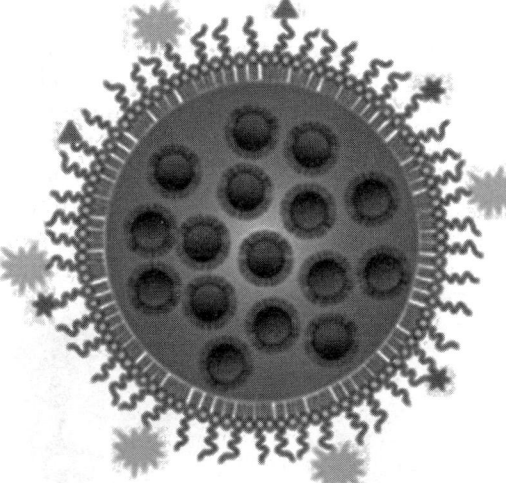

Fig. 8.11: Nanoemulsions and microemulsion herbal formulations

Transdermal Systems (Fig. 8.12)

Transdermal drug delivery devices are the polymeric formulations which are applied over the skin and deliver the drug at predetermined rate and for predetermined time. There are various types of the transdermal delivery devices which can be formulated by using the polymer matrix, adhesive bandage and permeation enhancers. Transdermal delivery system provides the advantage of controlled drug delivery, enhanced bioavailability, reduction in side effects and easy application. Transdermal drug delivery systems are potentially used for the sustained delivery of the drugs up to several days or even months. The herbal formulations nanoemulsions and microemulsion with their biological activity are given in Table 8.7.

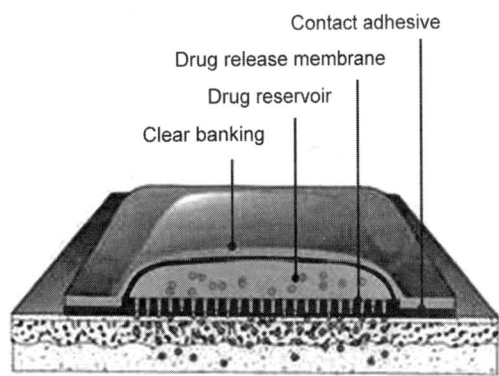

Fig. 8.12: Transdermal system

Table 8.7: Nanoemulsions and microemulsion herbal formulations

Name of bioactive component	Target site/ biological activity
Norcantharidin microemulsion	Liver
Puerarin Micro-emulsion	Cardiovascular and cerebrovascular disease
Silybin nanoemulsion	Liver
Berberine Nano-emulsion	Tumor
Matrine Nanoemulsion	Anti-bacterial, anti-inflammatory, anti-virus

Implants (Fig. 8.13)

These are the polymeric devices which are used for the controlled and sustained delivery of the drugs. These are directly placed in the body fluids/cavities and are fabricated by using biodegradable polymers. A microsurgery is always required for the insertion of these devices. Implants of the extract of Danshen (*Radix Salviae Miltiorrhizae*) have been developed using chitosan and gelatin. This drug is used for healing of muscles and tissues in abdominal cavities.

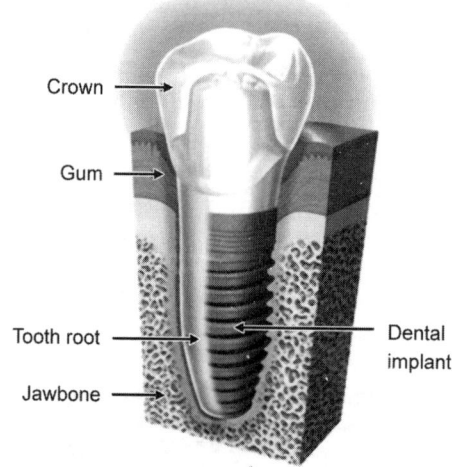

Fig. 8.13: Implants

Micropellets (Fig. 8.14)

These are the solid particles which fall in the range of 1–1000 µm. Controlled release pellets are used for the delivery of drugs to specific sites and for the extended period of time. Used for the delivery of two incompatible drugs-simultaneously at same or different sites. It prevents dose dumping which occurs with the conventional dosage forms, i.e. vomiting, loss of appetite and nausea.

Pellets are also used for the coating and taste masking of the formulations. Pectin-hydroxypropyl methylcellulose (HPMC) coated curcumin pellets were prepared for delivery of the curcumin in the colon to treat the inflammatory disease. Andrographolide (*Andrographis paniculata wall*) micropellets can

be prepared by sodium alginate to release the drug away from the upper part of GIT and prevent the GIT irritation problems.

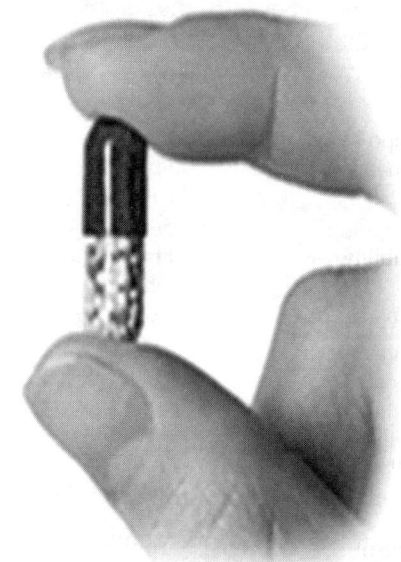

Fig. 8.14: Micropellets

Complexation

Complexation is the association between the two or more molecules to form a nonbonded entity with a well-defined stochiometry. Various complexing agents such as EDTA, cyclodextrins and polymers have been used for the complexation. Curcumin is a poorly soluble drug, its solubility has been increased by formation of curcumin soya lecithin complex for hepatoprotective activity. Complexation increase permeability of the curcumin.

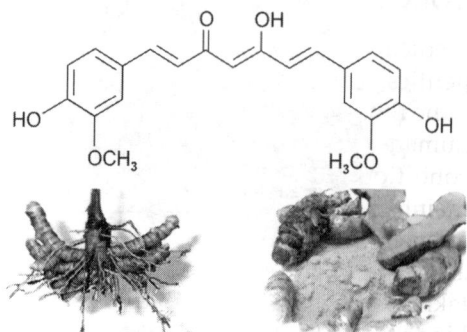

Fig. 8.15: Curcumin

Table 8.8: Assessment of the drug carrier

Characters	Liposomes	Transferosome	Ethosomes	Microsphere	Nanoparticles	Phytosomes	Nanoemulsions/Microemulsions
Size	0.05–5.0 μm	0.05–10.0 μm	0.05–10.0 μm	1–300 μm	10 to 1000 μm	0.05–5.0 μm	0.01 to 50 μm
Composition	Phospholipids and cholesterol	Phospholipids surfactant	Phospholipids ethanol	Polymers	Polymers	Phospholipids and cholesterol surfactant	Oil phase and aqueous phase
Flexibility	Rigid in nature	High deformability due to surfactant	High deformability and elasticity due to ethanol	Rigid and hard in nature, bigger in size	Small and rigid with hard nature	Similar to liposomes	High deformability (globules)
Mechanism	Diffusion/ Fusion/ Lipolysis	Deformation of vesicle	Lipid Perturbation	Diffusion/ erosion	Diffusion/ erosion	Diffusion/ Fusion/ Lipolysis	Diffusion/ fusion/ deformation of globules
Route of administration	Oral, topical and transdermal parenteral	Topical and transdermal	Topical and transdermal	Oral, topical and transdermal parenteral	Oral, topical and transdermal parenteral	Oral, topical and transdermal	Oral, topical and transdermal parenteral
Marketed products	**VincaXome** Vincristine solid tumours NeXstar, USA				**Abraxane** Paclitaxel Abraix bioscience cancer treatment AstraZeneca USA	**Meriva-SR** Curcumin Anti-inflammatory, detoxification, cardiovascular Thorne Research, USA	

CONCLUSION

Medicinal herbs as potential source of therapeutics aids has attained a significant role in health system all over the world for both humans and animals not only in the diseased condition but also as potential material for maintaining proper health. Herbs are staging a comeback, herbal 'renaissance' is happening all over the globe and more and more people are taking note of herbal therapies to treat various kinds of ailments in place of mainstream medicine. There are three main reasons for the popularity of herbal medicines as there is a growing concern over the reliance and safety of drugs and surgery. Modern medicine is failing to effectively treat many of the most common health conditions. Many natural measures are being shown to produce better results than drugs or surgery without the side effects. Novel drug delivery system is a novel approach to drug delivery that addresses the limitations of the traditional drug delivery systems. Modern medicine cures a particular disease by targeting exactly the affected zone inside a patient's body and transporting the

Table 8.9: Recent patents on novel herbal formulations

US patent No.	Active ingredient	Novel system
US 5948414	Opioid analgesic and aloe	Nasal Spray
US 6340478 B1	Ginsenosides	Microencapsulated and controlled release formulations
Us6890561 B1	Isoflavones	Microencapsulated formulation
US6896898 B1	Alkaloids of Aconitum species	Transdermal delivery system
US patent 2005/0142232 A1	Oleaginous oil of *sesamum indicum* and *alcoholic extract* of centella asiatica	Brain tonic
US patent 2007/0042062 A1	Glycine max containing form globulin protein extract, curcumin, ginger officinalis	Herbal tablet dosage form
US patent 2007/0077284A1	Opioid analgesic (phenanthrene gp)	Transdermal patch
US patent 7569236132	Flavonoids (such as quercetin) and Terpenes (ginkgolide A, B, C and J)	Microgranules

drug to that area. Drug delivery system is the method by which an optimum amount of the concerned drug is administered to the patient in such a way that it reaches exactly the 'site of action' and starts working then and there. Novel drug delivery system attempts to eliminate all the disadvantages associated with conventional drug delivery systems.

Evaluation, Intellectual Property Right and Regulatory Issues of Herbal Drugs

☞ Evaluation of Drugs

☞ Patenting and Regulatory Requirements of Natural Products

☞ Regulatory Issues

9 Evaluation of Drugs

INTRODUCTION

WHO Guidelines for the Assessment of Herbal Medicines

Definitions of Relevant Terms

i. *Quality:* It is status of the drug that is determined by identity, purity, content and various chemical, physical and biological properties.

ii. *Safety:* To assure that drug has no side and hazardous effect.

iii. *Purity:* Freedom from adulteration or contamination.

iv. *Potency:* Amount of drug required to produce a given percentage of its maximal effect, irrespective of the size of maximal effect

v. *Identity:* The herb as it should be.

vi. *Quality control:* The term quality control refers to the sum of all procedures undertaken to ensure the identity and purity of a particular pharmaceutical.

vii. *Herbal medicine:* These include herbs, herbal materials, herbal preparations and finished herbal products.

viii. *Herbal materials:* Herbal materials are either whole plant or part of medicinal plants in the crude state. These include herbs, fresh juices, gums, fixed oils, essential oil, resins and dry powders of herbs.

ix. *Herbal preparations:* These are finished herbal products produced with extraction, distillation, expressions, fractionation, purification, concentration and fermentation.

History of Development of WHO Guidelines

⮑ In 1991, the Director-General of WHO, in a report to the forty-fourth World Health Assembly, emphasized the great importance of medicinal plants to the health of individuals and communities.

⮑ Earlier, in 1978, the thirty-first World Health Assembly had adopted a resolution (WHA31.33) that called on the Director-General to compile and periodically update a therapeutic classification of medicinal plants, related to the therapeutic classification of all drugs.

⮑ Subsequently resolution WHA40.33, adopted in 1987, urged Member States to ensure quality control of drugs derived from traditional plant remedies by using modern techniques and applying suitable standards and good manufacturing practices.

⮑ Resolution WHA42.43, of 1989, urged member states to introduce measures for the regulation and control of medicinal plant products and for the establishment and maintenance of suitable standards.

⮑ Moreover, the international conference on Primary Health Care, held in Alma-Ata,

USSR, in 1978, recommended, inter alia, the accommodation of proven traditional remedies in national drug policies and regulatory measures.

➥ In developed countries, a resurgence of interest in herbal medicines has resulted from the preference of many consumers for products of natural origin. In addition, manufactured herbal medicines often follow in the wake of migrants from countries where traditional medicines play an important role.

➥ In both developed and developing countries, consumers and health care providers need to be supplied with up-to-date and authoritative information on the beneficial properties, and possible harmful effects, of all herbal medicines.

➥ The fourth International Conference of Drug Regulatory Authorities, held in Tokyo in 1986, organized a workshop on the regulation of herbal medicines moving in international commerce. Another workshop on the same subject was held as part of the Fifth International Conference of Drug Regulatory Authorities, held in Paris in 1989. Both workshops confined their considerations to the commercial exploitation of traditional medicines through over-the-counter labelled products.

➥ The Paris meeting concluded that the World Health Organization should consider preparing model guidelines containing basic elements of legislation designed to assist those countries wishing to develop appropriate legislation and registration.

Objectives

The objectives of these guidelines are as follows:

1. To define basic criteria for the evaluation of quality, safety and efficacy of herbal medicines and thereby to assist national regulatory authorities, scientific organizations and manufacturers to undertake an assessment of the documentation/submissions/dossiers in respect of such products.

2. As a general rule in this assessment, traditional experience means that long-term use as well as the medical, historical and ethnological background of those products shall be taken into account. The definition of long-term use may vary according to the country but should be at least several decades. Therefore, the assessment should take into account a description in the medical/pharmaceutical literature or similar sources, or a documentation of knowledge on the application of a herbal medicine without a clearly defined time limitation. Marketing authorizations for similar products should be taken into account.

3. Prolonged and apparently uneventful use of a substance usually offers testimony of its safety. In a few instances, however, investigation of the potential toxicity of naturally occurring substances widely used as ingredients in these preparations has revealed previously unsuspected potential for systematic toxicity, carcinogenicity and teratogenicity. Regulatory authorities need to be quickly and reliably informed of these findings. They should also have the authority to respond promptly to such alerts, either by withdrawing or varying the licences of registered products containing suspect substances, or by rescheduling the substances to limit their use to medical prescription.

Assessment of Quality

Pharmaceutical Assessment

This assessment covers all important aspects of the quality assessment of herbal medicines. It is sufficient to make reference to a pharmacopoeial monograph if one exists. If no such monograph is available, a monograph must be supplied and should be set out as in an official pharmacopoeia. All procedures should be in accordance with good manufacturing practices.

Crude Plant Material

The botanical definition, including genus, species and authority, should be given to ensure correct identification of a plant. A definition and description of the part of the plant from which the medicine is made (e.g. leaf flower, root) should be provided, together with an indication of whether fresh, dried or traditionally processed material is used. The active and characteristic constituents should be specified and, if possible, content limits should be defined. Foreign matter, impurities and microbial content should be defined or limited. Voucher specimens, representing each lot of plant material processed, should be authenticated by a qualified botanist and should be stored for at least a 10-year period. A lot number should be assigned and this should appear on the product label.

Plant Preparations

Plant preparations include comminuted or powdered plant materials, extracts, tinctures, fatty or essential oils, expressed juices and preparations whose production involves fractionation, purification or concentration. The manufacturing procedure should be described in detail. If other substances are added during manufacture in order to adjust the plant preparation to a certain level of active or characteristic constituents or for any other purpose, the added substances should be mentioned in the manufacturing procedures. A method for identification and, where possible, assay of the plant preparation should be added. If identification of an active principle is not possible, it should be sufficient to identify a characteristic substance or mixture of substances (e.g. "chromatographic fingerprint") to ensure consistent quality of the preparation.

Finished Product

The manufacturing procedure and formula, including the amount of excipients, should be described in detail. A finished product specification should be defined. A method of identification and, where possible, quantification of the plant material in the finished product should be defined. If the identification of an active principle is not possible, it should be sufficient to identify a characteristic substance or mixture of substances (e.g. "chromatographic fingerprint") to ensure consistent quality of the product. The finished product should comply with general requirements for particular dosage forms.

For imported finished products, confirmation of the regulatory status in the country of origin should be required. The WHO Certification Scheme on the Quality of Pharmaceutical Products Moving in International Commerce should be applied.

Stability

The physical and chemical stability of the product in the container in which it is to be marketed should be tested under defined storage conditions and the shelf-life should be established.

Assessment of Safety

This should cover all relevant aspects of the safety assessment of a medicinal product. A guiding principle should be that, if the product has been traditionally used without demonstrated harm, no specific restrictive regulatory action should be undertaken unless new evidence demands a revised risk–benefit assessment.

A review of the relevant literature should be provided with original articles or references to the original articles. If official monograph/ review results exist, reference can be made to them. However, although long-term use without any evidence of risk may indicate that a medicine is harmless, it is not always certain how far one can rely solely on long-term usage to provide assurance of innocuity in the light of concern expressed in recent years over the long-term hazards of some herbal medicines.

Reported side-effects should be documented according to normal pharmaco-vigilance practices.

Toxicological Studies

Toxicological studies, if available, should be part of the assessment. Literature should be indicated as above.

Documentation of Safety Based On Experience

As a basic rule, documentation of a long period of use should be taken into consideration when assessing safety. This means that, when there is no detailed toxicological studies, documented experience of long-term use without evidence of safety problems should form the basis of the risk assessment. However, even in cases of drugs used over a long period, chronic toxicological risks may have occurred but may not have been recognized. The period of use, the health disorders treated, the number of users and the countries with experience should be specified. If a toxicological risk is known, toxicity data must be submitted. The assessment of risk, whether independent of dose or related to dose, should be documented. In the latter case, the dosage specification must be an important part of the risk assessment. An explanation of the risks should be given, if possible. Potential for misuse, abuse or dependence must be documented. If long-term traditional use cannot be documented or there are doubts on safety, toxicity, data should be submitted.

Assessment of Efficacy

This should cover all important aspects of efficacy assessment. A review of the relevant literature should be carried out and copies provided of the original articles or proper references made to them. Research studies, if they exist, should be taken into account.

Activity

The pharmacological and clinical effects of the active ingredients and, if known, their constituents with therapeutic activity should be specified or described.

Evidence Required Supporting Indications

The indication(s) for the use of the medicine should be specified. In the case of traditional medicines, the requirements for proof of efficacy should depend on the kind of indication. For treatment of minor disorders and for non-specific indications, some relaxation in requirements for proof of efficacy may be justified, taking into account the extent of traditional use. The same considerations may apply to prophylactic use. Individual experiences recorded in reports from physicians, traditional health practitioners or treated patients should be taken into account.

Where traditional use has not been established, appropriate clinical evidence should be required.

Combination Products

As many herbal remedies consist of a combination of several active ingredients, and as experience of the use of traditional remedies is often based on combination products, assessment should differentiate between old and new combination products. Identical requirements for the assessment of old and new combinations would result in inappropriate assessment of certain traditional medicines.

In the case of traditionally used combination products, the documentation of traditional use (such as classical texts of Ayurveda, traditional Chinese medicine, Unani, Siddha) and experience may serve as evidence.

An explanation of a new combination of well-known substances, including effective dose ranges and compatibility, should be required in addition to the documentation of traditional knowledge of each single ingredient. Each active ingredient must contribute to the efficacy of the medicine.

Clinical studies may be required to justify the efficacy of a new ingredient and its positive effect on the total combination.

Intended Use

Product information for the consumer: Product labels and package inserts should be understandable to the consumer or patient. The package information should include all necessary information on the proper use of the product.

The following elements of information will usually suffice:
- ➲ Name of the product
- ➲ Quantitative list of active ingredient(s)
- ➲ Dosage form

➲ Indications
- Dosage (if appropriate, specified for children and the elderly)
- Mode of administration
- Duration of use
- Major adverse effects, if any
- Over dosage information
- Contraindications, warnings, precautions and major drug interactions
- Use during pregnancy and lactation

➲ Expiry date
➲ Lot number
➲ Holder of the marketing authorization.

Identification of the active ingredient(s) by the Latin botanical name, in addition to the common name in the language of preference of the National Regulatory Authority, is recommended.

Sometimes not all information that is ideally required may be available, so Drug Regulatory Authorities should determine their minimal requirements.

Promotion: Advertisements and other promotional material directed to health personnel and the general public should be fully consistent with the approved package information.

Utilization of These Guidelines

These guidelines for the assessment of herbal medicines are intended to facilitate the work of regulatory authorities, scientific bodies and industry in the development, assessment and registration of such products. The assessment should reflect the scientific knowledge gathered in that field. Such assessment could be the basis for future classification of herbal medicines in different parts of the world. Other types of traditional medicines in addition to herbal products may be assessed in a similar way.

The effective regulation and control of herbal medicines moving in international commerce also requires close liaison between national institutions that are able to keep under regular review all aspects of production and use of herbal medicines, as well as to conduct

or sponsor evaluative studies of their efficacy, toxicity, safety, acceptability, cost and relative value compared with other drugs used in modern medicine.

WHO Guidelines for the Assessment of Herbal Drugs (Fig. 9.1)

The various guidelines of WHO are as follows:

WHO's mission in essential drugs and medicines policy is to help save lives and improve health by closing the huge gap between the potential that essential drugs have to offer and the reality that for millions of people particularly the poor and disadvantaged medicines are unavailable, unaffordable, unsafe or improperly used. It does this by carrying out a number of core functions: Articulating policy and advocacy positions; working in partnership; producing guidelines and practical tools; developing norms and standards; stimulating strategic and operational research; developing human resources; and managing information.

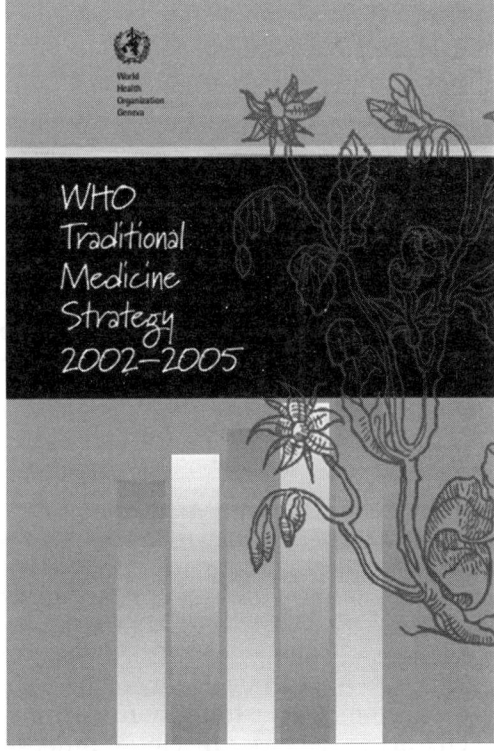

Fig. 9.1: Cover page of WHO traditional medicine strategy (2002–2005)

WHO Traditional Medicines Strategy 2002–2005

The WHO Traditional Medicines Strategy 2002–2005 reviews the status of traditional medicine/complementary and alternative medicine (TM/CAM) globally, and outlines WHOs own role and activities in TM/CAM. But more importantly it provides a framework for action for WHO and its partners, aimed at enabling TM/CAM to play a far greater role in reducing excess mortality and morbidity, especially among impoverished populations. The strategy incorporates four objectives:

1. **Policy:** Integrate TM/CAM with national health care systems, as appropriate, by developing and implementing national TM/CAM policies and programmes.

2. **Safety, efficacy and quality:** Promote the safety, efficacy and quality of TM/CAM by expanding the knowledge base on TM/CAM, and by providing guidance on regulatory and quality assurance standards.

3. **Access:** Increase the availability and affordability of TM/CAM, as appropriate, with an emphasis on access for poor populations.

4. **Rational use:** Promote therapeutically sound use of appropriate TM/CAM by providers and consumers. Implementation of the strategy will initially focus on the first two objectives. Achieving the safety, efficacy and quality objective will provide the necessary foundation for achieving the access and rational use objectives.

WHO Guidelines On Safety Monitoring of Herbal Medicines in Pharma-covigilance Systems (Fig. 9.2)

The objectives of these guidelines are:

1. To support member states, in the context of the WHO International Drug Monitoring Programme, to strengthen national pharmacovigilance capacity in order to carry out effective safety monitoring of herbal medicines.

2. To provide technical guidance on the principles of good pharmacovigilance and the inclusion of herbal medicines in existing national drug safety monitoring systems; and where these systems are not in place, to facilitate the establishment of an inclusive national drug safety monitoring system.

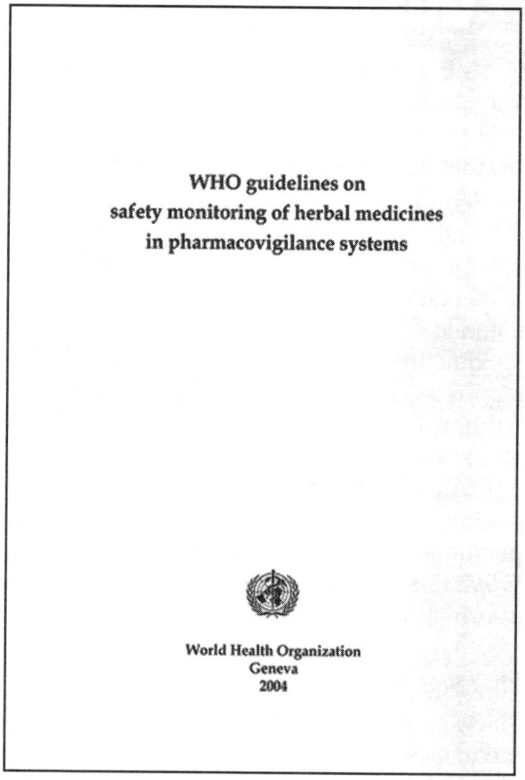

WHO guidelines on safety monitoring of herbal medicines in pharmacovigilance systems

World Health Organization
Geneva
2004

Fig. 9.2: Front page of WHO guidelines on safety monitoring of herbal medicines in pharmacovigilance systems (2004)

3. To provide standard definitions of terms relating to pharmacovigilance, and safety monitoring of herbal medicines.

4. To promote and strengthen internationally coordinated information exchange on pharmacovigilance, and safety monitoring of herbal medicines among member states.

5. To promote the safe and proper use of herbal medicines. The regulation of herbal medicines and their place in national health-care systems differs from country to country, and these guidelines will therefore

need to be adapted to meet the needs of the local situation.

Quality Control Methods For Medicinal Plant Material (Fig. 9.3)

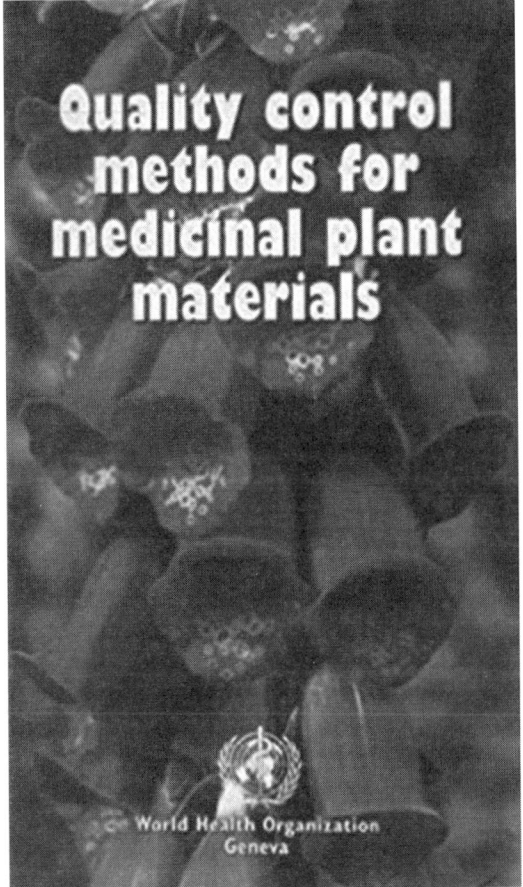

Fig. 9.3: Cover page of quality control methods for medicinal plant materials (1998)

It is a collection of test procedures to support the development of national standards based on local market conditions, with due regard to existing national legislation and national and regional norms. The test methods described in this manual are the best methods currently available. In addition to the test methods, some suggestions regarding general limits for contaminants are included. They should be considered as a basis for establishing national limits.

The methods for analysis of medicinal plant materials frequently employed in this manual are volumetric analysis, gravimetric determinations, gas chromatography, column chromatography, high-performance liquid chromatography and spectrophotometric methods.

WHO Guidelines On Good Manufacturing Practices (GMP) for Herbal Medicines (Fig. 9.4)

The core requirements for GMP for herbal medicines are common to GMP for pharmaceutical products. In 1996, WHO issued "Good manufacturing practices: Supplementary guidelines for the manufacture of herbal medicinal products".

The present consolidated guidelines include, "Core WHO GMP" and "WHO updated GMP: Supplementary guidelines for manufacture of herbal medicines", which are reproduced from the respective annexes of the WHO Technical

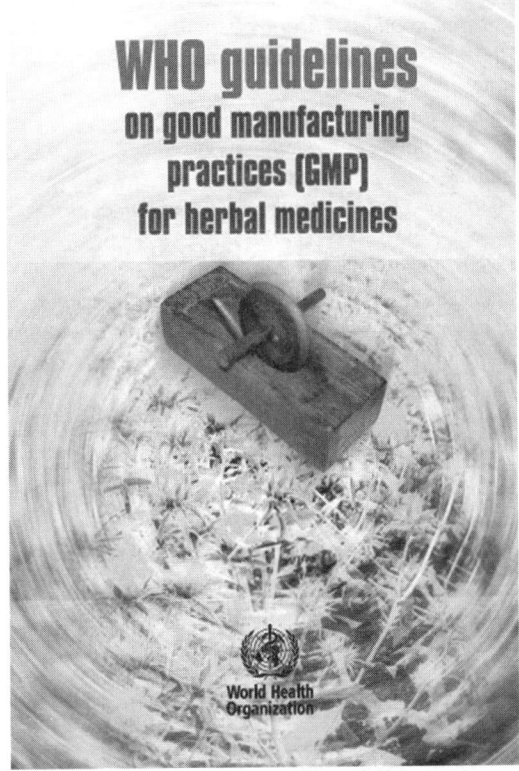

Fig. 9.4: Cover page of WHO guidelines on good manufacturing practices (GMP) for herbal medicines (2005)

Reports. This volume also contains the contents page of the "Quality Assurance Compendium Vol. 2, 2nd update (2007)", a publication which includes all of the GMP texts published to date, in order to enable full cross-referencing to the WHO GMP, as the GMP guidelines on validation and water, in particular, might also be necessary to those manufacturing herbal medicines.

A series of volumes, the *WHO monographs on selected medicinal plants* (Fig. 9.5, Table 9.1) aims to provide scientific information on the safety, efficacy, and quality control of widely used medicinal plants; provide models to

Table 9.1: List of selected medicinal plants mentioned in WHO monographs

Vol. 1	Vol. 2	Vol. 3	Vol. 4
Bulbus allii cepae	Radix althaeae	Fructus ammi majoris	Fructus agni casti
Bulbus allii sativi	Herba andrographidis	Fructus ammi visnagae	Cortex berberidis
Aloe	Radix angelicae sinensis	Fructus anethi	Gummi boswellii
Aloe vera gel	Flos calendulae	Aetheroleum anisi	Semen cardamomi
Radix astragali	Flos caryophylli	Fructus anisi	Fructus chebulae
Fructus bruceae	Rhizoma cimicifugae racemosae	Semen armenicae	Semen cucurbitae
Radix bupleuri	Folium-cum-flore crataegi	Flos arnicae	Folium cynarae
Herba centellae	Radix eleutherococci	Folium azadirachti	Cortex granati
Flos chamomillae	Aetheroleum eucalypti	Oleum azadirachti	Pericarpium granati
Cortex cinnamomi	Folium eucalypti	Flos carthami	Folium guavae
Rhizoma coptidis	Cortex frangulae	Stigma croci	Lichen islandicus
Rhizoma curcumae longae	Folium et cortex hamamelidis	Fructus foeniculi	Fructus macrocarponii
Radix echinaceae	Semen hippocastani	Radix gentianae luteae	Cortex magnoliae
Herba echinaceae purpureae	Herba hyperici	Radix gentianae scabrae	Herba millefolii
Herba ephedrae	Aetheroleum melaleucae alternifoliae	Gummi gugguli	Fructus momordicae
Folium ginkgo	Folium melissae	Radix harpagophyti	Fructus myrtilli
Radix ginseng	Aetheroleum menthae piperitae	Rhizoma hydrastis	Radix panacis quinquefolii
Radix glycyrrhizae	Folium menthae piperitae	Radix ipecacuanhae	Cortex phellodendron
Radix paeoniae	Folium ocimi sancti	Aetheroleum lavandulae	Rhizoma picrorhizae
Semen plantaginis	Oleum oenotherae biennis	Flos lavandulae	Oleum ricini
Radix platycodi	Rhizoma piperis methystici	Strobilus lupuli	Aetheroleum rosmarini
Radix rauwolfiae	Cortex pruni africanae	Gummi myrrha	Folium rosmarini
Rhizoma rhei	Cortex rhamni purshianae	Herba passiflorae	Cortex salicis
Folium sennae	Flos sambuci	Testa plantiginis	Fructus tribuli
	Radix senegae	Radix rehmanniae	Flos trifolii
	Fructus serenoae repentis	Fructus schisandrae	Ramulus-cum-uncis uncariae
	Fructus silybi mariae	Radix scutellariae	Cortex viburni prunifolii
	Herba tanaceti parthenii	Radix-cum-herba taraxaci	Radix withaniae
	Radix urticae	Semen trigonellae foenugraeci	
		Cortex uncariae	
		Fructus zizyphi	

assist member states in developing their own monographs or formularies for these and other herbal medicines; and facilitate information exchange among member states. WHO monographs, however, are not pharmacopoeial monographs; rather they are comprehensive scientific references for drug regulatory authorities, physicians, traditional health practitioners, pharmacists, manufacturers, research scientists and the general public.

Each monograph follows a standard format with information presented in two parts followed by a reference list. The first part presents pharmacopoeial summaries for quality assurance. The second part includes sections on medicinal uses, pharmacology, safety issues, and dosage forms. The descriptions under the medicinal uses section merely represent, for purposes of information exchange, the systematic collection of scientific information available at the time of each volume's preparation and should not be taken as having WHO's official endorsement or approval.

Volume 1 contains 28 monographs published in 1999. *Volume 2*, published in 2003, includes 30 monographs. *Volume 3* in this series was published in 2007 and includes 31 monographs. *Volume 4*, which was published in 2009, includes 28 monographs (Table 9.2).

Each volume after *Volume 1* has a *general technical notice* and two cumulative indexes to facilitate referencing; one lists the monographs

Table 9.2:	List of annexures in different volumes in WHO monographs
Vol. 1: Annex.	Participants in the WHO consultation on selected medicinal plants
Vol. 2: Annex:	Participants in the second WHO consultation on selected medicinal plants
Vol. 3: Annex 1:	Participants in the third WHO consultation on selected medicinal plants, the Governmental Conference Centre, Ottawa, Canada, 16–19 July, 2001
Annex 2:	Cumulative index (in alphabetical order of plant name)
Annex 3:	Cumulative index (in alphabetical order of plant material of interest)
Vol. 4: Annex 1:	Participants of the fourth WHO consultation on selected medicinal plants Salerno-Paestum, Italy, 3–6 October 2005
Annex 2:	Cumulative index (in alphabetical order of plant name)
Annex 3:	Cumulative index (in alphabetical order of plant material of interest)
Annex 4:	Cumulative index of medicinal plants (in alphabetical order of Latin binomial plant name)
Annex 5:	Cumulative index of major chemical constituents (by compound name in alphabetical order)

Contd.

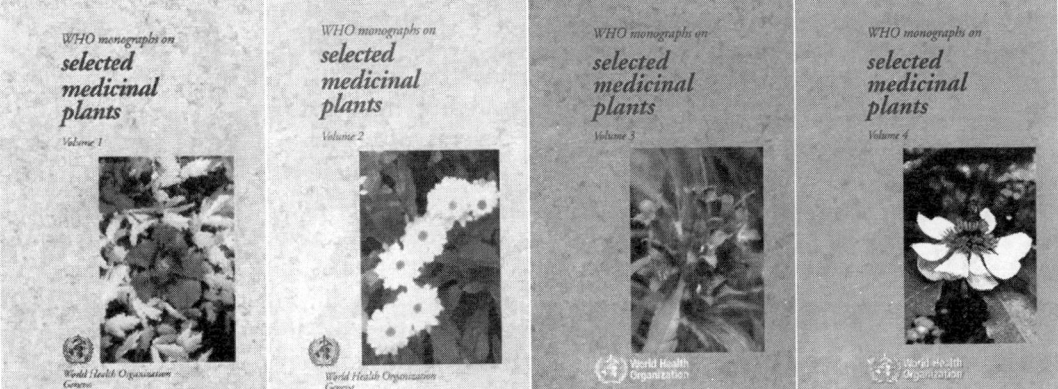

Fig. 9.5: WHO monographs on selected medicinal plants. Vol. 1 (1999); Vol. 2 (2004); Vol. 3 (2007); Vol. 4 (2009)

Table 9.2: List of annexures in different volumes in WHO monographs (*Contd.*)

Annex 6: Cumulative index of major chemical constituents (ordered by CAS number)

Annex 7: Cumulative index of major chemical constituents (ordered by molecular formula)

in alphabetical order by plant name and the other according to the plant material of interest.

WHO Guidelines for Assessing Quality of Herbal Medicines with Reference to Contaminants and Residues (Fig. 9.6)

The objectives of these guidelines are to provide:

⊃ Guiding principles for assessing the quality in relation to the safety of herbal medicines, with specific reference to contaminants and residues;

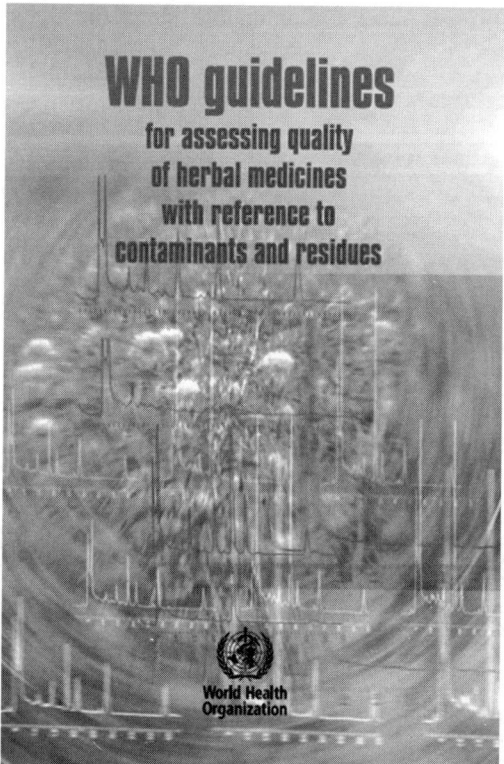

WHO guidelines
for assessing quality
of herbal medicines
with reference to
contaminants and residues

World Health
Organization

Fig. 9.6: Cover page of WHO guidelines for assessing quality of herbal medicines with reference to contaminants and residues (2007)

⊃ Model criteria for use in identifying possible contaminants and residues;

⊃ Examples of methods and techniques; and

⊃ Examples of practical technical procedures for controlling the quality of finished herbal products.

Basic Tests for Drugs—Pharmaceutical Substances, Medicinal Plant Materials and Dosage Forms

This book provides a step-by-step guide to simple methods for verifying the identity of commonly used pharmaceutical substances and dosage forms. The basic tests described can also be used to detect mislabeled, substandard, or counterfeit products when the labeling or physical attributes give rise to doubt. Intended for use in developing countries, where resources and specialized skills may be scarce, all tests rely on a limited range of easily available reagents and equipment and need not be performed in a fully equipped laboratory or by persons with specialized training in pharmacy or chemistry. The book describes tests for 23 pharmaceutical substances and 58 pharmaceutical dosage forms, most of which are included in the WHO model list of essential drugs. Basic tests for confirming the identity of four commonly used medicinal plant materials are also included. As stressed in the text, these tests, which merely confirm identity, are intended for use as primary screening tools and may need to be followed, in cases of adverse test results, by a full pharmacopoeial analysis. The book opens with a brief description of the importance of basic tests as one of the many steps needed to ensure a supply of safe and effective drugs. Chapter two describes several collections of more sophisticated tests, including volumetric or spectrophotometric analysis and thin-layer chromatography, that can be useful in the primary screening of imported pharmaceutical substances, and dosage forms. Information on how to obtain and use these guides to tests, which have not been published by WHO is also provided. Against this background, the main part of the book sets out test procedures for verifying the identity of selected pharmaceutical substances, pharmaceutical dosage forms, and medicinal plant materials. The book concludes with a cumulative index of test procedures described here and in the related WHO publications "Basic Tests for Pharmaceutical Substances" and "Basic Tests for Pharmaceutical Dosage Forms". This manual, which is complementary to WHO's Basic Tests for pharmaceutical substances (1986) and Basic Tests for pharmaceutical dosage forms (1991), describes simple and readily applicable tests for verifying the identity of a number of pharmaceutical substances and dosage forms, and medicinal plant materials in common use. These include:

➲ *Ipecacuanhae radix*
➲ *Podophylli resina*

➲ *Sennae folium*
➲ *Sennae fructus*

It also presents tests to indicate gross degradation of less stable substances. The methods described use a limited range of easily available reagents and equipment, and do not require a fully equipped laboratory. They need not be carried out by a qualified pharmacist, but should be performed by persons with some understanding of analytical chemistry.

Basic tests are not, in any circumstances, intended to replace the requirements of pharmacopoeial monographs, which give an assurance of quality, as opposed to merely confirming identity.

General Guidelines for Methodologies on Research and Evaluation of Traditional Medicine (Fig. 9.8)

WHO has developed these general guidelines in response to the question: What types of academic research approaches and methods can be used to evaluate the safety and efficacy of traditional medicine? The guidelines consist of sections on herbal medicines, traditional procedure-based therapies, clinical research, and related issues including ethics, education and training, and surveillance systems.

The specific objectives of the guidelines are to: Harmonize the use of certain accepted and important terms in traditional medicine; summarize key issues for developing methodologies for research and evaluation of traditional medicine; improve the quality and value of research in traditional medicine; and provide appropriate evaluation methods to facilitate the development of regulation and registration of traditional medicine.

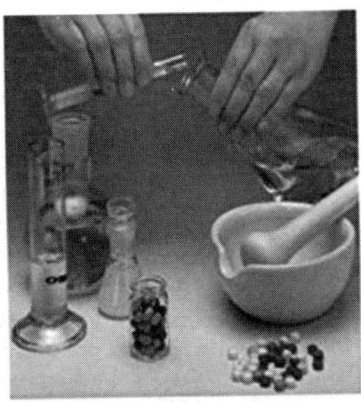

BASIC TESTS FOR DRUGS

Pharmaceutical substances, medicinal plant materials and dosage forms

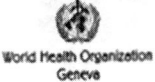

World Health Organization
Geneva

Fig. 9.7: Cover page of basic tests for drugs—pharmaceutical substances, medicinal plant materials and dosage forms (1998)

Methodologies for research and evaluation of traditional procedure—based therapies

Clinical research

Other issues and considerations

Annexes

Annex I. Guidelines for the assessment of herbal medicines

Annex II. Research guidelines for evaluating the safety and efficacy of herbal medicines

Contd.

Annex III. Report of a WHO consultation on traditional medicine and AIDS: Clinical evaluation of traditional medicines and natural products

Annex IV. Definition of levels of evidence and grading of recommendation

Annex V. Guidelines for levels and kinds of evidence to support claims for therapeutic goods

Annex VI. Guidelines for good clinical practice (GCP) for trials on pharmaceutical products

Annex VII. Guidance for Industry: Significant scientific agreement in the review of health claims for conventional foods and dietary supplements

Annex VIII. Guideline for good clinical practice

Annex IX. WHO QOL (Quality of life) User Manual: Facet definitions and response scales

Annex X. Participants in the WHO consultation on methodologies for research and evaluation of traditional medicine

----

WHO Guidelines on Good Agricultural and Collection Practices (GACP) for Medicinal Plants (Fig. 9.9)

Within the overall context of quality assurance, the WHO guidelines on good agricultural and collection practices (GACP) for medicinal plants are primarily intended to provide general technical guidance on obtaining medicinal plant materials of good quality for the sustainable production of herbal products classified as medicines. They apply to the cultivation and collection of medicinal plants, including certain post-harvest operations. Raw medicinal plant materials should meet all applicable national and/or regional quality standards. The guidelines therefore may need to be adjusted according to each country's situation.

The main objectives of these guidelines are to contribute to the quality assurance of medicinal plant materials used as the source for herbal medicines, which aim to improve

WHO/EDM/TRM/2000.1
Distr.: General
Original: English

General Guidelines for Methodologies on Research and Evaluation of Traditional Medicine

World Health Organization
Geneva

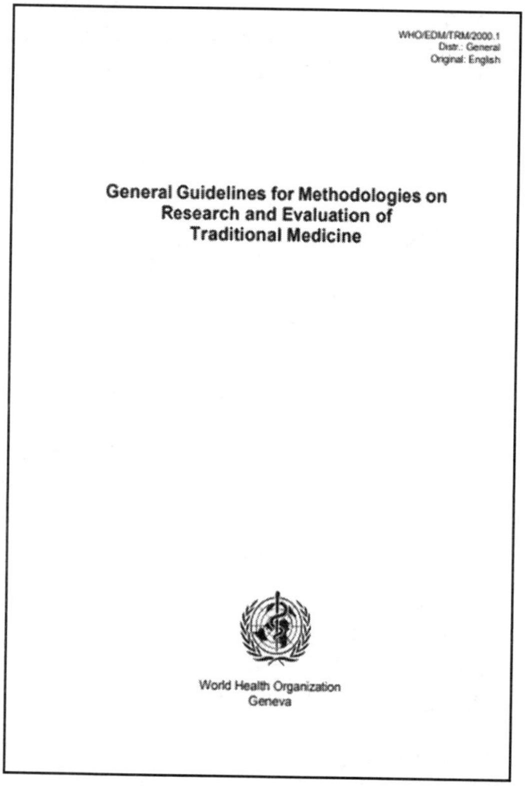

Fig. 9.8: Front page of general guidelines for methodologies on research and evaluation of traditional medicine (2000)

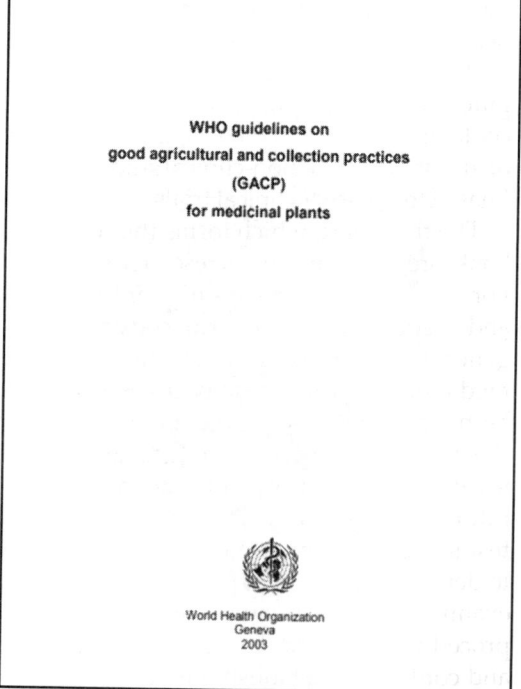

WHO guidelines on

good agricultural and collection practices

(GACP)

for medicinal plants

World Health Organization
Geneva
2003

Fig. 9.9: Front page of WHO guidelines on good agricultural and collection practices (GACP) for medicinal plants (2003)

the quality, safety and efficacy of finished herbal products; guide the formulation of national and/or regional GACP guidelines and GACP monographs for medicinal plants and related standard operating procedures; and encourage and support the sustainable cultivation and collection of medicinal plants of good quality in ways that respect and support the conservation of medicinal plants and the environment in general.

Research Guidelines for Evaluating the Safety and Efficacy of Herbal Medicines (Fig. 9.10)

The guidelines, which reflect the consensus reached by 17 experts in pharmacology, biochemistry, and traditional medicine, respond to the need to assure the safety of widely used herbal medicines while also facilitating the search for new pharmaceutical products. Specific research criteria are covered together with general principles of investigation, including ethical concerns.

The book has three parts. The first discusses the special properties of herbal medicines that need to be considered when designing research protocols. The second part provides detailed guidance on the objectives of research, the contents of a research protocol, and the methods of investigation for non-clinical studies and for Phase I to Phase IV clinical trials.

The third part, which forms the core of the book, presents three sets of research guidelines: For quality specifications of plant materials and preparations, for pharmacodynamic and general pharmacological studies of herbal medicines, and for toxicity investigation of herbal medicines. Topics covered range from the information required to establish the identity and quality of plant materials or preparations, through the selection of appropriate test systems for pharmacodynamic studies, to detailed advice on the many different tests, examinations, observations, and experimental procedures required, in experimental animals and controls, to establish the safety of herbal medicines.

The guidelines are intended to facilitate the work of research scientists and clinicians

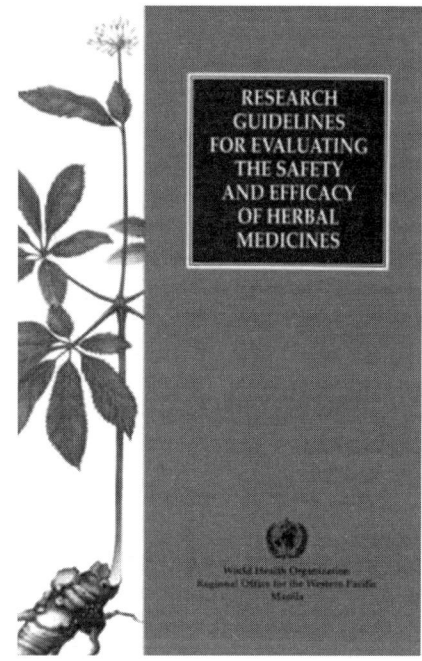

Fig. 9.10: Cover page of research guidelines for evaluating the safety and efficacy of herbal medicines (1993)

while also furnishing some reference points for the governmental, industrial, and non-profit organizations providing financial support.

Regulatory Situation of Herbal Medicines: A Worldwide Review

These guidelines contain basic criteria for the assessment of quality, safety, and efficacy and important requirements for labelling and the package insert for consumers' information. The requirements for pharmaceutical assessment cover issues such as identification, galenical forms, analysis and stability. Safety assessment should at least cover the documented experience of safety and toxicological studies, where indicated. The assessment of efficacy and intended use includes evaluation of traditional use through appraisal of the literature and evidence to support the indication claims. Special chapters on combination products and on requirements for product information for consumers are included. The WHO guidelines are intended to facilitate the work of regulatory authorities, scientific bodies and industry in the development, assessment and registration of herbal medicines, reflecting scientific results which could be the basis for future classification of herbal medicines and would also accommodate cross-cultural transfer of traditional herbal medicinal knowledge between different parts of the world.

HERBAL DRUGS AND ITS SPECIFICATIONS (Fig. 9.11)

HERBAL MATERIALS AND CONTAMINANTS (Fig. 9.12)

Herbal ingredients of high quality should be free from insects, animal matter and excreta. It is usually not possible to remove completely all contaminants. Contaminants in herbal medicines are classified into physicochemical contaminants and biological contaminants. Quality assurance measures such as good agricultural and collection practices (GACP)

for medicinal plants, and good manufacturing practices (GMP) for herbal medicines should be adopted to avoid and control contamination. Chemical and microbiological contaminants can result from the use of human excreta, animal manures and sewage as fertilizers.

Contamination of Herbal Materials (Fig. 9.14)

Herbal materials should be entirely free from visible signs of contamination by moulds or insects, and other animal contamination, including animal excreta. No abnormal odour, discolouration, slime or signs of deterioration should be detected. During storage, products should be kept in a clean and hygienic place, so that no contamination occurs. Special care should be taken to avoid formation of moulds, since they may produce aflatoxins.

1. Toxic substances such as arsenic can be attributed to causes like environmental pollution like emissions and contaminated water from industries which is finally moved to sea, lakes and rivers.

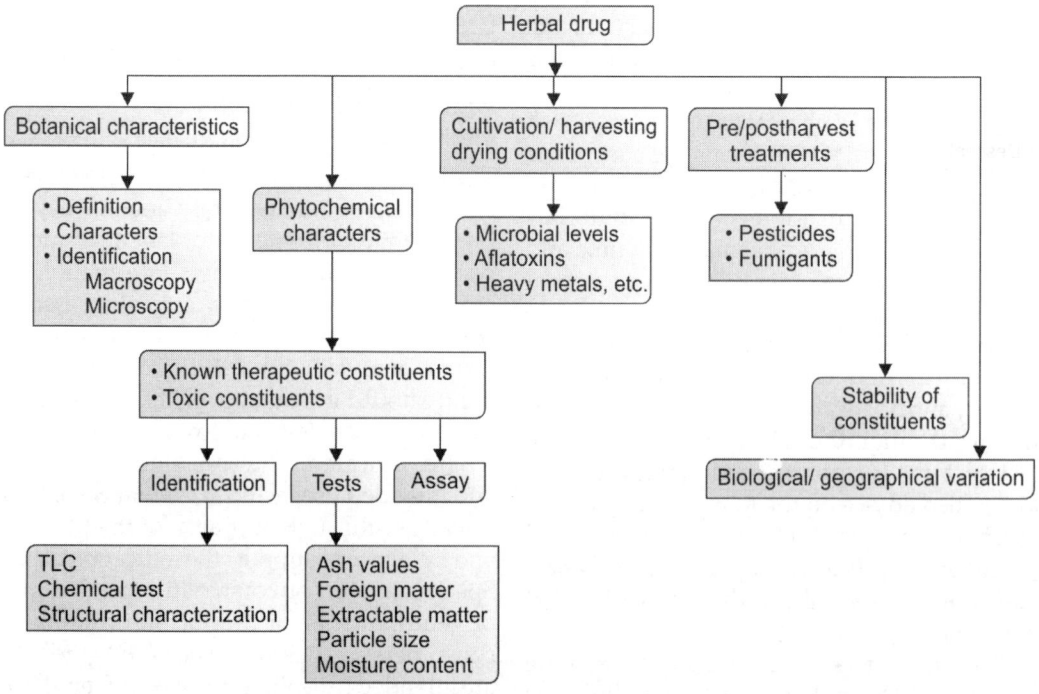

Fig. 9.11: Specifications of herbal drugs

2. Persistent Organic Pollutants (POPs) includes organic chemicals were extensively used in agriculture as pesticides
   a. Synthetic aromatic chlorinated hydrocarbons, which are only slightly soluble in water and are persistent or stable in the presence of sunlight, moisture, air and heat.

b. Persistent pesticides, such as DDT and benzene hexachloride (BHC), were previously used and often contaminate medicinal plants growing nearby.

3. Radioactive contamination including of radionuclides may be consequence of a nuclear accident or may arise from other sources. Examples of such radionuclides

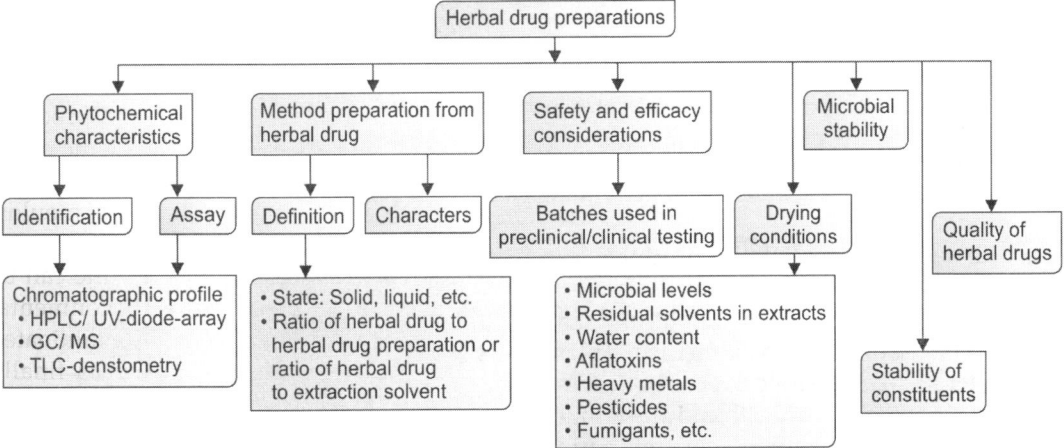

Fig. 9.12: Specifications of herbal drug preparations

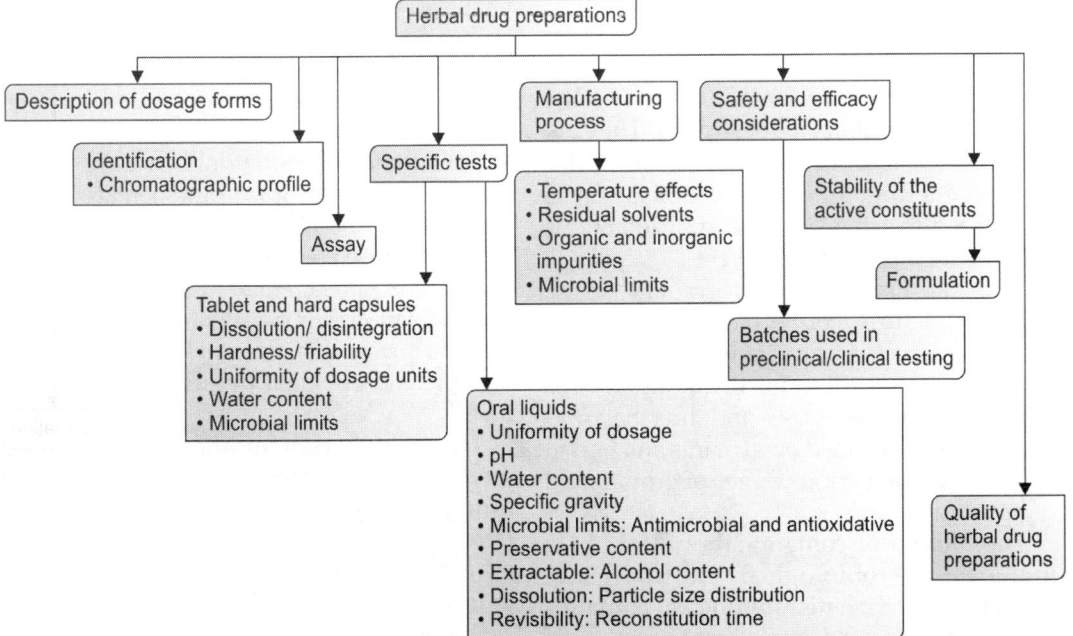

Fig. 9.13: Specifications of herbal medicinal products

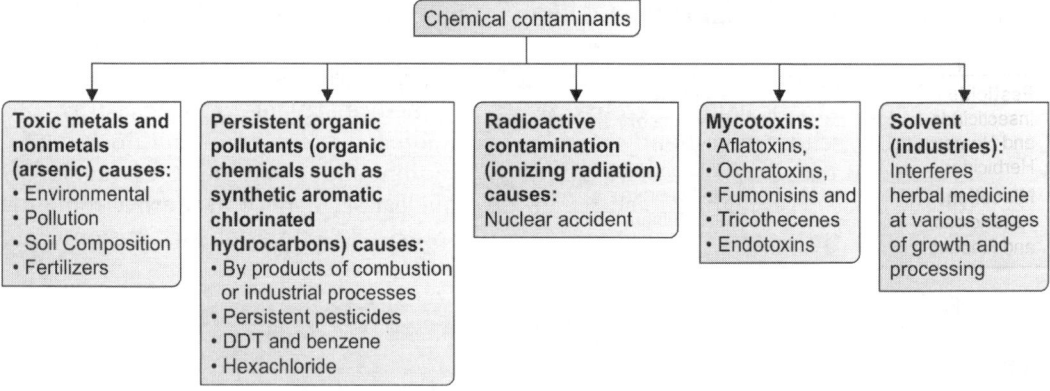

Fig. 9.14: Contamination of herbal materials

include long-lived and short-lived fission products, actinides and activation products.

4. The secondary metabolic products like mycotoxins are non-volatile, have a relatively low molecular weight, and may be secreted onto or into the medicinal plant material. Mycotoxins can pose both acute and chronic risks to health and are thought to play a dual role, firstly, in eliminating other microorganisms competing in the same environment and secondly, helping parasitic fungi to invade host tissues.

5. Endotoxins are found mainly in the outer membranes of certain Gram-negative bacteria and are released only when the cells are disrupted or destroyed. They are complex lipopolysaccharide molecules that elicit an antigenic response, cause altered resistance to bacterial infections and have other serious effects.

6. Solvents used in industries other than the manufacturing of herbal medicines, are often detected as contaminants in water used in irrigation, for drinking and for 15 industrial purposes and thus they find their way into medicinal plants and herbal materials at various stages of growth and processing.

The biological contamination (Fig. 9.15) includes microbiological and parasitic contaminants. The **microbiological contamination** may be caused for current practices of harvesting, production, transportation and

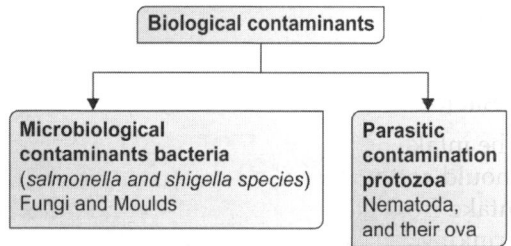

Fig. 9.15: Biological contaminants

storage. While cultivation of herbs and herbal materials normally carry a large number of bacteria and moulds, often originating in soil or derived from manure. These range of bacteria and fungi form the naturally occurring microflora of medicinal plants, aerobic spore-forming bacteria frequently predominate.

Parasitic contamination is mainly due to parasites such as protozoa and nematoda, and their ova, may be introduced during cultivation and may cause zoonosis, especially if uncomposted animal excreta are used. This type of contamination can arise during processing and manufacturing of herbs and herbal material if appropriate personal hygiene has not been taken.

The main agrochemical residues in herbal medicines are derived from pesticides and fumigants (Fig. 9.16). Pesticides may be classified on the basis of their intended use, for example, as follows:

➲ Insecticides;

➲ Fungicides and nematocides;

➲ Herbicides; and

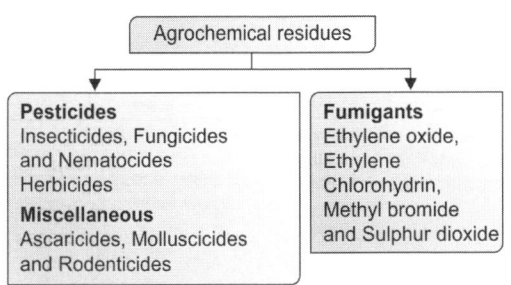

Fig. 9.16: Agrochemical residues

➲ Other pesticides (e.g. ascaricides, mollusci-
cides and rodenticides).

Examples of fumigants include ethylene
oxide, ethylene chlorohydrin, methyl bromide
and sulphur dioxide.

Pesticide Residues

The intake of residues from herbal materials
should account for no more than 1% of total
intake from all sources, including food and
drinking water. Since the level of pesticide
residues may change during the production
process, it is vital to determine the actual
quantity of residues consumed in the final
dosage form.

Acceptable Residue Level

An ARL (in mg of pesticide per kg of medicinal
plant material) can be calculated on the basis of
the maximum ADI of the pesticide for humans,
as recommended by FAO and WHO, and the
mean daily intake (MDI) of the medicinal plant
material.

$$ARL = ADI \times E \times 60 / MDI \times 100$$

Residual Solvents

A range of organic solvents are used for manufacturing herbal medicines, and can be detected
as residues of such processing in herbal preparations and finished herbal products. They
should be controlled through GMP and quality
control. Solvents are classified by ICH (CPMP/
ICH 283/95), according to their potential risk,
into: • class 1 (solvents to be avoided such as
benzene); • class 2 (limited toxic potential such
as methanol or hexane); and • class 3 (low toxic
potential such as ethanol).

Foreign Matter

Foreign matter found in a sample of herbs and
herbal materials should not exceed limits set
in national, regional or international pharmacopoeias. Foreign matter includes insects and
other animal contamination including animal
excreta, as well as other species of plants. In
general, any substance other than the acceptable sample of good quality medicinal plant
material is regarded as foreign matter. A pure
sample is seldom found and there is always
some foreign matter present. However, no
poisonous, dangerous or otherwise harmful
foreign matter should be allowed. Thus
following the GACP should help to ensure that
contamination is kept to a minimum. Removal
of larger pieces of foreign matter from whole
and cut plants is often done by hand-sorting
after macroscopic examination. Finished
products should also be examined for foreign
materials.

Analytical Methods

Determination of Arsenic and Toxic Metals

➲ Determination of radioactive contaminants
➲ Determination of aflatoxins
➲ Determination of microbiological contami-
nants

Microbial contamination limits in herbal
materials, preparations and finished products.
Different limits are set according to the
intended use of the herbal material and the
medicines themselves. Some examples are
given here.

Raw medicinal plant and herbal materials
intended for further processing. For contamination of raw medicinal plant, and herbal
materials intended for further processing
(including additional decontamination by
a physical or chemical process), the limits,
adapted from the provisional guidelines
established by an international consultative
group, are given for untreated herbal material
harvested under acceptable hygienic conditions:

➲ *Escherichia coli*, maximum 104 per gram
➲ *Mould propagules*, maximum 105 per gram
➲ Shigella, absence per gram or ml.

STANDARDIZATION OF HERBAL DRUGS (FIG. 9.17)

Determination of Foreign Matter

Weigh a sample of herbal material, taking the quantity indicated above unless otherwise specified in the test procedures for the herbal material concerned. Spread it in a thin layer and sort the foreign matter into groups either by visual inspection, using a magnifying lens (6× or 10×), or with the help of a suitable sieve, according to the requirements for the specific herbal material. Sift the remainder of the sample through a No. 250 sieve; dust is regarded as mineral admixture. Weigh the portions of this sorted foreign matter to within 0.05 g. Calculate the content of each group in grams per 100 g of air-dried sample.

Macroscopic and Microscopic Examination (Fig. 9.18)

Herbs are categorized according to sensory, macroscopic and microscopic characteristics to establish, purity and possibly quality.

Macroscopic Examination

1. *Size:* Graduated ruler
2. *Colour:* Daylight and artificial light source.
3. Surface texture and fracture: Magnifying lens.
4. Odour
5. Taste

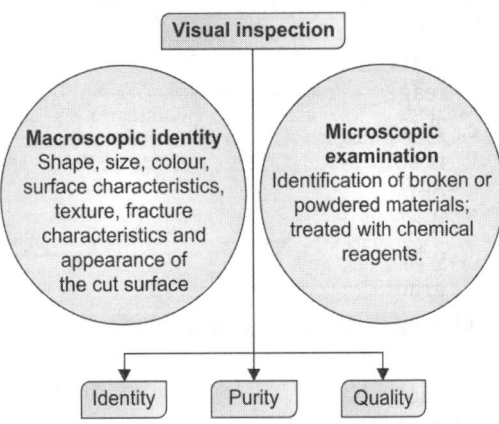

Fig. 9.18: Macroscopic and microscopic examination

1. **Size:** The measurement of length, width and thickness of herbal material is done by graduated ruler in millimetres.
   Example: Small seeds and fruits are aligned 10 in number for the measurements on a sheet of calibrated paper, with 1 mm spacing between lines, and dividing the result by 10.

2. **Colour:** The colour of the sample is examined under daylight compared with reference sample. If required, an artificial light source with wavelengths may be used.

3. **Surface texture and fracture characteristics**
   a. A magnifying lens (6x to 10x) may be used to examine the untreated sample.

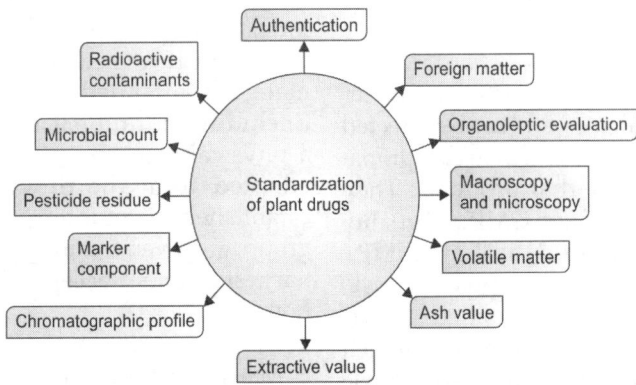

Fig. 9.17: Standardization of herbal drugs

b. To observe the characteristics of a cut surface wetting of sample with water or reagents can be done if required.

c. Touch the material to determine if it is soft or hard; bend and rupture it to obtain information on brittleness and the appearance of the fracture plane whether it is fibrous, smooth, rough, granular, etc.

4. **Odour**

a. If the material is expected to be innocuous, place a small portion of the sample in the palm of the hand or in a beaker of suitable size, and slowly and repeatedly inhale the air over the material. If no distinct odour is perceptible, crush the sample between the thumb and index finger or between the palms of the hands using gentle pressure.

b. If the material is known to be dangerous, crush by mechanical means and then pour a small quantity of boiling water onto the crushed sample in a beaker.

First, determine the strength of the odour (none, weak, distinct, strong) and then the odour sensation (aromatic, fruity, musty, mouldy, rancid, etc.). A direct comparison of the odour with a defined substance is advisable (e.g. peppermint should have an odour similar to menthol, cloves should have an odour similar to eugenol).

5. **Taste:** This test should be applied only if specifically required for a given herbal material.

Microscopic Examination (Fig. 9.3)

Microscopic identification of the herbal material is carried out with the microscope equipped with the magnification lenses, condenser, mechanical stage and objective magnification, polarizing filters, stage micrometer, and ocular micrometer. Set of drawing attachments for the microscope, a micro burner (Bunsen type), slides and cover-glasses of standard size and botanical dissecting instruments.

Preliminary treatment before microscopy

1. Selection of sample
2. Softening of dried parts of herbal plant by being placed in a moist atmosphere or by soaking in water.

   a. The procedure for *softening small quantities of material* is to use a test-tube, place a wad of cotton-wool moistened with water into the bottom of a test-tube and cover with a piece of filter-paper; allow it to stand overnight or until the material is soft and suitable for cutting.

   b. The procedure for *softening* for larger quantities of material, use of desiccators placing water into the lower part instead of the drying agent.

3. Softening of bark, wood and other dense and hard materials usually need to be soaked in water or in equal parts of water, ethanol and glycerol for a few hours or overnight until they are soft enough to be cut. Sometimes boiling in water for a few minutes may be required.

Preparation of specimens for microscopy

1. **Powdered materials**

   a. On a glass slide place one or two drops of water, glycerol/ethanol TS or chloral hydrate TS.

   b. Moisten the tip of a needle with water and dip into the powder.

   c. Transfer a small quantity of the material that adheres to the needle tip into the drop of fluid on the slide.

   d. Stir thoroughly, and apply a cover-glass.

   e. Press lightly on the cover-glass with the handle of the needle, and remove excess fluid from the margin of the cover-glass with a strip of filter paper.

2. **Surface tissues of leaves and flowers:** Thin leaves transparent:

   a. To clarify leaves and to render pieces of thin leaves transparent, boil them directly on a slide.

   b. Cut a piece of leaf into two portions, turn one piece upper side down and add chloral hydrate TS.

c. Boil the specimen carefully over a small flame of a microburner and, as soon as bubbles escape, remove the slide from the flame.

d. When the bubbles have ceased to appear, boil again until the fragments are transparent.

For slightly thicker but still papery leaves,

a. Cut square pieces, about 6 mm from the edge of the leaf, if not otherwise specified.

b. The pieces should be taken one-third to one-half of the way from the leaf-base and should include a midrib or large vein.

c. In addition, cut 1 or 2 pieces from the edge including 1 or 2 indentations, where appropriate.

For broken or cut leaves take suitable fragments as described above.

Place the fragments in a test-tube containing chloral hydrate TS and boil for a few minutes until they become transparent. Transfer a fragment to a slide and cut it into two equal portions. Turn one piece upper side down and align the two pieces so that both upper and lower surfaces can be observed under the microscope. Add 1–2 drops of chloral hydrate TS and apply a cover glass. For thicker leaves, that do not become transparent enough when prepared by the method described above, clarify fragments by boiling with chloral hydrate TS in a test-tube. Transfer a fragment onto a slide, cut it into two equal portions and turn one portion upper side down. Scrape the surface of the two portions using a scalpel until only a single layer of epidermis remains. Wash the epidermis with drops of chloral hydrate TS or glycerol/ethanol TS to remove any residues. If possible, turn both parts of the epidermis upper side down, and add one of the above fluids. For very thick or fleshy leaves, pull off the upper and lower parts of epidermis by winding the softened leaf around the index finger, pressing with the thumb and the middle finger against the index finger and carefully incising, catching the incised part with forceps, and carefully bending the epidermis backwards. Petals and sepals of flowers may be treated in a similar manner.

Sections

Select representative pieces of the material being examined and cut into suitable lengths, one end of which is softened and smoothed. Prepare cross or transverse sections by cutting with a razor blade or microtome at a right angle to the longitudinal axis of the material. Prepare longitudinal sections by cutting in parallel with the longitudinal axis, either in a radial direction (radial section) or in a tangential direction (tangential section).

a. Thick materials, such as wood, woody stems, rhizomes and roots can be cut by holding the softened material between the thumb and index finger, supported by the middle finger or by holding it in the central hole of a hand microtome.

b. Thin materials such as leaves, petals and slender stems should be bound between two halves of a piece of elder-pith or other suitable support. If necessary, moisten the surface to be cut and the blade with ethanol (~375 g/l) TS. Cut the sections as thinly and evenly as possible. Transfer the sections with a brush moistened with ethanol (~150 g/l) TS to a dish containing ethanol (~150 g/l) TS. Select satisfactory sections for the preparation of the slides. For certain materials a sliding microtome may be used.

c. Seeds and fruits that are very flat, or that are small and spherical, and cannot be held in the manner described above may be inserted into a notch cut into a small rubber stopper or embedded in hard paraffin (paraffin wax) as shown in Table 9.3.

Prepare a hard paraffin block, rectangular in shape, measuring about $7 \times 7 \times 15$ mm, and melt a small hole in the centre of one end using a heated needle or thin glass rod. Press the material, which should be dry or softened by exposure to moisture, into this hole. Then prepare sections with a microtome.

For slightly thicker but still papery leaves, cut square pieces, about 6 mm from the edge of the leaf, if not otherwise specified. The pieces should be taken one-third to one-half of the way from the leaf-base and should include a midrib

Table 9.3: Reagents with properties and uses

S. No.	Reagents	Properties	Uses
1.	Chloral hydrate TS	Refractive index (nD 20) of 1.44–1.48.	On gentle heating chloral hydrate TS dissolves starch grains, aleurone grains, plastids, and volatile oils, and expands collapsed and delicate tissue without causing any undue swelling of cell walls or distortion of the tissues. It is the best reagent for rendering calcium oxalate clearly evident and is particularly useful for small crystals.
2.	Lactochloral TS	Lactochloral TS has a similar use to chloral hydrate TS	It is usually applied to sections that are difficult to clarify. It may be used cold. Before use, any air present in the specimen should be removed by placing in a desiccator and applying a vacuum.
3.	Lactophenol TS	Lactophenol TS may be used cold or with heating. It has a refractive index (nD 20) of 1.44	It is useful for the preparation of fungi, pollen grains, most non-oily powders, and parasites such as mites and nematode worms. This reagent dissolves calcium carbonate deposits with a slow effervescence, owing to the presence of lactic acid.
4.	Sodium hypochlorite TS	The bleached sections give a negative reaction to lignin.	Sodium hypochlorite TS is used for bleaching deeply coloured sections. Immerse the sections in the solution for a few minutes until sufficiently bleached, wash with water and prepare the mount with glycerol/ethanol TS.
5.	Xylene R and light petroleum R	Solvents for fats and oils	It is used to remove fats and oils from oily powders or sections.

or large vein. In addition, cut 1 or 2 pieces from the edge including 1 or 2 indentations, where appropriate. For broken or cut leaves take suitable fragments as described above. Place the fragments in a test-tube containing chloral hydrate TS and boil for a few minutes until they become transparent. Transfer a fragment to a slide and cut it into two equal portions. Turn one piece upper side down and align the two pieces so that both upper and lower surfaces can be observed under the microscope. Add 1–2 drops of chloral hydrate TS and apply a cover glass.

For thicker leaves, that do not become transparent enough when prepared by the method described above; clarify fragments by boiling with chloral hydrate TS in a test-tube. Transfer a fragment onto a slide, cut it into two equal portions and turn one portion upper side down. Scrape the surface of the two portions using a scalpel until only a single layer of epidermis remains. Wash the epidermis with drops of chloral hydrate TS or glycerol/ethanol TS to remove any residues. If possible, turn both parts of the epidermis upper side down, and add one of the above fluids. For very thick or fleshy leaves, pull off the upper and lower parts of epidermis by winding the softened leaf around the index finger, pressing with the thumb and the middle finger against the index finger and carefully incising, catching the incised part with forceps, and carefully bending the epidermis backwards. Petals and sepals of flowers may be treated in a similar manner.

Sections

Select representative pieces of the material being examined and cut into suitable lengths, one end of which is softened and smoothed. Prepare cross or transverse sections by cutting with a razor blade or microtome at a right angle to the longitudinal axis of the material. Prepare longitudinal sections by cutting in parallel with the longitudinal axis, either in a radial direction (radial section) or in a tangential direction (tangential section). Thick materials, such as wood, woody stems, rhizomes and roots can be cut by holding the softened material between the thumb and index finger, supported by the middle finger or by holding it in the central hole of a hand microtome. Thin materials such as leaves, petals and slender stems should be bound between two halves of a piece of elder-pith or other suitable support. If necessary, moisten the surface to be cut and the blade with ethanol (~375 g/l) TS. Cut the sections as thinly and evenly as possible. Transfer the sections with a brush moistened with ethanol (~150 g/l) TS to a dish containing ethanol (~150 g/l) TS. Select satisfactory sections for the preparation of the slides. For certain materials a sliding microtome may be used.

Seeds and fruits that are very flat, or that are small and spherical, and cannot be held in the manner described above may be inserted into a notch cut into a small rubber stopper or embedded in hard paraffin (paraffin wax) as follows.

Prepare a hard paraffin block, rectangular in shape, measuring about $7 \times 7 \times 15$ mm, and melt a small hole in the centre of one end using a heated needle or thin glass rod. Press the material, which should be dry or softened by exposure to moisture, into this hole. Then prepare sections with a microtome.

Histochemical Detection of Cell Walls and Contents (Table 9.4)

Reagents can be applied to a powdered sample or a section on a slide by the following methods:

Add drops of the reagent to the sample and apply a cover glass, then irrigate using a strip of filter paper as described below.

Place drops of the reagent on one edge of the cover-glass of a prepared specimen. Place a strip of filter paper at the opposite edge of the cover glass to remove the fluid under the cover glass by suction, causing the reagent to flow over the specimen.

Using the second method, the progress of the reaction may be observed under a microscope. Care should be taken to avoid using reagents or vapours that could attack the lenses or stages of the microscope.

Disintegration of Tissues

Cut the material into small pieces about 2 mm thick and 5 mm long, or into slices about 1 mm thick (tangential longitudinal sections are preferred for woods or xylem from stems). Use one of the following methods depending on the nature of the cell walls. For tissues with ligni-fied cell walls use either method 1 or method 2. For tissues where lignified cells are few or occur in small groups, use method 3.

Method 1: Nitric Acid and Potassium Chlorate

Place the material in a test tube containing about 5 ml of nitric acid (~500 g/l) TS and heat to boiling. Add a small quantity of powdered potassium chlorate R and allow to react, warming gently if necessary to maintain a slight effervescence; add fresh quantities of powdered potassium chlorate R as needed. When the tissue appears to be almost completely bleached and shows a tendency to disintegrate, apply pressure with a glass rod to the material. If the material breaks, interrupt the reaction by pouring the contents of the test tube into water. Allow the material to settle, decant it and wash it with fresh water until the acidity is removed. Transfer the material onto a slide and tease it out with a needle. Add 1 drop of glycerol/ethanol TS and apply a cover glass. The disintegrated material gives a negative reaction for lignin.

Method 2. Nitric Acid and Chromic Acid

Place the material in a small dish and heat with nitro-chromic acid TS until the material breaks easily when pressure is applied with a glass rod. Wash the material repeatedly with water and transfer onto a slide. Tease out the material, add 1 drop of glycerol/ethanol TS and apply a cover glass. The disintegrated material gives a negative reaction for lignin.

This treatment can also be carried out on a slide. Place a moderately thick section of the material on a slide, add the reagent and allow it to stand for about 20 minutes. Separate the cells by applying gentle pressure, or with a sliding movement of the cover glass. This process is especially useful when the disintegration of the tissues of a section under the microscope needs to be observed to ascertain where isolated cells come from.

Method 3. Caustic Alkali Method

Place the material in a test tube containing about 5 ml of potassium hydroxide (~110 g/l) TS or sodium hydroxide (~80 g/l) TS, and heat on a water-bath for 15–30 minutes until a portion breaks easily when pressure is applied with a glass rod. Decant the liquid and wash the softened material several times with fresh quantities of water. This method is particularly useful for the disintegration of bark, seeds,

Table 9.4: Techniques of histochemical detection

S. No.	Particulars	Method
1.	Cellulose cell walls	Add 1–2 drops of iodinated zinc chloride TS and allow to stand for a few minutes; alternatively, add 1 drop of iodine (0.1 mol/l) VS, allow to stand for 1 minute, remove excess reagent with a strip of filter paper and add 1 drop of sulphuric acid (~1160 g/l) TS; cellulose cell walls are stained blue to blue-violet. On the addition of 1–2 drops of cuoxam TS, the cellulose cell walls will swell and gradually dissolve.
2.	Lignified cell walls	Moisten the powder or section on a slide with a small volume of phloroglucinol TS and allow to stand for about 2 minutes or until almost dry. Add 1 drop of hydrochloric acid (~420 g/l) TS and apply a cover glass; lignified cell walls are stained pink to cherry red.
3.	Suberized or cuticular cell walls	Add 1–2 drops of sudan red TS and allow to stand for a few minutes or warm gently; suberized or cuticular cell walls are stained orange-red or red.
4.	Aleurone grains	Add a few drops of iodine/ethanol TS; the aleurone grains will turn yellowish brown to brown. Then add a few drops of ethanolic trinitrophenol TS; the grains will turn yellow. Add about 1 ml of mercuric nitrate TS and allow to dissolve; the colour of the solution turns brick red. If the specimen is oily, render it fat-free by immersing and washing it in an appropriate solvent before carrying out the test.
5.	Calcium carbonate	Crystals or deposits of calcium carbonate dissolve slowly with effervescence when acetic acid (~60 g/l) TS or hydrochloric acid (~70 g/l) TS is added.
6.	Calcium oxalate	Crystals of calcium oxalate are insoluble in acetic acid (~ 60g/l) TS but dissolve in hydrochloric acid (~70 g/l) TS without effervescence (if applied by irrigation the acid should be more concentrated); they also dissolve in sulfuric acid (~350 g/l) TS, but needle-shaped crystals of calcium sulphate separate on standing after about 10 minutes. In polarized light, calcium oxalate crystals are birefringent. Calcium oxalate is best viewed after the sample has been clarified (e.g. with chloral hydrate TS).
7.	Fats, fatty oils, volatile oils and resins	Add 1–2 drops of sudan red TS and allow to stand for a few minutes or heat gently, if necessary. The fatty substances are stained orange-red to red. Irrigate the preparation with ethanol (~750 g/l) TS and heat gently; the volatile oils and resins dissolve in the solvent, while fats and fatty oils (except castor oil and croton oil) remain intact.
8.	Hydroxyan-thraquinones	Add 1 drop of potassium hydroxide (~55 g/l) TS; cells containing 1,8-dihydroxy-anthraquinones are stained red.
9.	Inulin	Add 1 drop each of 1-naphthol TS and sulfuric acid (~1760 g/l) TS; spherical aggregations of crystals of inulin turn brownish red and dissolve.
10.	Mucilage	Add 1 drop of Chinese ink TS to the dry sample; the mucilage shows up as transparent, spherically dilated fragments on a black background. Alternatively, add 1 drop of thionine TS to the dry sample, allow to stand for about 15 minutes, then wash with ethanol (~188 g/l) TS; the mucilage turns violet-red (cellulose and lignified cell walls are stained blue and bluish violet respectively).
11.	Starch	Add a small volume of iodine (0.02 mol/l) VS; a blue or reddish blue colour is produced. Alternatively, add a small volume of glycerol/ethanol TS and examine under a microscope with polarized light; birefringence is observed giving a Maltese cross effect with the arms of the cross intersecting at the hilum.
12.	Tannin	Add 1 drop of ferric chloride (50 g/l) TS; it turns bluish black or greenish black.

leaves and flowers, facilitating the elimination of fibres, scleroids, lactiferous tissues and epidermis. The disintegrated material gives a negative reaction for lignin.

Leaf Stomata (Fig. 9.19)

Stomata are specialized cells which respond to environmental and endogenous signals and change shape to allow gas exchange. The cells are structurally adapted for movement that occurs as a result of increasing osmotic potential and turgor pressure.

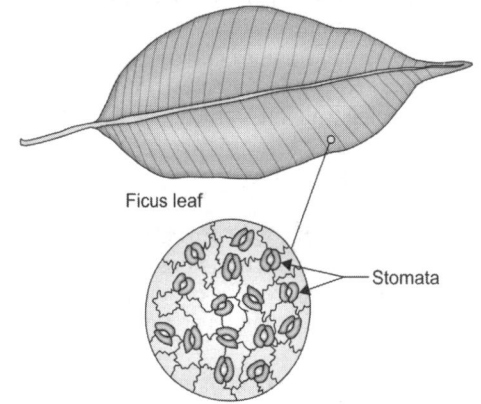

Fig. 9.19: Leaf stomata

Types of Stomata

In the mature leaf, four significantly different types of stoma are distinguished by their form and the arrangement of the surrounding cells, especially the subsidiary cells, as follows:

i. *Anomocytic or ranunculaceous (irregular-celled) type:* The stoma is surrounded by a definite number of cells that are not different from the remainder of the epidermis.

ii. *Anisocytic or cruciferous (unequal celled) type:* The stoma is surrounded by three cells of which one is distinctly smaller than the other two.

iii. *Diacytic or caryophyllaceous (cross-celled) type:* The stoma is enclosed by a pair of subsidiary cells whose common wall is at right angles to the guard cells.

iv. *Paracytic or rubiaceous (parallel celled) type:* The stoma is accompanied on either side by one or more subsidiary cells parallel to 30 the long axis of the pore and guard cells.

Determination of the Stomatal Index

a. *Clearing of leaves:* In a test tube containing about 5 ml of chloral hydrate TS place 5 × 5 mm fragments of leaves. Heat it on a water-bath for approx 15 minutes or until the fragments turned transparent.

b. *Mounting:* Transfer a transparent fragment to a slide; to prevent material from drying place a small drop of glycerol/ethanol TS at one side of the cover glass.

c. Examine under a microscope with a 40 × objective and a 6× eyepiece, equipped with a drawing apparatus. Mark on the drawing paper a cross (x) for each epidermal cell and a circle (o) for each stoma.

   Calculate the stomatal index as follows:
   It is the average number of **stomata** per square mm of the epidermis of the leaf. **Stomatal index** is the percentage which the number of stomata forms to the total number of epidermal cells, each **stomata** being counted as one cell.
   Stomatal index = $S*100/E+S$
   where S = the number of stomata in a given area of leaf;
   E = the number of epidermal cells (including trichomes) in the same area of leaf.

Thin Layer Chromatography

Thin layer chromatography (TLC) is a chromatography technique used to separate mixtures and particularly valuable for the qualitative determination of small amounts of impurities. As it is effective and easy to perform, and the equipment required is inexpensive, the technique is frequently used for evaluating herbal materials and their preparations. It involves a stationary phase consisting of a thin layer of adsorbent material, usually silica gel, aluminum oxide, or cellulose immobilized onto a flat, inert carrier sheet. A liquid phase consisting of the solution to be separated is then dissolved in an appropriate solvent and is drawn up the plate via capillary action, separating the experimental solution based on the polarity of the components of the compound.

Principle

TLC has been included under both adsorption and partition chromatography. As different materials of different adsorptive power are used in TLC, the separation of components is not always by adsorption phenomenon. Separation may results due to adsorption and partition or by both phenomenon depending upon the nature of adsorbents used plates and solvent system used for developments.

Advantages

TLC has the following advantages over paper chromatography:

a. Greater speed
b. Greater sensitivity for many substances than paper
c. Small sample requirement
d. Usually sharper preparation
e. Different kinds of reagents can be applied without damaging the plate.
f. Require very little equipment.
g. Require very little time
h. Spraying with corrosive solvent for identification is also permitted.

i. The individual samples do not get diffuse.
j. Separated component can be easily recovered.

The following parameters should be determined for the analysis of each individual herbal material:

a. Type of adsorbent and method of activation (heat at 110°C for 30 minutes);
b. Method of preparation and concentration of the test and reference solutions;
c. Volume of the solutions to be applied on the plate;
d. Mobile phase and the distance of migration;
e. Drying conditions (including temperature) and method of detection;
f. For the spots obtained: Number and approximate position (or the Rf values if necessary), and fluorescence and colour.

TLC Basic Operations (Fig. 9.20)

A small spot of solution containing the sample is applied to a plate, about one centimeter from the base. The plate is then dipped into a suitable solvent, such as ethanol or water, and placed in a sealed container. The solvent moves up the plate by capillary action and meets the sample mixture, which is dissolved and is carried up

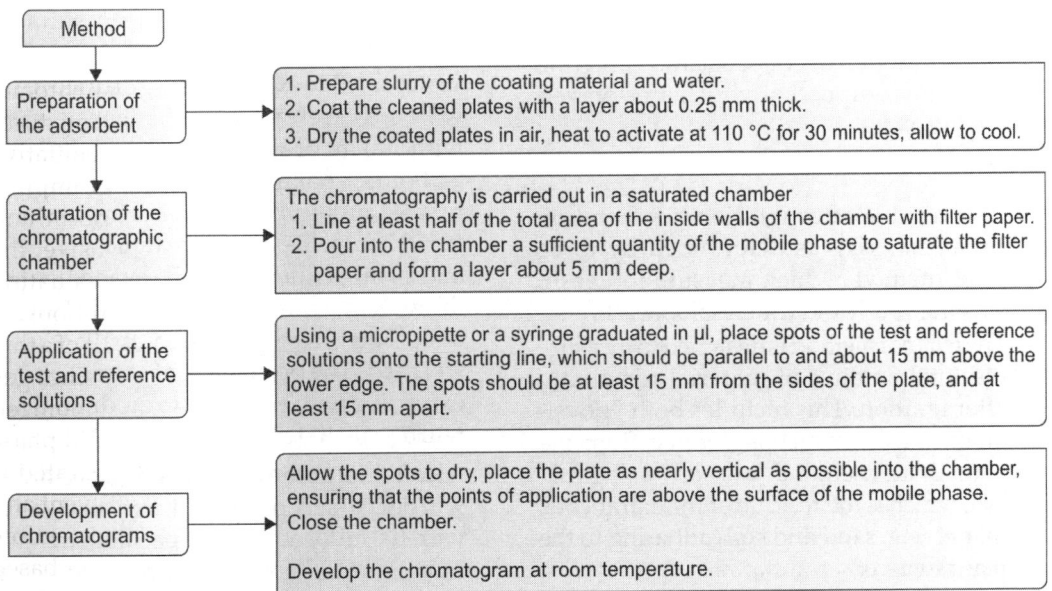

Fig. 9.20: Basic operations for TLC

the plate by the solvent. Different compounds in the sample mixture travel at different rates due to the differences in their attraction to the stationary phase, and because of differences in solubility in the solvent.

Plate Preparation

TLC plates are made by mixing the adsorbent, such as silica gel, with a small amount of inert binder like calcium sulphate (gypsum) and water. This mixture is spread as thick slurry on an unreactive carrier sheet, usually glass, thick aluminum foil, or plastic, and the resultant plate is dried and activated by heating in an oven for thirty minutes at 110 °C. The thickness of the adsorbent layer is typically around 0.1–0.25 mm for analytical purposes and around 1–2 mm for preparative TLC.

Analysis

As the chemicals being separated may be colourless, several methods exist to visualize the spots:

- ⮑ Often a small amount of a fluorescent compound, usually manganese-activated zinc silicate, is added to the adsorbent that allows the visualization of spots under a blacklight (UV254).
- ⮑ Iodine vapors are a general unspecific colour reagent.
- ⮑ Specific colour reagents exist into which the TLC plate is dipped or which are sprayed onto the plate.

Ash Values

The ash residue after ignition/incineration of herbal materials is determined by three different methods which measure total ash, acid-insoluble ash and water-soluble ash.

1. The *total ash* method is designed to measure the total amount of material remaining after ignition. This includes both "physiological ash", which is derived from the plant tissue itself, and "non-physiological" ash, which is the residue of the extraneous matter (e.g. sand and soil) adhering to the plant surface.
2. *Acid-insoluble ash* is the residue obtained after boiling the total ash with dilute hydrochloric acid, and igniting the remaining insoluble matter. This measures the amount of silica present, especially as sand and siliceous earth.
3. *Water-soluble ash* is the difference in weight between the total ash and the residue after treatment of the total ash with water.

Determination of Ash

Total ash (Fig. 9.21)

Acid-insoluble ash (Fig. 9.22)

Water-soluble ash

To the crucible containing the total ash, add 25 ml of water and boil for 5 minutes. Collect the insoluble matter in a sintered-glass crucible or on an ashless filter paper. Wash with hot water and ignite in a crucible for 15 minutes at a temperature not exceeding 450°C. Subtract the weight of this residue in mg from the weight of total ash. Calculate the content of water-soluble ash in mg per g of air-dried material.

Determination of Extractable Matter

This method determines the amount of active constituents extracted with solvents from a given amount of herbal material. It is employed for materials for which as yet no suitable chemical or biological assay exists.

i. **Water soluble extractives:** 5 g of dried drug will be, coarsely powdered, and macerated with 100 ml of water in a closed flask for 24 hours, shaking frequently during the first 6 hours and will be allowing to stand for 18 hours, then it will be rapidly filtered and 25 ml of filterate will be evaporated to dryness in a tared flat-bottomed shallow dish. Then it will be dried at 105°C and weighed. The percentage of water-soluble extractive with reference to air dried drug will be calculated.

ii. **Alcohol soluble extractives:** 5 g dried drug, will be coarsely powdered, and macerated with 100 ml. of ethanol of specified strength in a closed flask for 24 hours, shaking frequently during the first 6 hours and allowing to stand for 18 hours thereafter,

Place about 2–4 g of the ground air-dried material, accurately weighed, in a previously ignited and tared crucible (usually of platinum or silica).

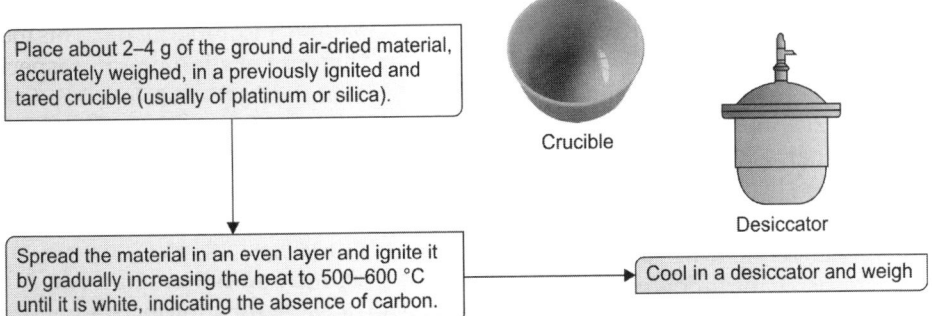

Crucible

Desiccator

Spread the material in an even layer and ignite it by gradually increasing the heat to 500–600 °C until it is white, indicating the absence of carbon.

Cool in a desiccator and weigh

If carbon-free ash cannot be obtained in this manner, cool the crucible and moisten the residue with about 2 ml of water or a saturated solution of ammonium nitrate R. Dry on a water-bath, then on a hot-plate and ignite to constant weight. Allow the residue to cool in a suitable desiccator for 30 minutes, and then weigh without delay. Calculate the content of total ash in mg per g of air-dried material.

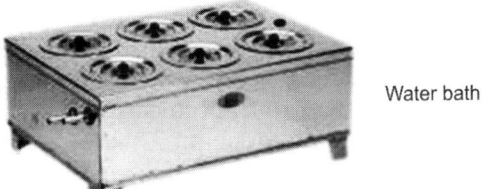

Water bath

Fig. 9.21: Determination of total ash

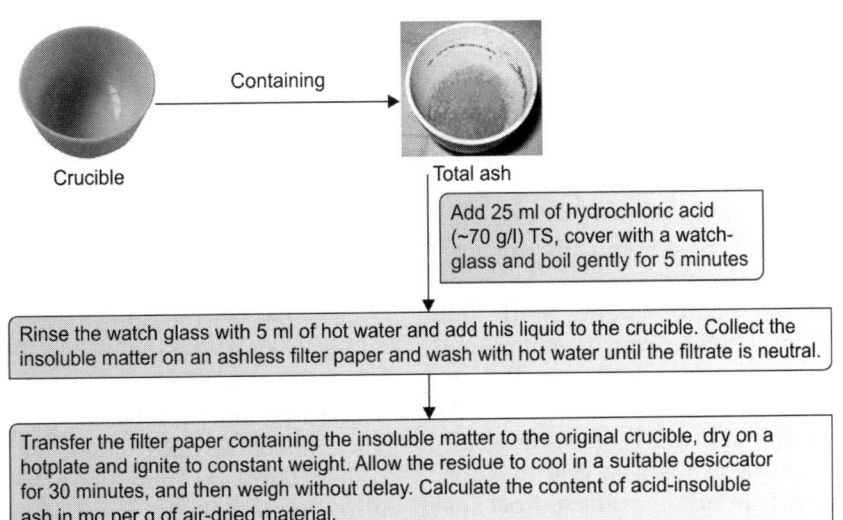

Crucible   Containing

Total ash

Add 25 ml of hydrochloric acid (~70 g/l) TS, cover with a watch-glass and boil gently for 5 minutes

Rinse the watch glass with 5 ml of hot water and add this liquid to the crucible. Collect the insoluble matter on an ashless filter paper and wash with hot water until the filtrate is neutral.

Transfer the filter paper containing the insoluble matter to the original crucible, dry on a hotplate and ignite to constant weight. Allow the residue to cool in a suitable desiccator for 30 minutes, and then weigh without delay. Calculate the content of acid-insoluble ash in mg per g of air-dried material.

Fig. 9.22: Determination of acid insoluble ash

it will be filtered rapidly taking precaution against loss of ethanol, and evaporated to 25 ml of the filterate to dryness in a tared flat-bottomed shallow dish, then it will be dried at 105°C and weighed. The percentage of ethanol-soluble extractive with reference to air dried drug will be calculated.

The percentage yield of each extract was calculated by using the following formula:

$$\text{Percentage yield} = \frac{\text{Weight of extract}}{\text{Weight of powder drug taken}} \times 100$$

Determination of Water and Volatile Matter

An excess of water in herbal materials will encourage microbial growth, the presence of fungi or insects, and deterioration following hydrolysis. Limits for water content should therefore be set for every given herbal material. This is especially important for materials that absorb moisture easily or deteriorate quickly in the presence of water.

The test for *loss on drying* determines both water and volatile matter. Drying can be carried out either by heating to 100–105°C or in a desiccator over phosphorus pentoxide R under atmospheric or reduced pressure at room temperature for a specified period of time. The desiccation method is especially useful for materials that melt to a sticky mass at elevated temperatures.

Determination of Volatile Oils

Volatile oils are characterized by their odour, oil-like appearance and ability to volatilize at room temperature. Chemically, they are usually composed of mixtures of, for example, monoterpenes, sesquiterpenes and their oxygenated derivatives. Aromatic compounds predominate in certain volatile oils. Because they are considered to be the 'essence' of the herbal material, and are often biologically active, they are also known as 'essential oils'. The term 'volatile oil' is preferred because it is more specific and describes the physical properties.

Determination of Volatile Oils (Fig. 9.23)

Procedure

A. *Method A:* This method is used to determine the volatile oils with relative density less than 1.0.

Take a quantity of the powdered sample which is expected to give 0.5–1.0 ml of volatile oil, weigh accurately to the nearest 0.01 g, and put into a round-bottomed flask. Add 300–500 ml of water (or appropriate amount) and a few glass beads, shake and mix well. Connect the round bottomed flask to a volatile oil determination tube and then connect the volatile oil determination tube to a reflux condenser. Add water through the top of reflux condenser until the graduated tube of volatile oil determination tube is filled and overflows to the round-bottomed flask. Heat the flask gently until boiling by using an electric heating jacket or other appropriate means. Continue the gentle boiling for about 5 h until the volume of oil does not increase. Stop heating; allow it to stand for a while. Open the stopcork at the lower part of volatile oil determination tube and run off the water layer slowly until the oily layer is 5 mm above the zero mark. Allow to stand for at least 1 h, open the stopcock again, run off the remaining water layer carefully until the oily layer is just on the zero mark. Record the volume of oil in the graduated tube of volatile oil determination tube and calculate the percentage of volatile oil in sample.

B. *Method B:* This method is used to determine the volatile oils with relative density more than 1.0.

Add 300 ml of water and a few pieces of glass beads into a round-bottomed flask. Connect the round-bottomed flask to volatile oil determination tube. Add water through the top of volatile oil determination tube until the graduated tube is filled and overflows to the round-bottomed flask.

Add 1 ml of xylene by using a pipette and then connect the reflux condenser to volatile oil determination tube. Heat the flask until boiling, continue the heating to allow the distillation proceed at a rate that will keep the middle part of the condenser cold. Stop heating

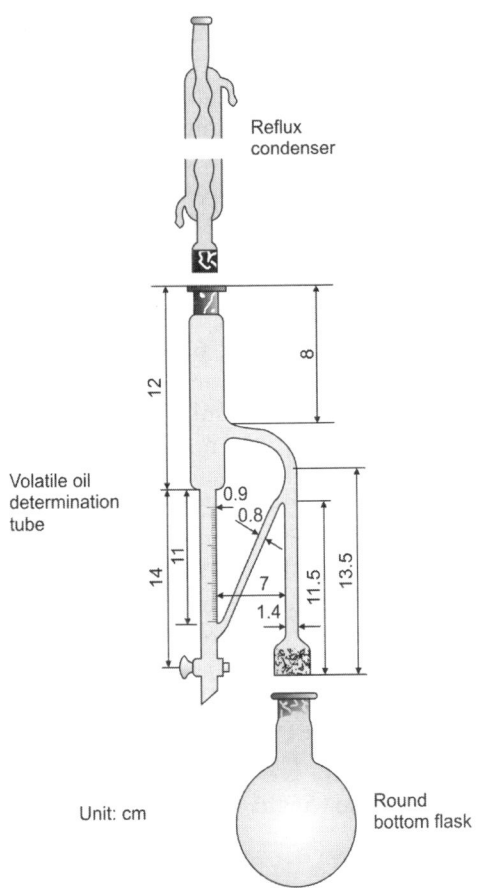

Reflux condenser

Volatile oil determination tube

Unit: cm

Round bottom flask

Fig. 9.23: Determination of volatile oils

after 30 min, and allow it to stand for at least 15 min.

Record the volume of xylene in the graduated tube of volatile oil determination tube. Carry out the procedure as described in method A beginning at the words "Take a quantity of the powdered sample". Subtract the volume of xylene previously observed from the volume of oily layer, the difference in volume is taken to the content of volatile oil, calculate the percentage of volatile oil in sample.

Determination of Bitterness Value

Bitter substances are mostly composed of two or more constituents with various degrees of bitterness, it is first necessary to measure total bitterness by taste. Herbal materials that have a strong bitter taste ("bitters") are therapeutically used as appetizing agents. Their bitterness stimulates secretions in the gastrointestinal tract, especially of gastric juice.

Method

1. After rinsing the mouth with safe drinking water, taste 10 ml of the most dilute solution swirling it in the mouth mainly near the base of the tongue for 30 seconds.
2. If the bitter sensation is no longer felt in the mouth after 30 seconds, spit out the solution and wait for 1 minute to ascertain whether this is due to delayed sensitivity.
3. Then rinse with safe drinking water.
4. The next highest concentration should not be tasted until at least 10 minutes have passed.
5. The threshold bitter concentration is the lowest concentration at which a material continues to provoke a bitter sensation after 30 seconds.
6. After the first series of tests, rinse the mouth thoroughly with safe drinking water until no bitter sensation remains.
7. Wait for at least 10 minutes before carrying out the second test. In order to save time in the second test, it is advisable to ascertain first whether the solution in tube no. 5 (containing 5 ml of ST in 10 ml) gives a bitter sensation. If so, find the threshold bitter concentration of the material by tasting the dilutions in tubes 1–4. If the solution in tube no. 5 does not give a bitter sensation, find the threshold bitter concentration by tasting the dilutions in tubes 6–10.
8. All solutions and the safe drinking-water for mouth washing should be at 20–25°C. Calculate the bitterness value in units per g using the following formula:

$$\frac{2000 \times c}{a \times b}$$

where a = the concentration of the stock solution (ST) (mg/ml); b = the volume of ST (in ml) in the tube with the threshold bitter concentration; c = the quantity of quinine hydrochloride R (in mg) in the tube with the threshold bitter concentration

Determination of Haemolytic Activity

The most characteristic part of saponins is their ability to cause haemolysis; when added to the suspension the saponins produce change in erythrocyte membranes causing haemoglobin to diffuse into the surrounding medium.

The haemolytic activity of herbal materials, or a preparation containing saponins, is determined by comparison with that of a reference material, saponin R, which has a haemolytic activity of 1000 units per g.

A suspension of erythrocytes is mixed with equal volumes of a serial dilution of the herbal material extract. The lowest concentration to effect complete haemolysis is determined after allowing the mixtures to stand for a given period of time. A similar test is carried out simultaneously with saponin R.

Calculate the haemolytic activity of the herbal material using the following formula:

$$1000 \times a/b$$

where 1000 = the defined haemolytic activity of saponin R in relation to ox blood; a = quantity of saponin R that produces total haemolysis (g); b = quantity of herbal material that produces total haemolysis (g).

Tannins

Tannins (or tanning substances) are polyphenolic plant secondary metabolites substances capable of turning animal hides into leather by binding proteins to form water-insoluble substances that are resistant to proteolytic enzymes. This process, when applied to living tissue, is known as an 'astringent' action and is the reason for the therapeutic application of tannins.

Determination of Tannins

1. Powder the herbal material weighed accurately, introduce into a conical flask. Add 150 ml of water and heat over a boiling water bath for 30 minutes.
2. Cool, transfer the mixture to a 250 ml volumetric flask and dilute to volume with water.
3. Allow the solid material to settle and filter the liquid through a filter paper, diameter 12 cm, discarding the first 50 ml of the filtrate.
4. To determine the total amount of material that is extractable into water, evaporate 50.0 ml of the plant material extract to dryness, dry the residue in an oven at 105°C for 4 hours and weigh ($T1$).
5. To determine the amount of herbal material not bound to hide powder that is extractable into water, take 80.0 ml of the herbal material extract, add 6.0 g of hide powder R and shake well for 60 minutes. Filter and evaporate 50.0 ml of the clear filtrate to dryness. Dry the residue in an oven at 105°C and weigh ($T2$).
6. To determine the solubility of hide powder, take 6.0 g of hide powder R, add 80.0 ml of water and shake well for 60 minutes. Filter and evaporate 50.0 ml of the clear filtrate to dryness. Dry the residue in an oven at 105°C and weigh ($T0$).

Calculate the quantity of tannins as a percentage using the following formula:

$$[T1 - (T2 - T0)] \times 500 \, w$$

where w = the weight of the herbal material in grams.

Determination of Swelling Index

The swelling index is the volume in ml taken up by the swelling of 1 g of herbal material under specified conditions. Swelling properties of materials provide them therapeutic or pharmaceutical utility especially gums and those containing an appreciable amount of mucilage, pectin or hemicellulose.

Its determination is based on the addition of water or a swelling agent as specified in the test procedure for each individual herbal material (either whole, cut or pulverized). Using a glass-stoppered measuring cylinder, the material is shaken repeatedly for 1 hour and then allowed to stand for a required period of time.

Procedure

1. Carry out simultaneously no fewer than three determinations for any given material. Introduce the specified quantity

of the herbal material concerned, previously reduced to the required fineness and accurately weighed, into a 25 ml glass-stoppered measuring cylinder.

2. The internal diameter of the cylinder should be about 16 mm, the length of the graduated portion about 125 mm, marked in 0.2 ml divisions from 0 to 25 ml in an upward direction.

3. Unless otherwise indicated in the test procedure, add 25 ml of water and shake the mixture thoroughly every 10 minutes for 1 hour.

4. Allow to stand for 3 hours at room temperature, or as specified. Measure the volume in ml occupied by the herbal material, including any sticky mucilage.

5. Calculate the mean value of the individual determinations, related to 1 g of herbal material.

Determination of Foaming Index

Many herbal plants contain saponins that can cause persistent form when aqueous decoction is shaken.

1. Weigh accurately, 1 g reduce herbal material to a coarse powder (sieve size no. 1250) and transfer to a 500 ml conical flask containing 100 ml of boiling water.

2. Maintain at moderate boiling for 30 minutes.

3. Cool and filter into a 100 ml volumetric flask and add sufficient water through the filter to dilute to volume.

4. Pour the decoction into 10 stoppered test tubes (height 16 cm, diameter 16 mm) in successive portions of 1 ml, 2 ml, 3 ml, etc. up to 10 ml, and adjust the volume of the liquid in each tube with water to 10 ml.

5. Stopper the tubes and shake them in a lengthwise motion for 15 seconds, two shakes per second.

6. Allow to stand for 15 minutes and measure the height of the foam. The results are assessed as follows:

   a. If the height of the foam in every tube is less than 1 cm, the foaming index is less than 100.

   b. If a height of foam of 1 cm is measured in any tube, the volume of the herbal material decoction in this tube (a) is used to determine the index. If this tube is the first or second tube in a series, prepare an intermediate dilution in a similar manner to obtain a more precise result.

   c. If the height of the foam is more than 1 cm in every tube, the foaming index is over 1000. In this case repeat the determination using a new series of dilutions of the decoction in order to obtain a result. Calculate the foaming index using the following formula:

$$1000/a$$

where a = the volume in ml of the decoction used for preparing the dilution in the tube where foaming to a height of 1 cm is observed.

Determination of Pesticide Residues

Determination of Total Chlorine and Phosphorus

Most pesticides contain organically bound chlorine or phosphorus.

Recommended Procedure

Preparation of samples

Reduce the herbal material to a fine powder, and extract with a mixture of water and acetonitrile R. Most pesticides are soluble in this mixture, while most cellular constituents (e.g. cellulose, proteins, amino acids, starch, fats and related compounds) are sparingly soluble and are thus removed. A number of polar and moderately polar compounds may also be dissolved; it is therefore necessary to transfer the pesticides to light petroleum R. For pesticides containing chlorine, further purification is seldom required, but for those containing phosphorus, further purification by column chromatography may be necessary, eluting with mixtures of light petroleum R and ether R.

Determination of Arsenic and Toxic Heavy Metals

Limit Test for Arsenic

Arsenic is abundant in nature and its presence in herbal materials should be no different to its wide occurrence in foods. A popular test method relies on the digestion of the herbal material matrix followed by subjection of the digestate to a comparative colourimetric test in a special apparatus. The test method described below uses colourimetry and does not use toxic mercuric bromide paper. The method uses N-N-diethylmethyldithiocarbamate in pyridine and it reacts with hydrogen arsenide to afford a red–purple complex. The limit is expressed in terms of arsenic (III) trioxide(As_2O_3).

The aim of the limit test for heavy metals is to control metal contaminants potentially originating from reagents, solvents, electrodes, reaction vessels, rubber seals. The test serves as a screening tool indicating the overall quality of the production process. The principle of the test is based on the precipitation of metal sulfides and assumes that all metals behave in a similar manner to a lead standard with which samples are compared. As investigations have shown, the test is effective for detecting Pb, Hg, Pd, Ag, V, Au and Cu which give dark brown or black precipitates. The color of other precipitates varies from pale yellow to orange.

The total viable aerobic count (TVC) of the herbal material being examined is determined, as specified in the test procedure below, using one of the following methods: Membrane-filtration, plate count or serial dilution. Aerobic bacteria and fungi (moulds and yeasts) are determined by the TVC.

Usually a maximum permitted level is set for certain products, but when the TVC exceeds this level then it is unnecessary to proceed with determination of specific organisms; the material should be rejected without being subjected to further testing.

Determination of Aflatoxins

Tests For Aflatoxins

These tests are designed to detect the possible presence of aflatoxins B1, B2, G1 and G2, which are highly toxic contaminants in any material of plant origin.

Recommended Procedure

The method described below does not require the use of toxic solvents, such as chloroform and dichloromethane. It uses a multifunctional column, which contains lipophilic and charged active sites, and high-performance liquid chromatography (HPLC) using fluorescence detection to determine aflatoxins B1, B2, G1 and G2. The advantages of employing a multifunctional column are:

- ➲ High total recoveries of aflatoxins B1, B2, G1 and G2 (more than 85%);
- ➲ The column can be kept (stocked) at room temperature and for a fairly long time prior to use.

Radioactive Contamination

Following a severe nuclear accident, the environment may be contaminated with airborne radioactive materials. These may deposit on the leaves of medicinal plants. Their activity concentration and the type of radioactive contamination can be measured by the radiation monitoring laboratories of most of the WHO Member States. The activity concentration of radioisotopes in herbs should be assessed by the competent national radio-hygiene laboratories taking into account the relevant recommendations of international organizations, such as Codex Alimentarius, the International Atomic Energy Agency (IAEA), the Food and Agriculture Organization of the United Nations (FAO) and WHO. Since radio-nuclides from accidental discharges vary with the type of facility involved, a generalized method of measurement is not yet available. However, should such contamination be a concern, suspect samples can be analysed by a competent laboratory.

STABILITY TESTING OF HERBAL PRODUCTS

Stability testing of herbal products is a complicated issue because the entire herb or herbal product is regarded as the active substance, regardless of whether constituents with defined therapeutic activity are known. The stability testing of herbal products checks the quality of herbal products which varies with the time under the influence of environmental factors, such as

a. temperature,
b. humidity,
c. light,
d. oxygen,
e. moisture, other ingredients or
f. excipient in the dosage form, particle size of drug, microbial contamination, trace metal contamination, leaching from the container, etc. and also provide statistics for the determination of shelf lives.

Therefore, evaluation of the parameters based upon chemical, physical, microbiological, therapeutic and toxicological studies can serve as an important tool in stability studies.

The most important aspect in the evaluation of the stability study of a product is its storage condition. Stability studies should be performed on at least three production batches of the herbal products for the proposed shelf-life, which is normally denoted as long term stability and is performed under natural atmospheric conditions. With the help of modern analytical techniques like spectrophotometry, HPLC, HPTLC and by employing proper guidelines it is possible to generate a sound stability data of herbal products and predict their shelf-life, which will help in improving global acceptability of herbal products.

Specific Characteristics of Herbal Medicinal Products

Herbal drugs and preparations are classified in their entirety like the Active Pharmaceutical Ingredient (API) in the HMP. From the chemical and analytical point of view, herbal drugs, herbal preparations and HMPs are complex in nature due to the high number of constituents belonging to different chemical classes and having different analytical behaviours (for example, flavonoids versus essential oils). In many cases, these constituents have only very low concentrations, especially in the finished product.

With regard to the constituents that are responsible for the pharmacological activity of a herbal preparation, the European Pharmacopoeia (6) and the "Quality Guideline" (2) subdivide them into:

➲ Standardised extracts
➲ Quantified extracts
➲ 'Other' extracts

Standardised extracts have a declared content of constituents with known therapeutic activity—for example, silymarines in *Silybum marianum*. Therefore, standardised extracts are generally treated in the same way as chemically defined APIs, including for example, dissolution testing for solid oral forms.

Quantified extracts are limited to a defined range of constituents that are known to contribute to therapeutic activity, for example, hypericines in *Hypericum perforatum*.

Other extracts without known effective constituents are essentially defined by their production process and their specifications—that is, the ratio of herbal substance to genuine herbal preparation (drug-extract-ratio, DER, genuine).

Choice of Markers

Herbal drugs/preparations are complex mixtures and, to calculate the quantity of a herbal substance or preparation in an HMP, single chemically-defined constituents or groups of constituents are used as 'markers'; these are also called 'active markers' for quantified extracts and 'analytical markers' for other extracts. The choice of marker should be justified by its ability to identify and assay in a selective and robust manner. It is generally recommended to take account of the following:

➲ Literature research about known constituents
➲ EP monograph or other pharmacopoeias and monograph drafts (Pharmeuropa)
➲ Analytical feasibility of the marker in the drug substance and drug product
➲ The marker's suitability for stability studies
➲ *Reference standards:* availability, quality and costs

Monographs may be a helpful tool to define a marker and can give helpful information about a suitable method. But it should be taken into consideration that these monograph methods can only be used for the purpose mentioned in the pharmacopoeia. Often, these methods are not applicable for a finished product containing this drug substance/preparation because the resulting concentration is too low, or matrix effects lead to a lack of selectivity. Methods and markers mentioned in pharmacopoeias are intended for batch release purposes only, not for stability studies and they are, therefore, not often considered for this kind of use. For this reason, the authorities should not bind the applicant to the markers mentioned in the monographs, and should allow alternative approaches in the sense of 'where applicable' and 'if justified'.

Role of Markers

Markers are chemically known compounds, which may or may not have therapeutic effect, used to calculate the quantity of herbal medicinal ingredients in herbal medicinal products. The choice of the marker has to be justified. Finding the "right" analytical marker is a crucial need for stability testing of HMPs. Typical sources for finding markers are:

1. Monographs and drafts (EDQM Pharmeuropa).
2. Experience, transfer from other plants/ constituents.
3. Literature research about known constituents.
4. Scientific research.

Analytical Methods for Herbal Products

The analysis of herbal preparations due to its complex composition is mostly done by running high performance liquid chromatography (HPLC) or gas chromatography (GC) and thin layer chromatography (TLC) methods, quantitative determinations by UV-visible spectroscopy or combinations of these. HPLC and GC methods have the benefit

that a specific fingerprint chromatogram for identification and purity testing, as well as the detection of single compounds for assay, is possible during one analysis. These specific methods are nowadays generally expected by the authorities. But especially in the case of a combined product with two, three or even more active ingredients, a specific determination and quantification of each drug preparation is often impossible. The use of highly sophisticated and expensive methods, for example, LC and GC mass coupling (LC-MS/GC-MS and so on) that have become part of the methods. An option to run the determination jointly, for example, by UV-visible spectroscopy, is expressly mentioned in the Guideline on Quality of Combination Herbals Medicinal Products/Traditional Herbal Medicinal Products. Although the group determination is a useful tool for an assay, the identity of all individual active substances should be proven by appropriate fingerprint chromatograms, or the proof of an individual specific constituent, for example by TLC. If applicable, the identification can be carried out at an earlier production stage, for example, in the primary bulk extract before blending and mixing. The necessity and appropriateness of the method combination has to be demonstrated by the applicant.

These general considerations particularly apply to so-called 'mixed extracts'. They originate from the preparation of tea from a mixture of different herbal drugs in the same way that herbal drugs are blended before a joint extraction using mostly organic solvents. The resulting product can be regarded as one extract, that is, one single substance.

THMPs are sometimes combinations of herbal preparations with vitamins and/or minerals. The (pharmacological) action of the vitamins and minerals should only be ancillary and linked to the indication(s) of the herbal preparation. If the vitamins and minerals are categorised as an API of the product, they should be analysed with regard to the effective requirements (chemical defined substances, vitamins, and so on).

Stability Studies

Stability is defined as the capacity of a drug substance or drug product to remain within the established specifications which maintains its identity, strength, quality and purity throughout the retest or expiration dating period. The objective of stability study is to determine the shelf life, namely the time period of storage at a specified condition within which the drug product still meets its established specifications.

Stability is an essential factor of quality, safety and efficacy of a drug product. A drug product, which is not of sufficient stability, can result in changes in physical (like hardness, dissolution rate, phase separation, etc) as well as chemical characteristics (formation of high risk decomposition substances).

The purpose of the stability testing is to provide evidence how the quality of a drug substance or drug product varies with time under the influence of a variety of environmental factors such as temperature, humidity and light.

Stability evaluation of drug substance or drug product is the key to drug quality as it determines the efficacy of any drug or dosage form.

Stability testing provides evidence that the quality of drug substance or drug product changes with time under the influence of various environmental conditions such as temperature, relative humidity etc.

The stability study consists of a series of tests in order to obtain an assurance of stability of a drug product, namely maintenance of the drug product packed in it specified packaging material and stored in the established storage condition within the determined time period.

Stability Protocol

Protocol include following elements
1. Information on batches tested (commercial formula)
2. Unit composition (or cross-reference)
3. Container-closure system (commercial)
4. Literature and/or supporting data
5. Stability specifications (only for finished pharmaceutical oroducts)
6. *Analytical methods:* Stability indicating (cross-reference)
7. Stability plan (schedule)
8. Tabulated test results (including specifications)
9. Analysis/discussion of data (statistical if negative trend)
10. Re-test or shelf-life proposal (including storage condition)
11. Post-approval commitments

REGULATORY GUIDELINES FOR STABILITY STUDY (FIG. 9.24)

There are many regulatory guidelines for stability study mainly International Conference on Harmonization (ICH), World Health Organization (WHO), Association of South East Asian Nations (ASEAN) and European Agency for Evaluation of Medicinal and Health Products (EMEA).

Importance of stability testing: It evaluates the efficacy of a drug. Stability studies are used to develop suitable packaging information for quality, strength, purity and integrity of product during its shelf life. It is used for determination of the shelf life.

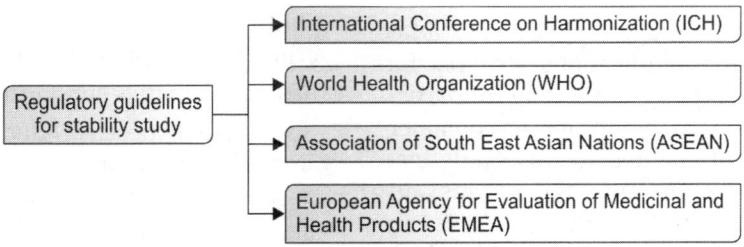

Fig. 9.24: Regulatory guidelines for stability study

ICH Guidelines For Stability

ICH guidelines given for drug substance and drug product is defined the stability data package for a new drug substance or drug product that is sufficient for a registration application within the three regions of the EC, Japan and the United States.

Q1A (R2)—Stability testing of new drug substances and products (Revision 2) (August 2003) CPMP/ICH/2736/99: Zone I and II

Objectives of the guideline

The following guideline is a revised version of the ICH Q1A guideline and defines the stability data package for a new drug substance or drug product that is sufficient for a registration application within the three regions of the EC, Japan, and the United States. It does not seek necessarily to cover the testing for registration in or export to other areas of the world. The guideline seeks to exemplify the core stability data package for new drug substances and products, but leaves sufficient flexibility to encompass the variety of different practical situations that may be encountered due to specific scientific considerations and characteristics of the materials being evaluated. Alternative approaches can be used when there are scientifically justifiable reasons.

Scope of the Guideline

The guideline addresses the information to be submitted in registration applications for new molecular entities and associated drug products. This guideline does not currently seek to cover the information to be submitted for abbreviated or abridged applications, variations, clinical trial applications, etc. Specific details of the sampling and testing for particular dosage forms in their proposed container closures are not covered in this guideline. Further guidance on new dosage forms and on biotechnological/biological products can be found in ICH guidelines Q1C and Q5C, respectively.

General principles

The purpose of stability testing is to provide evidence on how the quality of a drug substance or drug product varies with time under the influence of a variety of environmental factors such as temperature, humidity, and light, and to establish a re-test period for the drug substance or a shelf life for the drug product and recommended storage conditions.

Q1B—Photostability: Testing of new active substances and medicinal products (January 1998) CPMP/ICH/279/95

The intrinsic photostability characteristics of new active substances and medicinal products should be evaluated to demonstrate that, as appropriate, light exposure does not result in unacceptable change. Normally, photostability testing is carried out on a single batch of material selected as described under Selection of Batches in the Parent Guideline. Under some circumstances these studies should be repeated if certain changes are made to the product (e.g. formulation, packaging). Whether these studies should be repeated depends on the photostability characteristics determined at the time of first submission of an application and the type of change made. The guideline primarily addresses the generation of photostability information for submission in applications for marketing authorisations for new active substances and associated medicinal products. The guideline does not cover the photostability of medicinal products after administration (i.e. under conditions of use) and those applications not covered by the parent guideline. Alternative approaches may be used if they are scientifically sound and justification is provided. A systematic approach to photostability testing is recommended covering, as appropriate, studies such as:

i. Tests on the active substance;

ii. Tests on the exposed product outside of the immediate pack, and if necessary;

iii. Tests on the product in the immediate pack; and if necessary;

iv. Tests on the product in the marketing pack.

The extent of product testing should be established by assessing whether or not acceptable change has occurred at the end of the light exposure testing as described in the decision flow chart for photostability testing of medicinal products. Acceptable change is change within limits justified by the applicant. The formal labelling requirements for photolabile substances and products are established by national requirements.

Q1C—Requirements for New Dosage Forms (January 1998) CPMP/ICH/280/95

The ICH harmonised Tripartite Guideline on Stability Testing of New Active Substances and Medicinal Products was issued on October 27, 1993. This document is an annex to the ICH parent stability guideline and addresses the recommendations on the data which should be submitted regarding stability of new dosage forms by the owner of the original application, after the original submission for new active substances and medicinal products.

New dosage forms

A new dosage form is defined as a medicinal product which is a different pharmaceutical product type, but containing the same active substance as included in an existing product approved by the pertinent regulatory authority. Such pharmaceutical product types include products of a different route of administration (e.g. oral to parenteral), new specific functionality/delivery systems (e.g. immediate release tablet to modified release tablet) and different dosage forms of the same route of administration (e.g. capsule to tablet, solution to suspension). Stability protocols for new dosage forms should follow the guidance in the parent stability guideline in principle. However, a reduced stability database at submission time (e.g. 6 months accelerated and 6 months long-term data from ongoing studies) may be acceptable in certain justified cases.

Q1D—Bracketing and matrixing designs for stability testing of drug substances and drug products (August 2002) CPMP/ICH/4104/00.

Objectives of the guideline

This guideline is intended to address recommendations on the application of bracketing and matrixing to stability studies conducted in accordance with principles outlined in the ICH Q1A(R) Harmonised Tripartite Guideline on Stability Testing of New Drug Substances and Products (hereafter referred to as the parent guideline).

Scope of the guideline

This document provides guidance on bracketing and matrixing study designs. Specific principles are defined in this guideline for situations in which bracketing or matrixing can be applied. Sample designs are provided for illustrative purposes, and should not be considered the only, or the most appropriate, designs in all cases.

Q1E—Evaluation of stability data (August 2003) CPMP/ICH/420/02

Objectives of the guideline

This guideline is intended to provide recommendations on how to use stability data generated in accordance with the principles detailed in the ICH guideline "Q1A(R) Stability Testing of New Drug Substances and Products" (hereafter referred to as the parent guideline) to propose a retest period or shelf life in a registration application. This guideline describes when and how extrapolation can be considered when proposing a retest period for a drug substance or a shelf life for a drug product that extends beyond the period covered by "available data from the stability study under the long-term storage condition" (hereafter referred to as long-term data).

Scope of the guideline

This guideline addresses the evaluation of stability data that should be submitted in registration applications for new molecular entities and associated drug products. The guideline provides recommendations on establishing retest periods and shelf lives for drug substances and drug products intended for storage at or below 'room temperature'. It covers stability studies using single- or multi-factor designs and full or reduced designs.

Q1F—Stability data package for registration applications in climatic zones III and IV (August 2003) CPMP/ICH/421/02: Withdrawn on June 1st 2006.

Q5C—Stability testing of biotechnological and biological products (July 1996) CPMP/ICH/138/95

The guidance stated in this annex applies to well-characterised proteins and polypeptides, their derivatives and products of which they are components, and which are isolated from tissues, body fluids, cell cultures, or produced using rDNA technology. Thus, the document covers the generation and submission of stability data for products such as cytokines (interferons, interleukins, colony-stimulating factors, tumour necrosis factors), erythropoietins, plasminogen activators, blood plasma factors, growth hormones and growth factors, insulins, monoclonal antibodies, and vaccines consisting of well-characterised proteins or polypeptides. In addition, the guidance outlined in the following sections may apply to other types of products, such as conventional vaccines, after consultation with the appropriate regulatory authorities. The document does not cover antibiotics, allergenic extracts, heparins, vitamins or whole blood.

OBJECTIVES OF THE GUIDELINES

The objective of guidelines is to exemplify the core stability data package required for registration of active pharmaceutical ingredients (APIs) and finished pharmaceutical products (FPPs). These guidelines apply to new and existing APIs and address information to be submitted in original and subsequent applications for marketing authorization of their related FPP for human use. It is recommended that these guidelines should also be applied to products that are already being marketed,

with allowance for an appropriate transition period, e.g. upon re-registration or upon re-evaluation.

Stress Testing

Stress testing help to identify the degradation product, which can help to establish the degradation pathway. Stress tests are usually considered unnecessary for herbal drug and its preparation.

1. For herbal drugs and herbal drug preparations, a testing under accelerated or intermediate conditions may be omitted. This should apply to finished products as well, because it is known that most products fail at 30°C/65 per cent relative humidity (RH) and at 40°C/75 per cent RH in particular. Herbal drug substances at only 25°C/60 per cent RH, with no requirement for intermediate/accelerated testing.

2. If intermediate conditions are tested, the three-month time-point is omitted (that is, 0, 6, 9 and 12 months). In some cases of combination products, it is hardly possible to provide the required two batches of each extract at the same time due to different harvesting times.

Selection of Batches

Long-term testing is to be provided with on at least two batches of the drug substance and three batches of drug product. In some cases of

Table 9.5: Storage conditions in stability studies

Conditions of stability study	Storage conditions
General case	
Long term	25°C ± 2°C/60%Rh ± 5% Rh or 30°C ± 2°C/65%Rh ± 5% Rh
Intermediate	30°C ± 2°C/65% Rh ±5% Rh
Accelerated	40°C ± 2°C/75%Rh ± 5% Rh
For substance stored in refrigerator	
Long term	5°C ± 3°C
Accelerated	25°C ± 2°C/60%Rh ± 5% Rh
For substance stored in freezer	
Long term	−20°C ± 5°C

combination products, it is hardly possible to provide the required two batches of each extract at the same time due to different harvesting times. This should be taken into consideration when planning the schedule for stability study.

Predictable Changes in Herbal Medicinal Product

Following predictable changes may occur in herbal medicinal product during storage and in shelf life determination: Hydrolysis, oxidation, racemization, geometric isomerization, temperature, moisture and light

Hydrolysis: Reaction with water takes place which results in degradation of product.

Oxidation: Due to addition of electro-negative atom (o), removal of electro-positive atom, radical's formation results in decomposition of natural products.

Racemization: Racemization is the process in which one enantiomer of a compound, such as an L-amino acid, converts to the other enantiomer. The compound then alternates between each form while the ratio between the (+) and (−) groups approaches 1:1, at which point it becomes optically inactive.

Geometric Isomerization

Geometric isomerization: Products can be changed in *trans* or *cis* form. One form may be more therapeutically active.

Polymerization: There is combination of two or more identical molecule to form much larger and more complex molecule.

Temperature: The rate of most chemical increase with increase in temperature. So that "Tropical" area must be taken in consideration during preparation of the formula of the herbal substance.

Moisture: Moisture absorbed on to the surface of solid drug will often increase the rate of decomposition, if it is susceptible to the hydrolysis.

Light: Many type of chemical reaction induced by exposure to light of high energy. Autoxidation of volatile oil/fixed oil takes place and substance becomes coloured.

Stability testing of Herbal products with known chemical constituents is same as chemically defined APIs but the major herbal medicinal products are complex in nature. Major studies are same for both herbal medicinal and chemically defined products. The specific features for herbals are as follows:

1. Two batches of the drug substance and three batches of drug product.
2. No three-month testing-point at 30°C/65 per cent RH for the drug product
3. Herbal drug substance at only 25°C/60 per cent RH, with no requirement for intermediate/accelerated testing
4. Assay of marker substances for 'quantified' and 'other' extracts. Choice of methods, combination of methods and fingerprints.
5. Assay ±5 per cent or ±10 per cent from the initial value for quantified and other extracts (rather than for the declared value, as for standardized extracts and chemical APIs)
6. A requirement for ongoing stability studies.

WHO Guidelines

WHO guidelines derived from ICH parent guideline applies to new and existing API's and their related FPP's for human use. These guidelines have some significant differences in the parameters like selection of batches, storage conditions and statements and labelling which define its individuality as a separate guideline.

ASEAN (Association of South East Asian Nations) Guidelines

ASEAN guideline mainly focuses on the requirements for stability testing of drug products along with new chemical entities (NCEs). These guidelines have significant differences in stress testing, selection of batches and real time storage conditions.

These guidelines address the information to be submitted an application for marketing authorization of drug products in ASEAN countries including examples of a protocol of stability study, a report format, reduced design and extrapolation of data, and examples of types, thickness and permeability coefficient. The drug products covered in this guideline include NCE, Generics and Variation; exclude drug products containing vitamin and mineral preparations.

EMEA (European Agency for Evaluation of Medicinal and Health Products) Guidelines

EMEA guideline is an extension of EMEA/CVMP/VICH/899/99-Rev.1 on stability testing of new veterinary drug substances and medicinal products and sets out the stability testing requirements for existing active substances and related finished products. The guideline addresses the information to be submitted in registration applications for existing active substances and related finished products. It is applicable to chemical active substances and related finished products, herbal drugs, herbal drug preparations and related herbal medicinal products and not to radiopharmaceuticals, biological and products derived by biotechnology.

The guidelines have most of the parameters for drug substance and drug products same as the ICH guideline like stress testing, testing frequency, stability commitment, statement/labelling. The difference only lies with the parameters like selection of batches and storage conditions.

The guideline seeks to exemplify the core stability data package required for such active substances and finished products, but leaves sufficient flexibility to encompass the variety of different practical situations that may be encountered due to specific scientific considerations and characteristics of the materials being evaluated.

CONCLUSION

Stability study regulatory requirements are defined as the capacity of a drug substance or drug product to remain within the established specifications to maintain its identity, strength, quality and purity throughout the retest or expiration dating period. Various factors affect the stability of drugs are water, oxygen, temperature, pH, moisture and concentration.

The comparison of stability testing (ST) requirements of International Conference on Harmonization (ICH) with other international regulatory agencies like World Health Organization (WHO), Association of South East Asian Nations (ASEAN) and European Agency for Evaluation of Medicinal and Health Products (EMEA). ICH guideline is parent guideline defines stability testing requirements for new drug substances and drug products, whereas WHO guideline applies to both new and existing APIs and their related finished products and ASEAN guidelines mainly focuses on the stability testing requirements for drug products which include generics and variations along with NCEs.

10 Patenting and Regulatory Requirements of Natural Products

- Definition of the terms: Patent, IPR, farmers right, breeders right, bioprospecting and biopiracy
- Patenting aspects of traditional knowledge and natural products. Case study of curcuma and neem.

INTRODUCTION

Intellectual property rights (IPR) defined as ideas, inventions, and creative expressions based on which there is a public willingness to bestow the status of property. IPR provides exclusive rights to the inventors or creators of that property, in order to enable them to reap commercial benefits from their creative efforts or reputation. There are several types of intellectual property protection like patent, copyright, trademark, etc. IPR is prerequisite for better identification, planning, commercialization, rendering, and thereby protection of invention or creativity. Pharmaceutical industry currently has an evolving IPR strategy requiring a better focus and approach in the coming era.

TYPES OF INTELLECTUAL PROPERTIES AND THEIR DESCRIPTION

Originally, only patent, trademarks, and industrial designs were protected as 'Industrial Property', but now the term 'Intellectual Property' has a much wider meaning. IPR enhances technology advancement in the following ways:

(a) It provides a mechanism of handling infringement, piracy, and unauthorized use

(b) It provides a pool of information to the general public since all forms of IP are published except in case of trade secrets.

IP protection can be sought for a variety of intellectual efforts including

i. **Patents** are recognition for an invention, which satisfies the criteria of global novelty, non-obviousness, and industrial application.

ii. **Industrial designs** relate to features of any shape, configuration, surface pattern, composition of lines and colours applied to an article whether 2-D, e.g. textile, or 3-D.

iii. **Trademarks** relate to unique mark, name or logo under which trade is conducted for any product or service and by which the manufacturer or the service provider is identified. It can be bought, sold, and licensed, has no existence apart from the goodwill of the product or service it symbolizes. A trademark is a mark (i.e. the name of the product presented on signs or packages) which can be used to protect an herbal medicine's reputation. Manufacturers identify a federally registered trademark with a circled R symbol, i.e. "®". Trademarks are consumer oriented offer the end user a guarantee of quality, service, and product image.

iv. **Copyright** relates to expression of ideas in material form and includes literary, musical, dramatic, artistic, cinematography work, audio tapes, and computer software.

v. **Geographical indications** are indications, which identify as good as originating in the territory of a country or a region or locality in that territory where a given quality, reputation, or other characteristic of the goods is essentially attributable to its geographical origin.

IPR Laws in India

As a member of the various international conventions and agreements, India is bound to enact/amend relevant domestic laws to gear up and face the challenges of globalization. In order to confirm to the stipulations in the TRIPS (*Trade-Related* Aspects of *Intellectual Property Rights*) Agreement, IPRs related laws in India are undergoing changes.

A *Patent Act (1970)* which was one of the most important milestones in the history of IPR laws in India amendments by government in 1999, 2002 and 2005. The main changes brought through the amendments do not substantially affect traditional knowledge, farmers' rights and biodiversity. There are also a few provisions, which attempt to reduce biopiracy. As an example, the scope of an 'invention' has been expanded to cover all grounds of new scientific creations. Despite, new uses of known substances, including the duplication of traditional knowledge have been specifically excluded from patentability. In addition, the nondisclosure of the source of geographical origin of a traditionally known material has been made a basis for the challenge of a patent.

The Biological Diversity Act, 2002 was adopted following India's ratification of the Biodiversity Convention (CBD). It aims to conserve biodiversity, sustainable use of biological resources and equitable sharing of benefits that arise from their use or traditional knowledge. It mandates the setting up of institutions at national, state and local levels, for the purpose of regulation of biological diversity. The Act attempts to regulate access to biodiversity for commercial purposes, to fight biopiracy, and recognise community rights over traditional knowledge and biodiversity.

Plant Varieties Protection and Farmers Rights (PVPFR) Act, 2001 was enacted under the obligations set out in agreement on Trade Related Intellectual Property Rights (TRIPS) which mandates the protection of plant varieties either by patents. The Indian legislation on Plant Varieties Protection (PVP) is being perceived as a progressive legislation when compared to the PVP acts adopted by the other developing nations. The PVPFR Act of India, in addition to offering protection to plant breeders in the form of plant breeder's rights, also protects the rights of the farmers to save, use, sow, re-sow, exchange, share or sell farm produce including the seeds of any unprotected variety, with an exemption to prevent the sale of branded seeds. This law incorporates some principles of the Convention on Biological Diversity (CBD) like prior informed consent and sharing of benefits with farmers.

Patents

Patents may provide the strongest IP protection, most difficult to obtain for natural or herbal medicines. Patents provide the patentee the rights to exclude others from making, using, selling, offering for sale, or importing the patented invention. It is a grant by a state to an inventor or to his assignee, giving exclusive rights to make, use, exercise and vend the inventions for a limited period, in exchange for disclosure in a patent specification. According to Patent Act, 1970 it is defined as new invention which should be useful, new and non-obvious not used previously in use in India invention.

Objectives (Fig. 10.1)

1. Giving a legal monopoly to the patentee to reap the economic benefits from his invention.
2. Facilitating the improvements or providing the alternative approaches to develop the new ideas or/and products.
3. Invention of new drugs.

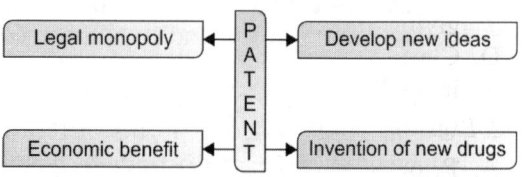

Fig. 10.1: Objective of patents

Rationale of Patent

Patent is recognition to the form of IP manifested in invention. Patents are granted for patentable inventions, which satisfy the requirements of *novelty* and *utility* under the stringent examination and opposition procedures prescribed in the Indian Patents Act, 1970, but there is not even a *prima-facie* presumption as to the validity of the patent granted. Most countries have established national regimes to provide protection to the IPR within its jurisdiction. Except in the case of copyrights, the protection granted to the inventor/creator in a country (such as India) or a region (such as European Union) is restricted to that territory where protection is sought and is not valid in other countries or regions. For example, a patent granted in India is valid only for India and not in the USA. The basic reason for patenting an invention is to make money through exclusivity, i.e., the inventor or his assignee would have a monopoly if,

a. the inventor has made an important invention after taking into account the modifications that the customer, and
b. If the patent agent has described and claimed the invention correctly in the patent specification drafted, then the resultant patent would give the patent owner an exclusive market.

The patentee can exercise his exclusivity either by marketing the patented invention himself or by licensing it to a third party.

Procedure For Patenting (Fig. 10.2)

1. Filling an application

A. Name, address and nationality of the applicant
B. Title, name, address and nationality of the inventor, if he is not the applicant or co-applicant
C. Specifications (provisional and complete) giving the details of the invention
D. Claims, definition and scope of the invention.

2. Examination of the application

A. Prior approved patents or applications filed

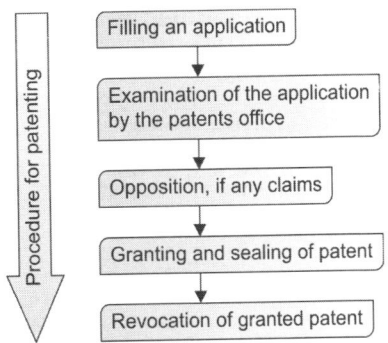

Fig. 10.2: Procedure of patent

B. Novelty
C. Usefulness
D. Nature of claims

3. Opposition

A three-month time period is given for any opposition. Contrary claims can be filed and contested.

4. Granting and sealing of patent

In case of no opposition or clearing satisfactorily all the objections by the applicant, patent is granted and sealed by the patent office by publishing in the official gazette.

5. Revocation

The validity of the patent can be challenged in High Court under specified grounds. The patent will be revoked if the court upholds the challenge.

6. Validity of a patent

Patent for food and medicines and drugs produced by chemical processes 5 years period from the date of granting the patent or 7 years period from the date of filing application or whichever is earlier.

Patent can be claimed by the following:

1. Any person claiming to be the true and first inventor of the invention
2. Any person being the assignee of the person claiming to be the true and first inventor in respect of the right to make such application
3. Any legal representative of any diseased person who immediately before his

death was entitled to make such an application (Fig. 10.3).

Patentable	Nonpatentable
• New process of manufacture • New chemical entities • New formulation processes • New composition of matter	• Discoveries • Methods of detection, diagnosis or treatment of diseases • Analytical methods • Methods of agriculture/ cultivation • The products made by chemical synthesis • Animal, plant, and biological methods for growing and rearing them.

Fig. 10.3: List of patentable and nonpatentable

The following would not qualify as patents:

1. An invention, which is frivolous or which claims anything obvious or contrary to the well-established natural law.
2. An invention, the primary or intended use of which would be contrary to law or morality or injurious to public health.
   ⊃ A discovery, scientific theory, or mathematical method.
   ⊃ A mere discovery of any new property or new use for a known substance or of the mere use of a known process, machine, or apparatus unless such known process results in a new product or employs at least one new reactant.
   ⊃ A substance obtained by a mere admixture resulting only in the aggregation of the properties of the components thereof or a process for producing such substance.
   ⊃ A mere arrangement or re-arrangement or duplication of a known device each functioning independently of one another in its own way
   ⊃ A method of agriculture or horticulture.
   ⊃ Any process for the medicinal, surgical, curative, prophylactic diagnostic, therapeutic or other treatment of human beings or any process for a similar treatment of animals to render them free of disease or to

increase their economic value or that of their products.
   ⊃ An invention relating to atomic energy
   ⊃ An invention, which is in effect, is traditional knowledge.

IPR and Farmer's Rights in India

India is one of the first countries in the world to have evolved an intellectual property rights legislation simultaneously granting rights to both breeders and farmers. The Protection of Plant Varieties and Farmers Rights Act, 2001, establishes a unique system by extending the concept of Plant Breeders' Rights (PBRs) currently applied to new varieties of breeders, to varieties held by farmers, NGOs and public sector institutions. The law emerged from a process that attempted to incorporate the interests of various stakeholders, including private sector breeders, public sector institutions, nongovernmental organizations and farmers, within the property rights framework. While the act is based on the important principle of distributing ownership rights in a fair and equitable manner, the assigning of multiple rights could pose several obstacles to useful utilization and exchange of resources. If the system is not carefully structured, a tragedy of the anti-commons situation could arise. The tragedy of the anti-commons refers to *underuse* of resources arising from multiple ownership or rights to exclude others from use. It occurs when governments grant too many people rights over a resource with no one having an effective privilege of use.

India's Policy on PBRS and Farmers' Rights

India's policy on IPR protection in agriculture has largely been governed by the following factors:

1. Common heritage or the principle of free exchange based on the view that the major food plants of the world are not owned by anyone and are a part of our human heritage.
2. A focus on ensuring access to technology and promoting economic development.

India did establish IPR laws to protect the rights of innovators, but attempted to balance this with the need for access to resources at reasonable prices.

3. A majority of agricultural research in India has largely been conducted by the public sector. India's seed policy until the 1980s restricted the role of the private sector in agriculture.

These factors promoted a system where India did not provide for plant breeders' rights as there was no real demand for such a system for decades. The absence of PBRs also meant that there was no requirement for farmers' rights as a counter to IPRs. Farmers were free to use, share and exchange seeds and since breeders could not acquire PBRs, there was no system of benefit sharing or compensation.

Policy Change

India's existing policy is undergoing substantial changes with the adoption of the Protection of Plant Varieties and Farmers' Rights Act. The law in India evolved through the incorporation of the interests of various actors and an analysis of this process provides the key to understanding its potential implications for stakeholder access. The enormous opposition against granting PBRs was overcome in India when mechanisms were created for assigning ownership rights over farmer's varieties and protection of resources with the public sector.

The farmer's right under this draft was defined as:

1. *Farmers' privilege:* Right to save, use, exchange, share and sell propagating material of seed except sale of branded seed

2. *Benefit sharing:* the Authority under the Act could require the breeder to pay reward/compensation to communities. There was no concept of farmers' rights as ownership rights or rights to register their varieties.

In spite of attempts by the government to take into account the various interests, the bill was opposed both by NGOs and industry. The Seed Association of India (SAI) criticized the bill stating that the very purpose of plant variety protection would be defeated if farmers start selling seed of a protected variety. If not amended this provision will be a disincentive to invest in research and development. SAI protested against several aspects of the bill and felt that the very purpose of plant variety protection would be defeated if farmers start selling seeds of a protected variety and suggested an almost complete removal of farmers' rights. Various NGOs voiced strong opposition against the bill mainly for not providing strong farmers' rights.

The Farmers Rights definition in the Act adopted and expanded all three aspects of Farmers' Rights:

1. Farmers' privilege as a right not only to save and exchange seeds but also to sell seeds (except branded)

2. Benefit sharing based on compensation and operating through a mechanism where communities/farmers can make claims for such compensation

3. Farmers Rights as ownership: The idea that farmers must be able to register their varieties.

The criteria for registration of extant varieties and farmers' varieties, however, are not entirely clear in the Act. The Act proposes that it would be based on distinctness, uniformity and stability *as defined by the Authority*. The Authority is yet to provide such definitions and this will be a crucial factor in determining whether farmers would actually be able to register their varieties.

Plant Variety and Farmer's Right Act

This is very important legislation enacted by the Parliament to honour India's obligation in TRIPs. This is *sui generis* law with respect of plant variety and farmer's right. The breeding activities move around genetic resources. The Act covers interplay of breeding, genetic resources and traditional knowledge.

The Act has the following important provisions for recognizing traditional knowledge. The Act recognized concept of benefit sharing between provider and recipient of the plant genetic resources. Applicant seeking registration of variety must disclose geographical location from where genetic material has been taken while evolving new variety.

Plant Breeders Rights

PBR is a patent-like system that allows the plant variety owner to prohibit specific unauthorized uses of the variety. PBR laws are special purpose systems apply only to plants. PBRs, like patents and other forms of IP law, are forms of national legislation. That is, protection applies only in countries where protection has been sought and granted. PBR under the TRIPS Agreement (Agreement on Trade-Related Aspects of Intellectual Property Rights) is a component of the World Trade Organization (WTO). Signatories of WTO (currently about 150) are committed to comply with the TRIPS requirements of a harmonized minimum level of IP rights protection.

Role of UPOV (International Union for the Protection of New Varieties of Plants)

Essentially, UPOV establishes a framework law that may be adopted by countries into their own national laws. UPOV does provide a mechanism for harmonizing national laws and providing standardized definitions/interpretations of terms. UPOV also requires nondiscrimination against foreign applicants of other Union members. UPOV member states have training and other technical support available to them, although an annual membership fee based on national income is imposed. Since its inception, UPOV has adopted four Acts (1961, 1972, 1978, and 1991). Members may at their discretion adopt a more recent Act, but older Acts are closed. Presently, the 1991 Act is the only one now opens to new members.

Biopiracy

Biopiracy is a situation where indigenous knowledge of nature, originating with indigenous people, is used by others for profit, without permission from and with little or no compensation or recognition to the indigenous people themselves. Developed countries are exploiting developing countries genetic resources and indigenous communities traditional knowledge in the name of patents on the inventions derived from those genetic resources.

It operates through unfair application of patents to genetic resources and traditional knowledge It is the theft or usurpation of genetic materials especially plants and other biological materials by the patent process, for example: Use of indigenous knowledge of medicinal plants for patenting by medical companies without recognizing the fact that the knowledge is not new, or invented by the patenter, And thereby the piracy deprives the indigenous community to the rights to commercial exploitation of the technology that they themselves had developed.

Meaning of Traditional Knowledge

Traditional Knowledge (TK), variously referred to as traditional ecological knowledge, local knowledge, and folk knowledge is knowledge developed by local and indigenous communities over time in response to the needs of their specific local environment. The World Intellectual Property Organization (WIPO) defines traditional knowledge as indigenous cultural and intellectual property, indigenous heritage, and customary heritage rights. The need to protect the traditional knowledge captured the attention of the international community only recently but the standard setting was left to the national governments. The absence of the international standards, that causes serious negligence for the protection of the traditional knowledge and the benefits of new technology.

PATENTS AND TRADITIONAL KNOWLEDGE IN INDIA

As a whole, the forests and its dwellers gives to India an abundant knowledge about the traditional value of various forest products. The way intellectual property rights have been designed in modern commerce, traditional knowledge cannot be protected. For instance, traditional knowledge cannot be patented because such knowledge lacks inventive character, because of the inherent lack of novelty. Traditional knowledge is also often held collectively by communities, rather than by individual owners. This traditional knowledge is information that is transmitted from generation to generation generally within the community or within families, within the community in an oral form without any adequate documentation. This has caused traditional knowledge to be undervalued and marginalized. In fact, one of the fears in these communities is that if the knowledge were to be documented it would have been lost to the community by expropriation. In India, the Forest Act itself acknowledges this fact and provides a framework for documentation of such knowledge and the nature of evidence required for recognition of the rights of these communities in the intellectual property in respect of such knowledge.

The provisions of the Biological Diversity Act and Forest Rights Act of 2006 both provide a shield for tribal traditional knowledge, by, on the one hand, respecting and protecting the knowledge of the local communities related to biodiversity and on the other, declaring that the intellectual property rights, in such knowledge belongs primarily to members of the community collectively. The TRIPS Agreement also has some provisions having limited application to the protection of Traditional Knowledge. The obligation to protect geographical indications can be used to protect traditional knowledge if associated with the indication used for production and sale of goods.

It is made clear that a given quality, reputation or other characteristics of the goods essentially attributable to its geographical origin are to be considered in identifying the geographical indications for protection. Thus it may be possible for protection through geographical indication the traditional knowledge associated with goods. Disclosing traditional knowledge which forms part of an invention and of the state of the art or prior art will promote the progress of science by creating an incentive for the maintenance of traditional knowledge systems. This will happen by traditional knowledge being widely and universally accepted within 'western' or "modern innovation

protection systems and becoming a reference point within the regular operations of the international patent system.

Traditional Knowledge in Danger

The national knowledge commission India recommended to protect traditional knowledge and said: Establish goals for conservation of natural resources: Natural populations of around 12% of the 6000 species of potentially medicinal plants are currently estimated to be under threat due to degradation and loss of habitats alongside unsustainable ways of harvesting and lack of cultivation. The problem of growing scarcity also leads to the danger of more counterfeit material being marketed. It is therefore necessary to support conservation and sustainable harvesting efforts in the forestry sector and cultivation in the agricultural sector. Direct support for conservation and cultivation as well as indirect methods through incentive policies should be pursued for nurturing these plant resources.

A. Support nongovernment and corporate initiatives for promotion of THS: The nongovernment and private sector have played an important role in building the public image of traditional health sciences. Nongovernmental research and education institutions, NGOs and corporate with a global vision must be strategically supported in the interest of enhancing national and international awareness of India's rich health system heritage.

B. Promote international cooperation: International cooperation in exploration of traditional health systems must be given a big boost through substantial initiatives like strategic research collaborations with reputed research centres and establishing wellness centres in countries that offer promising market opportunities. EXIM bank of India must be supported to work with industry to open world markets for these products and services.

C. Support primary healthcare in rural areas: With 70% of Indian population relying on traditional medicine for primary health care in the absence of adequate state primary health care, it becomes necessary to establish evidence-based guidelines for this informal-sector usage. A nation-wide network of Home Herbal Garden and Community Herbal Gardens (CHG) can be created to support the primary health care needs of rural communities for those plants and medications established as efficacious by evidence-based research.

D. Create a major re-branding exercise of Indian traditional medicine: Better branding of Indian traditional medicines proven to be effective in well-designed clinical trials can increase safe and effective healthcare options. Such proven medications should be integrated with the national healthcare system. Such evidence based well-validated and uniquely Indian holistic healthcare system combinations must be marketed extensively globally. The above mention facts show importance of protection of traditional knowledge in India and indicate traditional knowledge is in danger, some other reasons are following:

➲ **Encroachment, Bi-Prospecting and Bio-Piracy:** One of the biggest threats to biodiversity and related traditional knowledge is ever-increasingly bioprospecting activities on behalf of enthobotanists, pharmaceutical companies and others who wish to profit from the rich biodiversity and traditional knowledge in indigenous territories.

➲ **Devolution:** As demand for commercialization of biodiversity and traditional knowledge increases at a rapid pace and as the world globalizes, develops and modernizes, indigenous societies are being encroached upon faster than traditional knowledge can be protected. Their cultures and knowledge are being lost. In many parts of the world, the very existence of indigenous societies is under threat.

INADEQUACY OF LEGAL SYSTEM THAT ADDRESS TRADITIONAL KNOWLEDGE

This point is divided into two major sections.

General Issues Relating to the Protection of Traditional Knowledge

Devolution, encroachment, the bio prospecting rush, lack of appropriate legal systems and a clash of systems all make traditional knowledge highly vulnerable to biopiracy. Several traditional plants and related knowledge in Asia, specifically India, have also been allegedly falsely patented by the US patent office, including: Neem, haldi, pepper, harar, mustard, basmati rice, ginger, castor, jaramla, karela and jamun. Traditional knowledge is generally associated with biological resources and is invariably an intangible component of such a biological resource. Traditional knowledge has the potential of being translated into commercial benefits by providing leads/clues for development of useful practices and processes for the benefit of mankind. The valuable leads/clues provided by TK save time, money and investment of modern biotech and other industries into any research and product development. Some countries have specific legislation protecting this kind of knowledge while some other countries feel their existing IPR regime protects such knowledge. As of now, India does not have a specific *sui generis* legislation to protect such TK and folklore but is in the process of developing such legislation.

In the recent past, there have been several cases of bio-piracy of TK from India. First it was the patent on wound-healing properties of haldi (turmeric); now patents have been obtained in other countries on hypoglycaemic properties of karela (bitter gourd), brinjal, etc. An important criticism in this context relates to foreigners obtaining patents based on Indian biological materials without acknowledging the source of their knowledge or sharing the benefits. There is also the view that the TRIPS Agreement is aiding the exploitation of biodiversity by privatizing biodiversity expressed in life forms and knowledge.

A. **Neem:** A tree legendary to India has been used as a biopesticide and medicine in India for centuries. Ancient Indian Ayurvedic texts have described the Neem tree and its medicinal healing properties as far back as 5000 BC The European patent office (EPO) revoke in its entirety patent number 436257 which had been granted to the United States of America. Despite Neem's ancient tradition, over 12 US patents were recently taken out Neem-based emulsions and solutions.

B. **Turmeric:** In 1993, the US PTO granted the University of Mississippi Medical Center patent rights over a healing a wound by administering turmeric to a patient afflicted with a wound. But again, Turmeric has been used for centuries in India. Indians grow up with a constant awareness of turmeric, the tuber when dried keeps practically forever. The patent was eventually cancelled in 1998 after reexamination proceedings. But revealed to India and to indigenous societies around the world, again, how easy it was to falsely patent centuries-old traditional knowledge.

Traditional knowledge is being treated as a free input into research and commercial product development. When patents are falsely granted, equitable benefit sharing is not taking place either, while indigenous peoples remain subject to biopiracy and become ever more marginalized in the process. Recently amended patent law of ours contains provisions for mandatory disclosure of source and geographical origin of the biological material used in the invention while applying for patents in India. Provisions have also been incorporated to include non-disclosure or wrongful disclosure of the same as grounds for opposition and for revocation of the patents, if granted. To protect traditional knowledge from being patented, provisions have also been incorporated in the law to include anticipation of invention by available local knowledge including oral knowledge, as one of the grounds for opposition as also for revocation of patent. In order to further strengthen these

provisions, a new provision has been added to exclude innovations which are basically traditional or aggregation or duplication of known properties of traditionally known component or components from being patented. The view has been expressed that the granting to patents on traditional knowledge already in the public domain or without the content of indigenous peoples and local communities amount to unauthorized appropriation of the knowledge. It has been said that this occur particularly in the case where members do not appropriate definition of the criteria for penetrability or appropriate procedure. It has been said that the patent system is not working well enough in connection with the granting of patent covering traditional knowledge have been referred to definition of prior art used to determine wheather a claimed invitation meets the novelty stranded for patentability. The second concern the adequacy of the information on prior art available to patent examiners.

India as a free nation has not only updated some earlier legislations (e.g. Patents and Designs Act 1911) but has also enacted new laws aimed at protection of IPRs at the national as well as international level. India is one of the few countries in the world who has had a number of legislations on IPR protection. The Acts which have been enacted and are in force are: the Copyright Act, 1957, The Patents Act, 1970 (as amended in 2005), The Trademarks Act, 1999, The Geographical Indications of Goods (Registration and Protection) Act, 1999, the Designs Act, 2000, The Protection of Plant Varieties and Farmer's Right Act, 2001 and Biological Diversity Act, 2002. In the year 2008, India came out with Traditional Knowledge Digital Library (TKDL) in an effort to protect her traditional knowledge and traditional cultural expression. Also, the facility of electronic filing (in short, e-filing) of applications has been introduced since July, 2007 to bring the Indian Intellectual Property Regime in line with international requirements. Further, the Indian Innovation Bill, 2008; the Protection and Utilization of Public Funded Intellectual Property Bill, 2008; and the Copyright (Amendment)

Bill, 2010 are likely to give more strength to the IPR regime in India. If the Government is of the opinion that the applicant is seeking grant of patent for an invention which is important with viewpoint of safety or defense of the country, the Government may direct the person authorized to keep the application and all documents pertinent thereto as a secret until after such time as the Government deems fit.

279

1. India is rich in genetic resources and associated traditional knowledge and has been identified as one of the countries with mega biodiversity. Traditional knowledge has been used for centuries by Indian indigenous and local communities and has been the mainstay of their existence, especially in key sectors of food and health. In addition, TK also plays a vital role in the conservation of biodiversity in the country. For instance, some tribal populations in India, like the Garo and Khasi tribes of Northeastern India have created "sacred groves" in forest areas that help to conserve the forest and its inhabitants. Similarly the Onges of the little Andaman Island in the Andaman and Nicobars and the Cholanaickan tribals of Kerala have devised elaborate social procedures to conserve and sustainably exploit natural resources.

2. India, apart from her well-endowed biological resources, is also home to rich traditions of crafts. The Constitution of India does not directly address the issue of protection of traditional knowledge.

TK Documentation and Traditional Medicinal Knowledge

Documentation of traditional knowledge is one of the defensive forms of protection that has received a fair amount of attention in recent years. To tide over the problem of the open and freely accessible "public domain" and the concomitant instances of "poaching" on traditional knowledge without permission or benefit documentation, mostly in digital format has been seriously considered in recent years.

Case Study of Curcuma and Neem

Turmeric (*Curcuma longa* Linn): The rhizomes of turmeric are used as a spice for flavouring Indian cooking. It also has properties that make it an effective ingredient in medicines, cosmetics and as dyed. As a medicine, it has been traditionally used for centuries to heal wounds and rashes. In 1995, two expatriate Indians at the University of Mississippi Medical Centre were granted a US Patent (no. 5,401, 5045) on use of turmeric on wound healing. The Council of Scientific and Industrial Research (CSIR), India, New Delhi filed a re-examination case with the USPTO challenging the patent on the grounds of existing prior art. CSIR argued that turmeric has been used for thousands of years for healing wounds and rashes and therefore its medicinal use was not a novel invention. Their claim was supported by documentary evidence of traditional knowledge, including ancient Sanskrit text and a paper published in 1953 in the journal of the Indian Medical Association. Despite an appeal by the patent holders, the UPSTO upheld the CSIR objections and cancelled the patent. The turmeric case was a landmark judgment case as it was for the first.

Neem (*Azarirachta indica.*): Neem extracts can be used against hundreds of pests and fungal diseases that attach food crops; the oil extracted from its seed can be used to cure cold and flu; and mixed in soap, it provides relief from malaria, skin diseases and even meningitis. In 1994, European Patent Office (EPO) granted a patent (EPO Patent no. 436257) to use US Corporation WR Grace Company and US Department of Agriculture for a method for controlling fungi on plants by the aid of hydrophobic extracted Neem oil. In 1995, a group of international non-governmental organizations (NGOs) and representatives of Indian farmers filed legal opposition against the patent. They submitted evidence that the fungicidal effect of extracts of Neem seeds had been known and used for centuries in Indian agriculture to protect crops, and therefore was a prior art un-patentable. In 1999, the EPO determined that according to the evidence all features of the present claim were disclosed to the public prior to the patent application and the patent was not considered to involve an inventive step. The patent granted on Neem was revoked by the EPO in May 2000. EPO, in March 2006, rejected the challenge made in 2001 by the US Department of Agriculture and the chemicals multinational, WR Grace to the EPO's previous decision to cancel their patent on the fungicidal properties of the seeds extracted from the Neem tree.

Neem extracts can be used against hundreds of pests and fungal diseases that attack food crops; the oil extracted from its seeds can be used to cure cold and flu; and mixed in soap, it provides relief from malaria, skin diseases and even meningitis. In 1994, European Patent Office (EPO) granted a patent (EPO patent No.436257) to the US Corporation WR Grace Company and US Department of Agriculture for a method for controlling fungi on plants by the aid of hydrophobic extracted Neem oil. In 1995, a group of international NGOs and representatives of Indian farmers filed legal opposition against the patent. They submitted evidence that the fungicidal effect of extracts of Neem seeds had been known and used for centuries in Indian agriculture to protect crops, and therefore, were unpatentable. In 1999, the EPO determined that according to the evidence all features of the present claim were disclosed to the public prior to the patent application and the patent was not considered to involve an inventive step. The patent granted on was Neem was revoked by the EPO in May 2000.

CONCLUSIONS

Protections of the traditional knowledge of the local and indigenous communities seem to be one of the most contentious and complicated issue. The historical development of the protection of intellectual property in the wake of individual private property rights, pushed, the traditional knowledge and the innovative practice based on it outside the purview of the formal intellectual property protection regime. The new millennium poses serious challenge to the international legal community to set new international legal standard for tracking the problem of intellectual property protection throw open by the technology developments. Traditional knowledge was treated as knowledge in the public demeans for free exploitation without showing any respect or concern for the effort taken by the communities to preserve and promote the same. The new technological developments, particularly in biotechnology, clearly demonstrate the significance and usefulness of traditional knowledge for the development of new product of commercial importance. Traditional knowledge (TK) associated with the biological resources is the knowledge about a country's biodiversity; the applied uses and applications of biological resources and the prevalent practices. TK has direct correlation with the biodiversity of the country. It is an intangible component of the resource itself. TK has the potential of being transformed into commercial opportunity, providing useful leads for development of products and processes. Hence, a share of benefits must accrue to creators and holders of TK. TK valuable in global economy, Important for biotechnology based industries industry and agriculture, traditional societies depend on it for their food and healthcare needs, important for conservation and sustainable development of environment and management of biodiversity, Food security of the country is linked to protection of TK. Need to enable tribal communities to harness TK for their economic uplift and growth fast mobility of tribal societies.

11 Regulatory Issues

- Regulations in India (ASU DTAB, ASU DCC),
- Good Manufacturing Practices
- Regulation of manufacture of ASU drugs— Schedule Z of Drugs and Cosmetics Act for ASU drugs.

INTRODUCTION

According to **Drugs and Cosmetics Act** 'Ayur- vedic, Siddha or Unani drug' includes all medicines intended for internal or external use or in the diagnosis, treatment, mitigation or prevention of disease or disorder in human beings or animals, and manufactured exclusively in accordance with the formulae described in the authoritative books of Ayurvedic, Siddha and Unani Tibb systems of medicine, specified in the First Schedule.

Regulation of Manufacture of ASU Drugs— Schedule Z of Drugs and Cosmetics Act for ASU Drugs

Since Vedic age, herbal medicines are being used in India as well as documented in Rigveda. As per *Charak Samhita* people initially used traditional herbs from their experience and gradually a group of experts called apothecaries evolved to practice and explain the use of herbal medicines.

In India, herbal medicines are being used in Ayurveda, Siddha, and Unani and Homeopathic system of medicines. Ayurvedic system is being practiced since 6000 BC, whereas the modern system of medicines started since 1800 AD. Though Ayurveda has undergone many changes in the course of its long history, it still remains the mainstay of medical relief to a large section of population of the nation. In India these systems were popular due to

varied agro climatic zones and because of the experience and abundant availability of plants. We have around 45,000 species of plants, out of which 15,000–20,000 plants have proven to have medicinal value. The traditional system utilizes around 7,000–7,500 species in its formulations. Ayurveda uses 2000, Unani 1000, Siddha 1300, Tibetan 500 and 200 varieties in the modern medicine. A lot of big pharma companies started to turn aside their business strategy by investing large amount of finance in research and manufacturing of herbal medicines. According to the World Bank report herbal medicine has a global market of US $ 80–100 billion and this market is expected to reach US $2500 billion by the year 2010 and US$5 trillion by the year 2050. So now government institutions are also emphasizing on research on herbal medicines. The Indian herbal drug market is about $1 billion and the export of herbal crude extract is about $80 million. We have about 7800 manufacturing units engaged in manufacturing of herbal drugs in India, which are consuming 200 tons of herbs annually.

At the beginning there was no regulation for maintaining the quality of herbal medicines and the practitioners have faith on their experience on proper identification of the plant. In view of the new trend in Ayurvedic pharmaceutical field, Government of India considered it expedient to utilize the existing Drugs and Cosmetics Act 1940 and Drugs and Cosmetic

Table 11.1: Regulatory aspects of natural products based on Drugs and Cosmetics Act of India

Section	Item	Criteria
33 E	Misbranded drugs	**ASU drugs are considered to be misbranded** • If it so coloured coated or polished that damage is concealed or drugs are made to better or greater therapeutic value than it really is. • Not labelled in prescribed manner. • Label or container accompanying drug bears any misleading or false claim.
33EE	Adulterated drugs	**ASU drugs are deemed to be adulterated** • if it consists, in whole or in part, of any filthy, putrid or decomposed substance; or • if it has been prepared, packed or stored under insanitary conditions whereby it may have been contaminated with filth or whereby it may have been rendered injurious to health; or • if its container is composed, in whole or in part, of any poisonous or deleterious substance which may render the contents injurious to health; or • if it bears or contains, for purposes of colouring only, a colour other than one which is prescribed; or • If it contains any harmful or toxic substance which may render it injurious to health; or if any substance has been mixed therewith so as to reduce its quality or strength.
33EEA	Spurious drugs	**33EEA ASU drugs are deemed to be spurious** • if it is sold, or offered or exhibited for sale, under a name which belongs to another drug; or • if it is an imitation of, or is a substitute for, another drug or resembles another drug in a manner likely to deceive, or bears upon it or upon its label or container the name of another drug, unless it is plainly and conspicuously marked so as to reveal its true character and its lack of identity with such other drug; or • if the label or container bears the name of an individual or company purporting to be the manufacturer of the drug, which individual or company is fictitious or does not exist; or • if it has been substituted wholly or in part by any other drug or substance; or • if it purports to be the product of a manufacturer of whom it is not truly a product.
33EEB	Regulation of manufacture for sale of ASU drugs	No person shall manufacture for sale or distribution, Ayurvedic, Siddha or Unani drug except in accordance with prescribed standards

33EEC	Prohibition of manufacture and sale of certain ASU drug	a. Manufacture for sale or for distribution
		  i. Any misbranded, adulterated or spurious Ayurvedic, Siddha or Unani drugs;
		  ii. Any patent or proprietary medicine, unless there is displayed in the prescribed manner on the label or container there of the true list of all the ingredients contained in it; and
		  iii. Any Ayurvedic, Siddha or Unani drug in contravention of any of the provisions of this Chapter or any rule made thereunder;

Contd.

Table 11.1: Regulatory aspects of natural products based on Drugs and Cosmetics Act of India (*Contd.*)

Section	Item	Criteria
		b. Sell, stock or exhibit or offer for sale or distribute, any Ayurvedic, Siddha or Unani drug which has been manufactured in contravention of any of the provisions of this Act, or any rule made thereunder;
		c. Manufacture for sale or for distribution, any Ayurvedic, Siddha or Unani drug, except under, and in accordance with the conditions of, a licence issued for such purpose
33EED	Power of Central Government to prohibit manufacture of ASU drugs in public interest	Central government can prohibit manufacture of ASU if: • Drug involve any risk to human beings or animals • Drug does not have the therapeutic value claimed
33F	Government analysts	Central or state government can appoint any person with the prescribed qualification and do not have any financial interest in ASU drug
33G	Inspectors	Central or state government can appoint any person with the prescribed qualification and do not have any financial interest in ASU drug
33I	Penalty for manufacture, sale, etc, of Ayurvedic, Siddha or Unani drug	Manufactures for sale or for distribution of any ASU drugs deemed to be adulterated or without a valid licence as required
33J	Penalty for subsequent offences	Shall be punishable with imprisonment for a term not less than two years but which may extend to six years and with fine not less than 5000 INR
33K	Confiscation	Any person convicted under the Act, the respective stock of ASU drug can be confiscated
33M	Cognizance of offences	• No prosecution under this Chapter shall be instituted except by an Inspector • No court inferior to that of a [Metropolitan Magistrate] or of a [Judicial Magistrate] of the first class shall try an offence punishable under this Chapter
33N	Power of Central Government to make rules	The Central Government may, after consultation with, or on the recommendation of, the Board and after previous publication by notification in the Official Gazette, make rules for the purpose of giving effect to the provisions of this Chapter:
153	Application for licence to manufacture Ayurvedic (including Siddha) or Unani drugs	An application for the grant or renewal of a licence to manufacture for sale any ASU drugs shall be made in Form 24-D to the Licensing Authority along with a fee of rupees sixty
154	Form of licence to manufacture Ayurvedic (including Siddha) or Unani drugs	Subject to the conditions of rule 157 being fulfilled, a licence to manufacture for sale any ASU drugs shall be issued in Form 25-D
153-A	Loan Licence	An application for the grant of renewal of a loan licence to manu-facture for sale of any ASU drugs shall be made in Form 25-E to the Licensing Authority along with a fee of rupees thirty
155 B	Certificate of award of GMP of Ayurveda, Siddha and Unani Drugs	Shall be issued to licensees who comply with the requirements of GMP of ASU drugs as laid down in Schedule T
168	Standards to be complied with in manufacture for sale or for distribution of Ayurvedic, Siddha and Unani Drugs	**Single drugs:** The standards for identity, purity and strength as given in editions of Ayurvedic Pharmacopoeia of India **Asavas and Arishtas:** The upper limit of alcohol as self-generated alcohol should not exceed 12% v/v

Rules 1945. This act initially prescribed the standards of Ayurvedic, Siddha and Unani medicines and laid down rules and regulation on manufacturing.

The Act was accordingly amended in 1964, to ensure only a limited control over the production and sale of these medicines, namely:

I. The manufacture should be carried under prescribed hygienic conditions, under supervision of a person having a prescribed qualification;

II. The raw materials used in the preparation of drugs should be genuine and properly identified and

III. The formula or the true list of all the ingredients, contained in the drugs, should be displayed on the label of every container.

Ever since independence in 1947 there has been a sustained policy support for the development of Indian Systems of Medicine and Homeopathy, Government has taken a number of legislative and administrative measures to regulate the manufacture and sale of Ayurveda, Siddha and Unani (ASU) drugs. There is a separate Chapter IVA which regulates the manufacture and sale of ASU medicines in the Drugs and Cosmetics Act, 1940 Chapter IVA of the Indian Drugs and Cosmetics Act, 1940 has provisions for regulation of manufacture and sale of ASU drugs, packaging and labelling of ASU drugs for domestic use and export and penalty for manufacture and sale of ASU drugs in contravention of these rules and for misbranded, adulterated and spurious ASU drugs.

The Good Manufacturing Practices for ASU Drugs as described in Rule 157 of Drugs and Cosmetics Rules 1945 with conditions as specified in Schedule T/GMP are to ensure that:

I. Raw materials used in the manufacture of drugs are authentic, of prescribed quality and are free from contamination

II. The manufacturing process as has been prescribed to maintain the standards

III. Adequate quality control measures are adopted

IV. The manufactured drug which is released for sale is of acceptable quality

V. To achieve the objectives listed above, each licensee shall evolve methodology and procedures for following the prescribed process of manufacture of drugs which should be documented as a manual and kept for reference and inspection. However, under IMCC Act, 1970 registered Vaidyas, Siddhas and Hakeems who prepare medicines on their own to dispense to their patients and not selling such drugs in the market are exempted from the purview of Good manufacturing Practice (GMP).

The Act is enforced through the State Drug Licensing and Drug Control Authorities that a separate Ayurveda, Siddha and Unani Technical Advisory Board (ASU DTAB) has been constituted by the Central Government.

1. It comprises officials and nominees of Central Government, Pharmacogonists, Phytochemists and Members of the Ayurveda Pharmacopoeia Committee, Siddha Pharmacopoeia Committee and Unani Pharmacopoeia Committee and representatives of teachers, practitioners and ASU Drugs industry nominated by the Central Government to advise the Central and State Governments on technical matters relating to regulation of ASU drugs.

2. The Central Government has also constituted a Ayurveda, Siddha and Unani Drugs Consultative Committee (ASU-DCC) under the Act to advise the Central and State Governments and the ASUDTAB on any matter for the purpose of securing uniformity thoughout India in the administration of Drugs and Cosmetics Act, 1940 as it relates to ASU drugs.

3. Periodic meetings of these statutory bodies are held and all technical and regulatory issues arising out the enforcement of Chapter IVA of the Drugs and Cosmetics Act, 1940 relating to ASU drugs are referred to these bodies for advising the Central and State Governments.

4. A specific law, the Drugs and Magic Remedies Act, 1954, is also in place for prevention of objectionable advertisements

and publicity relating to certain drugs and magic remedies for treatment of certain identified diseases and disorders laying down of pharmacopoeial standards of drugs are mandatory as per Drugs and Cosmetics Act, which was amended in 1964 to bring under its purview Ayurveda, Siddha and Unani drugs.

5. For implementation of the Act and Rules thereunder, and as a first step the Pharmacopoeial Laboratory of Indian Medicine (PLIM) was set up in 1970 and the Homoeopathic Pharmacopoeial Laboratory (HPL) was set up in 1975 to facilitate drug standardization and testing of ASU drugs.

6. In addition 13 other reputed laboratories have been engaged to lay down pharmacopoeial standards and preparation of monographs and for evolving Standard Operating Procedures (SOPs) for ASU drugs Pharmacopoeial Committees have been constituted separately for ASU systems.

It is the responsibility of these Committees to lay down standards of quality, purity and strength of drugs and approve drug formularies. So far, 326 monographs of Ayurveda drugs in 4 volumes, 45 of Unani drugs, 916 of Homeopathic drugs have been published. Another 98 monographs on Ayurveda drugs are due for publication very soon. Formularies of Ayurveda, Siddha and Unani containing 636, 248 and 745 multi-ingredient classical formulations respectively have been published to facilitate manufacture of drugs with uniform composition and manufacturing procedures.

Parameters adopted for Quality control and Standardization Ayurveda, Siddha and Unani drugs which are mainly poly-herbal/herbo-mineral preparations are very different from synthetic molecules of the allopathic system which are produced under controlled laboratory conditions. Much depends on the quality and availability of raw materials of botanical origin. Keeping this in view, the National Medicinal Plants Board (NMPB) was established in the year 2000 with the objective of *in situ* conservation and *ex situ* cultivation

of quality medicinal plant raw materials. In view of environmental pollution the NMPB is examining how best to adopt Good Agricultural and Collection Practices for collection and cultivation of medicinal plants for ensuring quality raw material for ASU medicines. As a large number of our forest dwellers and small landholders are engaged in collection and cultivation, these norms have to be adopted in a way that livelihood is not affected.

Both traditional and modern parameters are used for quality testing and standardization of raw materials as well as finished products. Many methods from organoleptic standardization of drugs, chemical analysis, biological assaying for testing of heavy metals, pesticides and microbial load have been developed for quality control and standardi￼tion of ASU drugs. An effort has been made ￼ include Chromatographic fingerprint profile as a supplementary to Ayurvedic Pharmacopoeia Identification of active therapeutic ingredients and marker compounds with reference to which ASU drugs can be standardized are still evolving and all these parameters are being added to the ASU pharmacopoeia Pharmacopoeial Laboratories and laboratories of Central Council for Research in Ayurveda and Siddha (CCRAS), Central Council for Research in Unani Medicine (CCRUM), various laboratories of Council for Scientific and Industrial Research (CSIR) and private sector institutions and laboratories are doing a commendable job in evolving and laying down safety and quality standards for poly-herbal/herbo-mineral preparations including plant extracts. It needs to be emphasised that the work of quality control and standardization of herbal/herbo-mineral drugs is much more complex and standards are constantly evolving and this is not only true for ASU drugs, it is equally so in other traditional systems of medicine all over the world. While there is a need to speed up this work and for streamlining regulatory mechanism for ASU drugs, it will be inappropriate to term Ayurveda, Siddha and Unani drugs industry as being completely unregulated. It needs to be kept in mind that humanity has survived on traditional medicinal knowledge for thousands of years.

Standards of Drugs as per Existing Legislature of India

Drugs and Cosmetics Act 1940 contains standards of medicines and individual monographs are prescribed in the respective Pharmacopoeias.

The Government of India has released various Pharmacopoeia and Standard text which is given below:

1. Four volumes of Ayurvedic Pharmacopoeia consisting standards of 326 drugs, which is inadequate in comparison to the number of herbs used in the Ayurvedic system of medicines.
2. Herbal Pharmacopoeia was published having standards of 52 drugs. Unfortunately neither the herbal products nor the herbal Pharmacopoeias have any statutory standing in our country.
3. Some herbal drugs are also marketed as food or nutritional supplements, with medicinal claims. Keeping this problem in mind, status of herbal products was surveyed through different sources including pharmacopoeias of different countries.
4. In some countries herbal products are considered as drugs, e.g. China, UK, Canada, Germany, etc. while some countries do not grant herbal products, the status of drugs, e.g. USA, the Netherlands, etc. They consider it as nutritional supplements, and have framed definite legislation for it, e.g. USA.
5. In India there are some gray areas in case of status of herbal drugs and there exists no definite policies about food supplements. Recently Government of India has published Food Safety Act to resolve this problem.

As per the experts this said Act has not been implemented and failed to resolve the problem sometimes mere mentioning of a drug in some textbooks is considered sufficient as per existing legislature, whereas the texts are not properly defined.

Standards of Ayurvedic Drugs

Only four volumes of **Ayurvedic Pharmacopoeia** containing monographs of about 326 herbs have been published, which is insufficient with reference to the huge number of herbs used in the Ayurvedic System of Medicines.

There are many limitations of the available standards for ayurvedic drugs:

1. The monographs cover only a few parameters, which are considered to be quite inadequate for standardization.
2. Monographs of herbs in British Herbal Pharmacopoeia consist of detailed chemical characterization involving TLC, GC and PC electrophoresis, whereas no such modern methods are prescribed in the ayurvedic pharmacopoeia.
3. No standards for combination products are prescribed in statute, except asavas and aristas. Only alcohol content of these two products is given in D and C Act.
4. Minimum pharmacological characterization is required, which is quite inadequate, compared to characterization specified by other Pharmacopoeias.

All of these books are old texts except the Ayurvedic Formulary of India (Part I) and Ayurvedic Pharmacopoeia of India. There is ample scope of misuse of this provision, as 55 books out of 57 are not properly defined in the legislature.

Standards of Siddha Drugs

The Government of India has published Siddha Formulary of India (Part I). The Drugs Act only mention of manufacturing process in a list of 30 books. Amongst these 30 books, 29 are old texts.

Standards of Unani Tibetan System of Drugs

The Government of India has published National Formulary of Unani Medicine (Part I). The Drugs Act mere mentioning of manufacturing process in a list of 13 books allows production of Unani and Tibetan drugs. Amongst these 13 books, 12 are old texts.

Schedule T For Good Manufacturing Practice

To manufacture good quality ayurvedic, siddha and unani medicines good manufacturing practices have been made mandatory by incorporation of revised Schedule T in the year of 2003.

Important features of Schedule T are as follows:

The various stringent parameters needed to be considered for manufacture of medicines include:

1. Raw materials to be used in must be authentic, of prescribed quality and free from contamination.
2. Manufacturing process is as prescribed to maintain the standard.
3. Adequate quality control measures to be adopted.
4. Drugs released for sale shall be of acceptable quality.
5. To achieve the objectives listed above, the firm is required to maintain the following conditions stringently:
   - Premises should be well designed with sufficient space
   - Proper machineries require to be provided
   - Quality control laboratory require to be provided with required instruments
   - Well-qualified personnels are required in quality control laboratory.
   - Proper methodology and procedures for manufacturing.
   - Proper documentation to be maintained and kept for reference and inspection.

Standards of Homoeopathic Medicines

Standard of homeopathic medicines has been prescribed in second schedule of the Drugs and Cosmetics Act, 1940. The drugs included in homoeopathic pharmacopoeia of India need to compile with various standards of identity, purity and strength specified in Homeopathic Pharmacopoeia of India.

Schedule M1: In order to ensure proper quality of homeopathic medicines manufacture, Schedule M1 was introduced in 1987 specifying requirement of technical staff, manufacturing plants, testing equipment, etc. Experts feel that this is quite inadequate in this age of science.

The Government of India has taken an initiative to implement Good Manufacturing Practices (GMP) and a guideline has already been published, which is effective from 2nd October 2008. This guideline is more detailed and prescribed minimum requirement of manufacturing areas, equipment, minimum qualification required for the personnel engaged in manufacturing and quality control, documents to be maintained, etc for manufacturing quality medicines

Patent Protection To Be Exploited Fully

The Countries like China, Russia, Europe Japan and even USA have marched ahead with numerous international patents on medicinal plants but unfortunately despite of huge natural wealth, India has not shown assuring performance in the field of the global herbal market. Need of the hour is that if India can fully exploit its natural resources, skilled manpower and potential traditional knowledge and couple them with its technical powers then India can march ahead to compete with global players by partly substituting costly modern medicines with modern herbal drugs.

It is unfortunate that some of the Indian products have been patented by different companies which are being used in India since a long time like—Neem, Amla, Kurchi, Sarpagandha, Calendula, Sankhapushpi, Jamun, Anar, Bagbherenda, Karela.

Fortunately, Government of India has taken initiative to challenge the patent granted on turmeric to an US University and as a result US patent (No 5,401,504) on the use of turmeric (Curcuma longa L, Zingiberaceae) for healing was invalidated because it was not a novel invention. This is an encouraging victory for Indian activists campaigning to protect indigenous wisdom Under World Trade Organisation (WTO) rules, patents are provided for inventions that qualify for their novelty, non-obviousness, and utility. The turmeric patent failed to satisfy the criteria of novelty as turmeric paste has been used to treat wounds and stomach infections for centuries by Indians. The turmeric patent was just one of the hundreds that the developed countries have claimed by ignoring indigenous and existing knowledge.

Good Manufacturing Practices

AYUSH directs all the State Drug Licensing Authorities to take action against the defaulting ASU drug manufacturers for revocation of their licenses under Rules 157, 158 and 159 of the Drugs and Cosmetics Rules, 1945 for failure to comply with the Good Manufacturing Practices notified under Schedule 'T' of the Drugs and Cosmetics Rules, 1945 AYUSH directs the State Licensing Authorities of ASU drugs to ensure full compliance by all ASU drug manufacturers of the provisions of Rule 161 (1) and (2) relating to displaying on the label of the container or package of an Ayurveda, Siddha and Unani drug, the true list of all the ingredients (official and botanical names) used in the manufacture of the preparation together with the quantity of each of the ingredients incorporated therein. In case all the ingredients cannot be mentioned on the label because of their large number the same shall be indicated in the leaflet to be inserted in the package. Further that the container of a medicine shall conspicuously display the words 'Caution to be taken under medical supervision' if the list of ingredients contains a substance specified in Schedule E(1) of the Drugs and Cosmetics Rules, 1945.

The following major initiatives have been taken by the Central Government for ensuring safety and quality control of ASU drugs:

i. Good Manufacturing Practices (GMP) for ASU drugs were notified on 23rd June, 2000 under Schedule T of the Indian Drugs and Cosmetics Act, 1940 and Rules, 1945 which seeks mandatory compliance from the licensed manufacturers with regard to raw materials, manufacturing area, manufacturing processes, record keeping, storage of raw materials and finished products and quality testing State Governments and all State Licensing Authorities have been advised vide Department of AYUSH order dtd 13102005 to ensure strict compliance of GMP by ASU drugs manufactures and cancel the license of non-GMP compliant units.

ii. Provisions relating to proper labelling, packing and conspicuous display of all the ingredients along with the quantities contained in the formulations on the label/container or a leaflet inserted inside the container, have been reiterated for compliance by an order issued by the Department of AYUSH on 10102005 for strict compliance by State Drug Controllers/Licensing Authorities.

iii. To address domestic as well as international concerns on presence of heavy metals in ASU drugs exporters of purely herbal ASU drugs have been directed to either conspicuously display on the container of purely herbal ASU drugs words 'heavy metals within permissible limits' or furnish the above certificate from an appropriately equipped in-house laboratories or any other approved laboratories along with other consignment papers wef 112006. Mandatory testing for heavy metals on purely herbal ASU drugs will also be extended for sale of purely herbal ASU drugs within the country in phases keeping in view the testing infrastructure within the country.

iv. The issue of safety of herbo-mineral/herbo-metallic Bhasmas/Compounds is also being addressed by the Central Government. A project has been sanctioned for chemical analysis and safety studies of eight most widely used Rasaushadhis/Bhasmas, namely Kajjali, Rasmanikya, Nag Bhasma, Rasasindoor, Basantkusumkar Ras, Arogyavardhini Vati, Mahayograj Guggul and Mahalaxmi Vilas Ras by CSIR laboratories under the Golden Triangle Project within a time frame of 18 months.

v. Use of permissible excipients, preservatives for increasing the shelf-life of ASU drugs has been notified Draft rules for expiry date of ASU drugs have also been published in November, 2005 and a consultation process is on for finalizing these rules.

vi. Certain guidelines have also been issued to State Licensing Authorities with a view to curb the mushroom growth of irrational ASU combinations through the patent and proprietary route.

As mentioned above the issues concerning quality control and standardization of ASU drugs are very complex and very different from those concerning regulation of synthetic molecules produced under controlled laboratory conditions. This is a problem which is being faced by the regulators of traditional systems of medicine all over the world. Scientific methods and techniques for standardization and quality control of herbal/herbo-mineral drugs are constantly evolving all over the world. Regulators have to keep pace with the development taking place in the field of botany, phyto-chemistry, bio-chemistry apart from public and private sector research institutions. ASU drug industry itself is making an important contribution in the field of evolving methods and standards for drug standardization and quality control. Many private sector companies in India have made a notable contribution in the field of evolving standards and preparation of monographs on herbal plant extracts. Ministry of Health and Family Welfare, Department of AYUSH, apart from laying down pharmacopoeial standards and issuing guidelines under the Drugs and Cosmetics Act and rules from time to time, has initiated a process of consultation between Ayurveda, Siddha and Unani experts and experts in the field of Botany, Phytochemistry, Bio-chemistry and representatives of ASU drugs industry for making the regulatory framework responsive to the developments in the field of science and technology. It is as a result of these measures that use of techniques like Chromatographic fingerprint profiles and use of active therapeutic ingredients and marker compounds for standardization and quality control of herbal and herbo-mineral preparations are becoming popular in the ASU drugs industry. The Department of AYUSH will, in consultation with all concerned, come out with more detailed guidelines for licensing of classical and patent and proprietary ASU medicines based on a product dossier system very shortly with a view to further improve and strengthen the licensing framework for ASU drugs.

The department would like to reiterate that there are regulatory mechanisms in place for regulating standardization and quality control of ASU drugs and the regulatory framework is evolving in response to the developments in the field of science and technology. However, the general public should use ASU medicines as far as possible under medical supervision and they should be purchased on cash memos after proper verification of the ingredients mentioned on the label or on the leaflet inserted inside the container. In case of doubt, they should consult a qualified ayurveda/siddha/unani practitioner and any contravention with the labelling provisions should be brought to the notice of the district and state health authorities and the department. ASU drug industry associations should also motivate their members to move in the direction of self-regulation and self-certification and as a first step, start voluntarily printing indications and contra-indications of every formulation either on the label/container or in a leaflet to be inserted in the container for educating the general public regarding their products.

Regulatory Requirements for Establishing Herbal Drug Industry

☞ General Introduction to Herbal Industry

☞ Schedule T—Good Manufacturing Practices of Indian Systems of Medicine

12 | General Introduction to Herbal Industry

- Herbal drugs industry: Present scope and future prospects.
- A brief account of plant-based industries and institutions involved in work on medicinal and aromatic plants in India.

HERBAL DRUGS INDUSTRY: PRESENT SCOPE AND FUTURE PROSPECTS (FIG. 12.1)

According to reports of global industry analysts, the global herbal supplements and remedies market is forecast to reach $107 billion by the year 2017, spurred by growing aging population and increasing consumer awareness about general health and well being. According to the World Health Organization (WHO), more than 120 active compounds isolated from higher plants are widely used in modern allopathic medicine today and 80 per cent of them show a positive co-relation between their modern therapeutic use and the traditional use of the plants from which they are

derived. At least 7,000 medicinal compounds derived from plants, the ingredients of herbal medicine, are included in the modern pharmacopoeia of drugs.

Today, one-fourth of the world population depends on traditional medicines. Despite the introduction of antibiotics since the 1940s, even 80 per cent of the population today relies on indigenous medicinal plants and the drugs. It is estimated that the global traditional medicine market is growing at the rate of 7–15 per cent annually. The medicinal plant value is about ₹ 5000 crores in India and it is estimated that the country exports about ₹ 550 crore worth of herbal drugs. But with the rich and diverse botanical resources in our country,

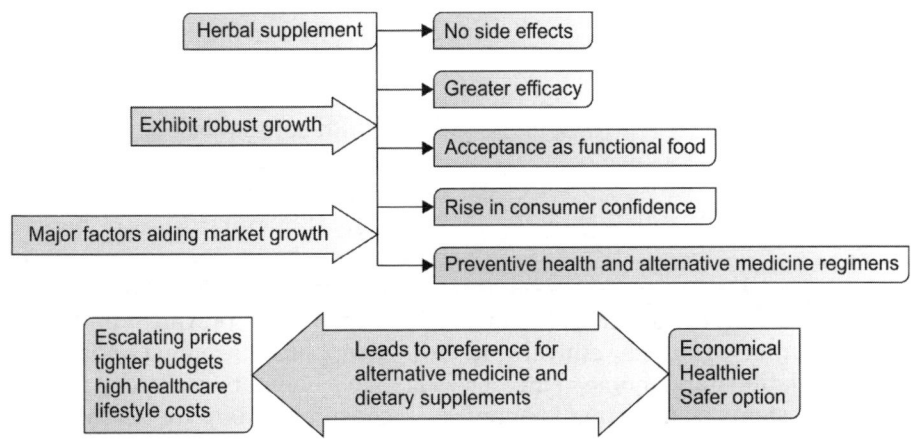

Fig. 12.1: Herbal drugs industry: Present scope and future prospects

this is not an impressive export performance considering the worldwide herbal market worth US 60 billion dollars.

SCENARIO OF INDIAN HERBAL TRADE IN WORLD

The utilization of herbal drugs is on the flow and the market is growing step by step. The annual turnover of the Indian herbal medicinal industry is about ₹ 2,300 crore as against the pharmaceutical industry's turnover of ₹ 14,500 crores with a growth rate of 15 percent. The export of medicinal plants and herbs from India has been quite substantial in the last few years. India is the second largest producer of castor seeds in the world, producing about 1,25,000 tonnes per annum. Major pharmaceuticals exported from India are enlisted in Table 12.1.

Table 12.1: Major pharmaceuticals exported from India

S.No.	Major pharmaceuticals exported from India
1.	Isabgol
2.	Opium alkaloids
3.	Senna derivatives
4.	Vinca extract
5.	Cinchona alkaloids
6.	Ipecac root
7.	Solasodine
8.	Diosgenine
9.	Menthol
10.	Gudmar herb
11.	Mehdi leaves
12.	Papain
13.	Rauwolfia
14.	Guar gum
15.	Jasmine oil
16.	Sandal wood oil

The turnover of herbal medicines in India as over-the-counter products, ethical and classical formulations and home remedies of traditional systems of medicine is about $ 1 billion and export of herbal crude extract is about $ 80 million. The herbal drug market in India is about $1 billion.

Market for Herbal Supplements

At the present time, the market for supplements of herbs differs by region based on various factors such as awareness of consumer, availability of product, and its delivery forms, product acceptance, and regional regulations.

⊃ **US and Europe:** Herbal medicines describe biggest share of the pharmaceutical market and covered in the regular medical practice. On the other hand, the market is highly regulated and tough to enter, before mass production companies need to pass through rigorous tests.

⊃ As stated by the market research report on Herbal Supplements and Remedies, **Europe** is the largest region for herbal supplements and remedies and accounting for the largest share of the world market.

⊃ On a global basis **Asia-Pacific and Japan** generate the other important markets for herbal supplements.

⊃ In terms of growth rate, the Asia-Pacific market, led largely by China and India is set to pave the way with the highest CAGR of 10.5% through 2017.

⊃ In countries such as France, Germany, UK and India, herbal supplements along with pharmaceuticals, are sold in drugstores.

Need of Herbal Supplements

The herbals are need of today's scenario, the various category of people need them for various problems such as:

1. The major consumer group women's particularly middle-aged, owing to rising health-consciousness, increased concern for diet, and emphasized towards preventive healthcare. Over the recent years, several manufacturers of herbal supplements have become prominent with various alternative therapies to relieve women from prevalent problems such as menopause, insomnia and hot flashes.

2. Baby boomers represent another major consumer group for herbal supplements and remedies.

3. **Emerging as alternatives to conventional synthetic supplements:** The rising demand

for natural health and food supplements such as fish oils, herbal supplements and other natural offerings such as probiotic.

4. **Substantial increase in the sale of food supplements:** Despite the slow economy, as large numbers of consumers perceive food supplements as an anti-medicinal, low-cost alternative to lead a healthy life style.

5. **Expanding healthy growth rates despite the economic downturn:** Food supplements including omega-3, herbal extracts, multivitamins, probiotics, chondroitin and glucosamine experienced.

6. **Increased demand for herbal and botanical products:** In multi formula and combo packed format, as well as for chewable capsules and tablets. Medicinal plants have been a major source of cure of human diseases since time immemorial.

To establish their products in the global markets, manufacturers in India have to stress on various standardization processes. Standardization starting from production of quality materials, analysis of raw materials for authentication, foreign matter, organoleptic evaluation, microscopic examination, extractive values, chromatographic profiles, pesticides residue, heavy metal detection, etc. Due to the need and emphasis on quality control of drugs, chemical assay, stability, safety assessment, pharmacokinetic studies, etc. have become necessary to establish the products and its efficacy in the global markets. Setting up of high profile and modern R&D quality control labs have become an unavoidable tool for herbal manufacturers to sell their products worldwide.

7. Meet international requirements: In order to supply to international requirements steps for quality in production and products, research and documentation are mandatory. However, to survive in domestic and international market global standards steps have to be taken to establish a good quality control mechanism and to met with various international pharmacopoeias like Ayurvedic Formulary of India, Herbal BP, China, Japanese Herbal, WHO Guidelines on Herbal Medicines.

Issue Faced by Herbal Industries

India is home to an amazing diversity of plants, with over 46 000 plant species recorded to occur there. As long as man has been on the earth herbs have been almost used by man. Early human tribal societies used elements of plants, trees, or shrubs as medicines. Many of these ancient humans chewed on grasses to ease the pain of stomach. Other early human tribes had herbalists who became their specialists when using herbs and plants as medicines. Many of these species are used for medicinal purposes,

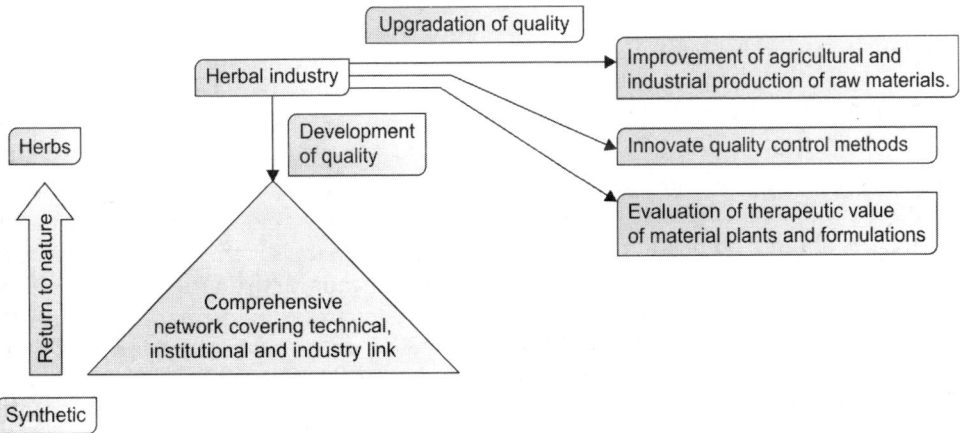

Fig. 12.2: Herbal drugs industry

with approximately 760 known to be harvested from the wild for use by India's large herbal medicine industry.

Herbs are the foundation of modern pharmacology and have been used to make many mainstream medicines. One of the most mainstream medicines made from herbs is aspirin which is derived from white willow back. Morphine is another herbal medicine and is a product of the opium poppy.

Herbs are also used as a method to fight cancer. It has been estimated that up to seventy-five percent of the human population of the earth still use herbal medicine techniques and preparations as either their only source or as a major source of healing. But the country from where the ayurvedic system of medicine originated is lagging far behind in the global herbal medicine market because of insufficient research back-up, lack of awareness and failure to prepare a road map for the production and promotion of quality medicines.

The Government of India had of late started organizing seminars in Europe and the USA but that was not enough. There was need to follow the strategy adopted by China which used acupuncture as a vehicle to promote its indigenous medicine system.

India could do the same by taking advantage of the popularity of yoga by integrating Ayurveda with it. So, Ayurveda could be given a boost only by a coordinated research and development effort involving premiere academic institutions and major pharmaceutical companies.

Laws Regulating Herbal Medicinal Industries in India (Fig. 12.3)

In India the sale of total herbal products is estimated at $1 billion and the export of herbal crude extract is about $80 million, of which 50% is contributed by Ayurvedic classical preparations. Particularly, herbal drugs are imported by several countries for their usage of traditional medicinal preparation from various parts of the country. In India, the traditional herbal medicines, such as ayurveda, siddha, and unani (ASU), are considered safe because of their long history of use. As such, no safety and efficacy studies are required for marketing approval, as per the Drugs and Cosmetics Act of 1940 (DCA). In 1959, the Government of India recognized the traditional Indian system of medicine and amended the Drug and Cosmetic Act to include the drugs derived from traditional Indian system. No product derived from traditional medicine may be manufactured without licence from state drug control authorities. Patent and proprietary medicines derived from the traditional systems must contain ingredients which are mentioned in the recognized books of the above systems as specified in Drug and Cosmetic Act. The government is advised by a special committee and an advisory board for ayurvedic, siddha and unani drugs. Pharmacopoeia committees have been constituted to prepare pharmacopoeias for all these systems.

Certification

As Scheduled for India's domestic markets certification is used as a tool to promote sustainable harvest and trade in medicinal plants. Through the generous support of the Rufford Foundation, initiated in early 2002 research on the use of certification within India was promoted, with a particular emphasis on the application to wild medicinal plant species. The primary focus is on 'independent, third-party certification' schemes, i.e. those where a party independent of those to be certified confirms that certification standards are met.

1. Forest Stewardship Council (FSC) is the best known certification scheme for sustainable forest management. In the 10 years of its existence, FSC has established itself internationally as the main third-party standard-setting and accrediting agency for this type of certification. While thus far primarily applied to timber, FSC includes medicinal plants and other NTFP within its remit. According to FSC, sustainable forest management is 'environmentally appropriate, socially beneficial, and economically viable management of the world's forests'.

2. Organic certification is another type of certification generally recognized both for harvested and wild-grown plants. Such type of certification is generally used in plants used in food and beverages like herbal teas, spices, etc. Other standards used for assessing and ensuring quality of medicinal plants, their possessing and end products include Good Manufacturing Practices (GMP) which was added under 2000 amendment to India's Drug and Cosmetics Act 1940. An international standardization body is ISO (International organization of standardization) whose ISO 9000 (management systems) and ISO 14000 (for environment) had a bearing on medical plants.

EU's Traditional Herbal Medicinal Products Directive (THMPD)

According to EU's Traditional Herbal Medicinal Products Directive (THMPD), companies making herbal products will have to provide clinical data to demonstrate its safety through use of those products within the EU for a minimum of at least 30 years, of which at least evidence of 15 years in an EU country should be there, if it is to be marketed as a non-prescription product. THMPD came into force in 2004, but was given a transition period till April 30, 2011. Under this regulation, all herbal medicinal products are required to obtain an authorization to market within EU. Previously, there was no formal authorization procedure across EU. Consequently, each EU member regulated these types of products at the national level. The only herbal medicines that are exempted from the provisions of THMPD are those unlicensed remedies that are made up for a patient following a consultation with a herbalist.

Role of WHO

In 1991 WHO developed guidelines for the assessment of herbal medicine, and the 6th International Conference of Drug Regulatory Authorities held at Ottawa in the same year ratified the same. The salient features of WHO guidelines are:

1. *Quality assessment:* Crude plant materials or extract plant preparation and finished product.
2. *Stability:* Shelf life.
3. *Safety assessment:* Documentation of safety based on experience and toxicological studies.
4. *Assessment of efficacy:* Documented evidence of traditional use and activity determination (Animals and human).

The legal protection accorded to traditional knowledge (relating ayurveda) in India is through its

➲ Patent laws with the amendment act of 2005, which contain provisions for mandatory disclosure of source and geographical origin of the biological material used in the invention while applying for patents and also allow the composition of a drug to be patented.

➲ The Indian Biodiversity Act 2002, which follows the convention for biological diversity's guidelines regarding benefit sharing.

➲ India has established a central authority 'National Biodiversity Authority' to monitor and control foreign access to Indian biological resources including traditional medicine.

Recommendations

In order to survive in the domestic and international markets, the Indian herbal industry, should take suitable steps to establish a good quality control mechanism, industry should set up a well-established unit which shall work towards excellence in standardization of drugs to meet international requirements in the coming years.

More so, stress on the upgradation of quality is by improvement of various techniques agricultural and industrial production of raw materials, preservation, innovate quality control methods, evaluation of therapeutic value of material plants and formulations.

Further, a comprehensive network covering technical, institutional and industry link for the development of quality of herbal drugs have to be developed industry stockholders.

Basically to address the issue of unsustainable collection of medicinal plants cultivation on private and government lands.

It will result in conservation of MAPs in its natural habitat, along with the improvement of socio-economic status of growers.

In this respect state or central government should provide training facilities in the villages to generate awareness of medicinal plants, their cultivation, harvesting, drying, storage and marketing. Final report on mechanism for sustainable development and promotion of herbal medicinal plants (H& MP).

Secondly, to meet the challenge of conservation of endangered medicinal plants, research institutions and State Forest Departments should make efforts for preserving these plants *in situ* by way of controlling over-exploitation, unscientific harvesting, protecting the plants in reserved forests and by enforcing legal channels so that endangered species do not become extinct. Some co-operative societies based on medicinal plant cultivation and its trading should also be established so that the problem of demand and supply of medicinal plants could be met.

Thirdly, in order to withstand competition in the global market, it is necessary to create a brand image, especially in cosmeceuticals and natural products. Craze among the people for a slim body, fair skin as a fashion is growing considerably. Out of the ₹ 12,000 crores industry, ₹ 700 crores belong to skincare products and ₹ 100 crores for general cosmetics. Over and above current herbal drugs used in cardiovascular is 27%; respiratory 15.3%, digestive 14.4%; hypnotics and sedatives 9.3%; miscellaneous 12%. The perfumery industry is also around ₹ 700 crores. So, the flavourists and perfume experts should face the challenging tasks of creating and developing complex compositions to meet the present and future consumer demand for which it is necessary to set up world standard research and development facilities in this sector. It is also necessary to integrate modern knowledge with traditional knowledge.

Fourthly, the agriculturists involved in herbal industry seldom understand the intricacies of processing the herbs or the certification issues or the type of marketing practices required in India and abroad. This situation has left the agriculturists often confused as they think that they frequently face dead end after the successful cultivation of the herbs. As agriculturists represent the nerve centre of the herbal industry, they need management support to give them confidence and to forge ahead. To meet such requirements, it is necessary to create MBA programmes that would exclusively meet the requirement of the herbal sector, with the herbal MBAs combining within themselves the knowledge about agricultural practices, technology issues, certification procedures, ecological aspects, marketing methodologies and the international regulations. There is need to build up specially trained cadre of management professionals for taking over the leadership role in the herbal industry.

Fifthly, the Eleventh Finance Commission of Orissa recommended that Preservation and cultivation of herbal/medicinal plants can be developed as a means for treatment of unemployment and debility in financial health of the State. India has only 0.5% share in the global export market of medicinal plants. It has been projected by the Planning Commission of India that there is a need to enhance our export by ₹ 5000 crores annually which can generate employment and income to approximately 2 crores families.

The Indian Council of Forestry Research and Education, Dehradun, Regional Research Laboratories, Central Institute of Medicinal and Aromatic Plants, other Universities and certain private research labs of major ayurvedic firms have developed standardized propagation techniques for medicinal herbs.

CONCLUSION

At present there is no straight forward Act on regulations both at national and international level that would favour growth of herbal medicinal industries in India. The EU's directives adversely are going to affect the Indian herbal industries and indirectly in Indian

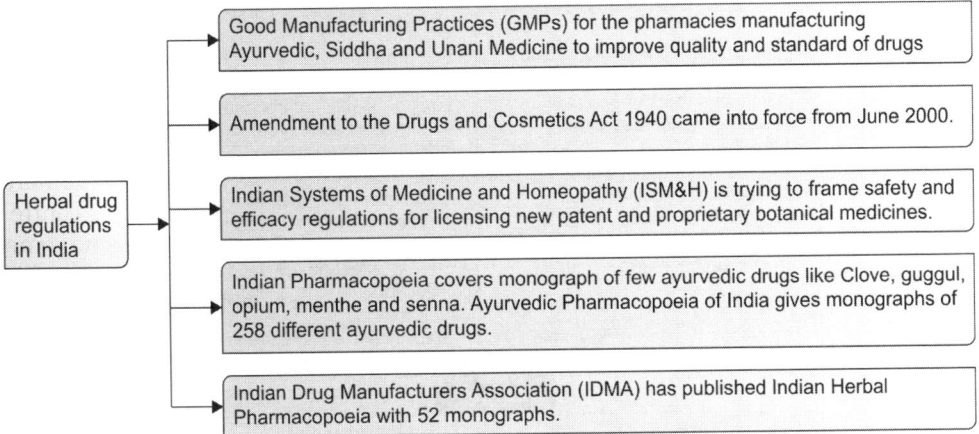

Fig. 12.3: Herbal drugs regulation in India

economy. In such situation the recommendations of different state level committees and workshops organized by states form the basis of future law or amendments to present laws. The proposed solutions to different challenges face by the herbal industries. Such solutions do not water tied may form the matrix of future Indian policies on herbal medicinal industries. India is sitting on a gold mine of well-recorded and well-practiced knowledge of traditional herbal medicine. The basic requirements for gaining entry into developed countries include well-documented traditional use, single-plant medicines, medicinal plants free from pesticides, heavy metals, etc., standardization based on chemical and activity profile and safety and stability. Herbal drug development is possible only through the development of standardized herbal products. The health care systems are going to become more and more expensive, therefore, we have to develop technologies to essentially introduce and integrate herbal medicine system in our health care. There is an enormous scope for India also to emerge as a major player in the global herbal product based medicine. The drug manufactured in accordance with principles of ayurveda, siddha and unani will reach new horizons and make them the best in the world if the quality of the herbal drugs is maintained, efficacy would it self be maintained and then there is nothing to stop them from competing with the modern medicine with added advantages of fewer side effects and lower costs.

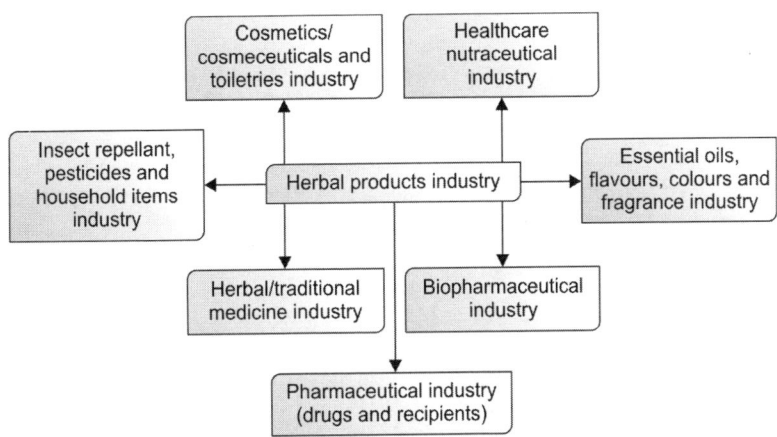

Fig. 12.4: Scope of herbal industry

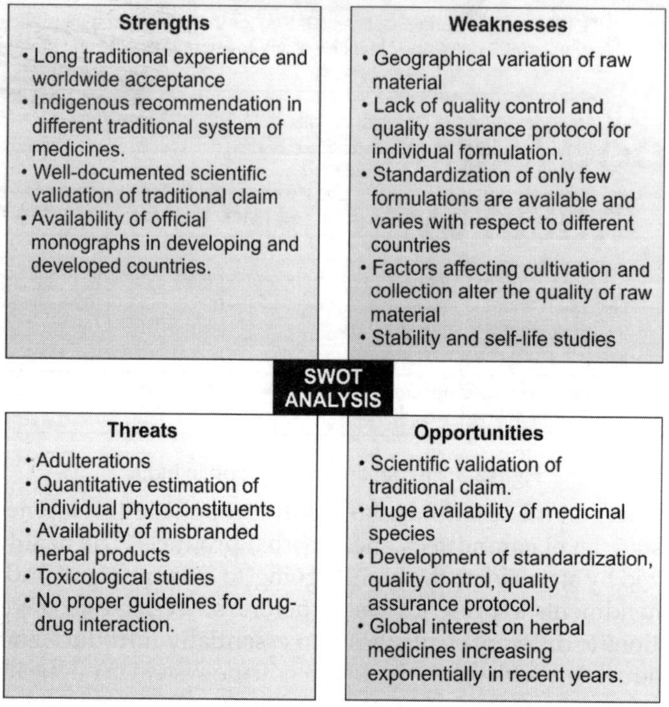

Strengths	Weaknesses
• Long traditional experience and worldwide acceptance • Indigenous recommendation in different traditional system of medicines. • Well-documented scientific validation of traditional claim • Availability of official monographs in developing and developed countries.	• Geographical variation of raw material • Lack of quality control and quality assurance protocol for individual formulation. • Standardization of only few formulations are available and varies with respect to different countries • Factors affecting cultivation and collection alter the quality of raw material • Stability and self-life studies
SWOT ANALYSIS	
Threats	**Opportunities**
• Adulterations • Quantitative estimation of individual phytoconstituents • Availability of misbranded herbal products • Toxicological studies • No proper guidelines for drug-drug interaction.	• Scientific validation of traditional claim. • Huge availability of medicinal species • Development of standardization, quality control, quality assurance protocol. • Global interest on herbal medicines increasing exponentially in recent years.

Fig. 12.5: SWOT analysis of herbal industry

Schedule T—
Good Manufacturing Practices of
Indian Systems of Medicine

GOOD MANUFACTURING PRACTICES FOR (INDIAN SYSTEMS OF MEDICINE) AYURVEDIC, SIDDHA AND UNANI MEDICINES (FIG. 13.1)

The good manufacturing practices are prescribed to ensure that:

i. Raw materials used in the manufacture of drugs are authentic, of prescribed quality and are free from contamination.

ii. The manufacturing process as has been prescribed to maintain the standards.

iii. Adequate quality control measures are adopted.

iv. The manufactured drug which is released for sale is of acceptable quality.

v. To achieve the objective listed above, each licensee shall evolve methodology and procedures for following the prescribed process of manufacturer of drugs which should be documented as a manual and kept for reference and inspection. However, teaching institutions and registered qualified Vaidyas, Siddha and Hakeems who prepare medicines on their own to dispense to their patients and not selling such drugs in the market are exempted from the purview of GMP.

Good Manufacturing Practices

Factory Premises

The manufacturing plant should have adequate space for: Manufacturing process areas, quality control section, finished goods store, receiving and storing raw material office, office for rejected goods/drugs store.

General Requirements

A. **Location and surroundings:** The factory for manufacture of Ayurvedic, Siddha and Unani medicines shall be so situated and constructed as to avoid contamination from open sewerage, drain, public lavatory or any factory which produces disagreeable or obnoxious odour or fumes or excessive soot, dust or smoke.

B. **Buildings:** The building used for factory shall be such as

➲ To permit production of drugs under hygienic conditions and

➲ It should be free from cobwebs and insects/rodents.

➲ It should have adequate provision of light and ventilation.

➲ The floor and the walls should not be damp or moist.

➲ The premises used for manufacturing, processing, packaging and labeling will be in conformity with the provisions of the Factory Act.

C. **Water supply:** The water used in manufacture shall be pure and of potable quality. Adequate provision of water for washing the premises shall be made.

D. **Disposal of waste:** From the manufacturing sections and laboratories the waste water and the residues which might be prejudicial to the workers or public health shall be disposed off after suitable treatment as per guidelines of pollution control authorities to render them harmless.

E. **Container's cleaning:** In factories where operations involving the use of containers such as bottles, vials and jars are conducted,

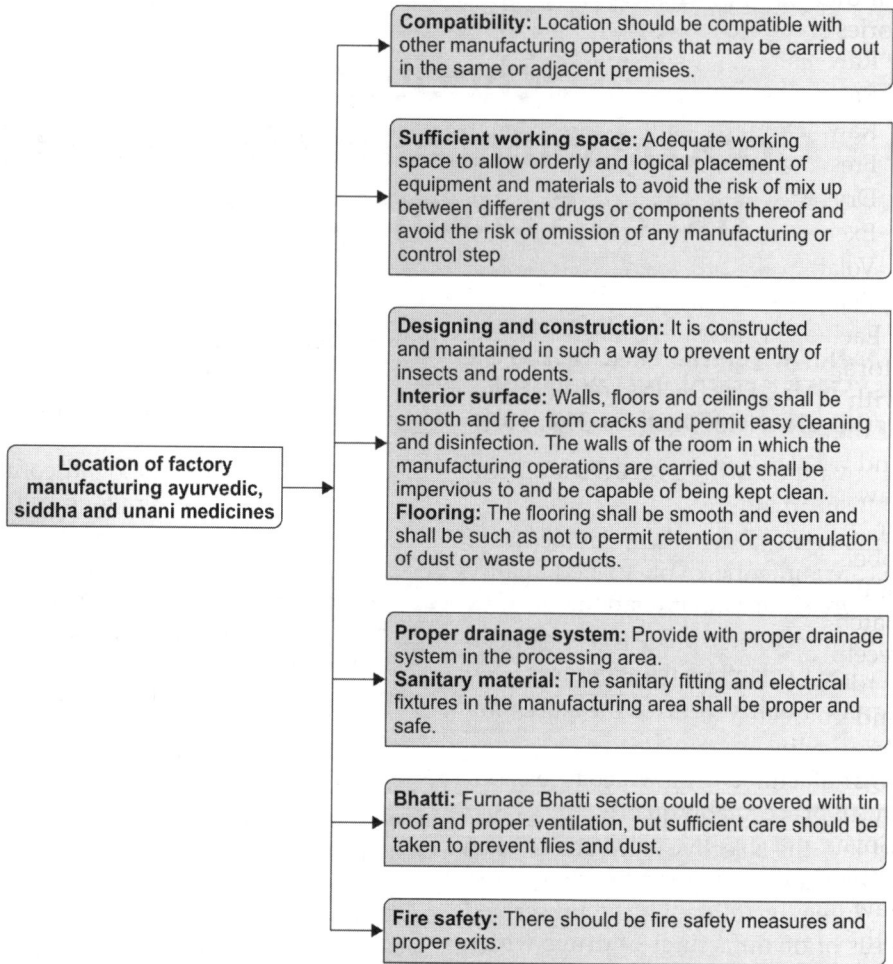

Fig. 13.1: Location of factory manufacturing ayurvedic, siddha and unani medicines

there shall be adequate arrangements separated from the manufacturing operations for washing, cleaning and drying of such containers.

F. **Stores:** Storage should have proper ventilation and shall be free from dampness. It should provide independent adequate space for storage of different types of material, such as raw material, packaging material and finished products.

  i. *Raw materials:* All raw materials procured for manufacturing will be stored in the raw materials store. The manufacture based on the experience and the characteristics of the particular raw material used in ayurveda, siddha and unani system shall decide the use of appropriate containers which would protect the quality of the raw material as well as prevent it from damage due to dampness, microbiological contamination or rodent and insect infestation, etc. If certain raw materials require such controlled environmental conditions, the raw materials stores may be sub-divide with proper enclosures to provide such conditions by suitable cabinization. While designing such containers, cabins or areas in the raw materials store, care may be taken to handle the following different categories of raw materials:

1. Raw material of metallic origin.
2. Raw material of mineral origin.
3. Raw material of animal source.
4. Fresh herbs.
5. Dry herbs or plant parts.
6. Excipients, etc.
7. Volatile oils/perfumes and flavours.
8. Plant extracts and exudates/resins.

Each container used for raw material storage shall be properly identified with the label which indicates name of the raw material, source of supply and will also clearly state the status of raw material such as 'UNDER TEST' or 'APPROVED' or 'REJECTED'. The labels shall further indicate the identity of the particular supply in the form of Batch No. or Lot. No. and the date of receipt of the consignment.

All the raw materials shall be sampled and got tested either by the in-house Ayurvedic, Siddha and Unani experts (Quality control technical person) or by the laboratories approved by the Government and shall be used only on approval after verifying. The rejected raw material should be removed from other raw material store and should be kept in a separate room. Procedure of 'First in first out' should be adopted for raw materials wherever necessary. Records of the receipt, testing and approval or rejection and use of raw material shall be maintained.

ii. *Packaging materials:* All packing materials such as bottles, jars, capsules, etc. should be stored properly. All container and closure lids should be properly cleaned and dried before packing the products.

iii. *Finished goods stores:* The finished goods transferred from the production area after proper packaging shall be stored in the finished goods stores within an area marked 'Quarantine'. After the quality control laboratory and the experts have checked the correctness of finished goods with reference to its packing/labeling as well as the finished product quality as prescribed, then it will be moved to "Approved Finished Goods Stock" area. Only approved finished goods shall be dispatched as per marketing requirements. Distribution records shall be maintained as required. If any Ayurvedic, Siddha and Unani drug needs special storage conditions, finished goods store shall provide necessary environments requirements.

G. **Working space:** The manufacturing area shall provide adequate space (manufacture and quality control) for orderly placement of equipment and material used in any of the operations. Facilities for easy and safe working.

➲ Facilities to minimize or eliminate mixing up of the drugs should be provided to prevent cross contamination of one drug by another drug that is manufactured, stored or handled in the same premises.

H. **Health clothing, sanitation and hygiene of workers:** All workers employed in the Factory shall be free from contagious diseases.

➲ The clothing of the workers shall consist of proper uniform suitable to the nature of work and the climate and shall be clean.

➲ The uniform shall also include cloth or synthetic covering for hands, feet and head wherever required.

➲ Adequate facilities for personal cleanliness such as clean towels, soap and scrubbing brushes shall be provided.

➲ Separate provision shall be made for lavatories to be used by men and women, and such lavatories shall be located at places separated from the processing rooms.

➲ Workers will also be provided facilities for changing their clothes and to keep their personal belongings.

I. **Medical services:** The manufacturer shall also provide:

a. Annual medical check-up of all employees should be done to ensure freedom from infectious diseases.

b. Medical examination of workers at the time of employment and periodical check up thereafter by a physician once a year, with particular attention being devoted to freedom from infections. Records thereof shall be maintained.

J. **Equipment:** Equipment should be according to the size of operation and nature of product manufactured.

➲ Suitable machinery manually operated, semi-automatic or automatic should be available in the manufacturing unit. These may include machines for use in the process.

K. **Batch manufacturing records:** The licensee shall maintain batch manufacturing record of each batch of Ayurvedic, Siddha and Unani drugs manufactured irrespective of the type of product manufactured (classical preparation or patent and proprietary medicines). The records are required to provide an account of the list of raw material and their quantities obtained from the store, tests conducted during the various stages of manufacture like taste, colour, physical characteristics and chemical tests as may be necessary or indicated in the approved books of Ayurveda, Siddha and Unani mentioned in the First Schedule of the Drugs and Cosmetics Act, 1940 (23 of 1940). These tests may include any in-house or pharmacopoeial test adopted by the manufacturer in the raw material or in the process material and in the finished product. These records shall be duly signed by Production and Quality Control Personnel respectively. Details or transfer of manufactured drug to the finished products store including dates and quantity of drugs transferred along with record of testing of the finished product, if any, and packaging, records shall be maintained. Only after the manufactured drugs have been verified and accepted quality shall be allowed to be cleared for sale. It should be essential to maintain the record of date, manpower, machine and equipments used and to keep in process record of various shodhana, bhavana, burning in fire and specific grindings in terms of internal use.

L. **Distribution records:** Records of sale and distribution of each batch of ayurvedic, siddha and unani drugs shall be maintained in order to facilitate prompt and complete recall of the batch, if necessary.

M. **Records of market complaints:** Manufactures shall maintain a register to record all reports of market complaints received regarding the products sold in the market. The manufacturer shall enter all data received on such market complaints investigations carried out by the manufacturers regarding the complaint as well as any corrective action initiated to prevent recurrence of such market complaints shall also submit the record of such complaints to the licensing authority. The Register shall also be available for inspection during any inspection of the premises. Reports of any adverse reaction resulting from the use of Ayurvedic, Siddha and Unani drugs shall also be maintained in a separate register by each manufacturer. The manufacturer shall investigate any of the adverse reaction to find if the same is due to any defect in the product, and whether such reactions are already reported in the literature or it is a new observation.

N. **Quality control:** Every licensee is required to provide facility for quality control section in his own premises or through government approved testing laboratory. The test shall be as per the ayurvedic, siddha and unani pharmacopoeial standard. Where the tests are not available, the test should be performed according to the manufacturer's specification or other information available. The quality control section shall verify all the raw materials monitor in process, quality checks and control the quality of finished product being released to finished goods store/warehouse. Preferably for such quality control there will be a separate expert. The quality control section shall have the following facilities:

1. There should be 150 sq feet area for quality control section.
2. For identification of raw drugs, reference books and reference samples should be maintained.
3. Manufacturing records should be maintained for the various process.
4. To verify the finished products controlled samples of finished products of each batch will be kept for 3 years.
5. To supervise and monitor adequacy of conditions under which raw material, semi-finished products and finished products are stored.
6. Keep record in establishing shelf life and storage requirements for the drugs.
7. Manufactures who are manufacturing patent proprietary Ayurveda, Siddha and Unani medicines shall provide their own specification and control references in respect of such formulated drugs.
8. The record of specific method and procedure of preparation, that is "Bhavana", "Mardana" and "Puta" and the record of every process carried out by the manufacturer shall be maintained.
9. The standards for identity, purity and strength as given in respective pharmacopoeias of Ayurvedic, Siddha and Unani systems of medicines published by Government of India shall be complied with.
10. All raw materials will be monitored for fungal, bacterial contamination with a view to minimize such contamination.
11. Quality control section will have a minimum of
    a. One person with degree qualification in ayurveda/siddha/unani (ASU) as per Schedule II of Indian Medicine Central Council Act, 1970 (84 of 1970) of a recognized university of Board.
    b. Provided that Bachelor of Pharmacy, Pharmacognosy and chemistry may be associated with the quality control section.

REQUIREMENT FOR STERILE PRODUCT

A. **Manufacturing areas:** For the manufacture of sterile Ayurvedic, Unani and Siddha drugs, separate enclosed areas specifically designed for the purpose shall be provided. These areas shall be provided with air locks for entry and shall be essentially dust free and ventilated with an air supply. For all areas where aseptic manufacture has to be carried out, air supply shall be filtered through bacteria retaining filters (HEPA filters) and shall be at a pressure higher than in the adjacent areas. The filters shall be checked for performance on installation and periodically thereafter the record of checks shall be maintained. All the surfaces in sterile manufacturing areas shall be designed to facilitate cleaning and disinfection. For sterile manufacturing routine microbial counts of all Ayurvedic, Siddha and Unani drug manufacturing areas shall be carried out during operations. Result of such count shall be checked against established in-house standards and record maintained.

Access to manufacturing areas shall be restricted to minimum number of authorized personnel. Special procedure to be followed for entering and leaving the manufacturing areas shall be written down and displayed.

For the manufacture of ayurvedic, siddha and unani drug that can be sterilized in their final containers, the design of the areas shall preclude the possibility of the products intended for sterilization being mixed with or taken to be products already sterilized. In case of terminally sterilized products, the design of the areas shall preclude the possibility of mix up between non-sterile and sterile products.

B. **Precautions against contamination and mix:**
    a. Carrying out manufacturing operations in a separate block of adequately isolated building or operating in an isolated enclosure within the building.

b. Using appropriate pressure differential in the process area.
c. Providing a suitable exhaust system.
d. Designing laminar flow sterile air systems for sterile products.
e. The germicidal efficiency of UV lamps shall be checked and recorded indicating the burning hours or checked using intensity.
f. Individual containers of liquids and ophthalmic solutions shall be examined against black-white background fitted with diffused light after filling to ensure freedom from contamination with foreign suspended matter.
g. Expert technical staff approved by the Licensing Authority shall check and compare actual yield against theoretical yield before final distribution of the batch.

All process controls as required under master formula including room temperature, relative humidity, volume filled, leakage and clarity shall be checked and recorded.

Table 13.1: List of recommended machinery, equipment and minimum manufacturing premises required for the manufacture of various categories of Ayurvedic, Siddha system of medicines

S. No.	Category of medicine	Minimum manufacturing space required	Machinery/equipment recommended
		1200 Square feet covered area with separate cabins or partitions for each activity. If Unani medicines are manufactured in same premises, an additional area of 400 sq. feet will be required	
1.	Churna and lepa	200 sq feet	Grinder/Disintegrator/Pulveriser/Powder mixer/Sieves/Shifter
2.	Pills, vati and tablets	100 sq. feet	Ball mill, mass mixer/powder mixer, granulator drier, tablet compressing machine, pill/vati cutting machine, stainless steel trays/container for storage and sugar coating, polishing pan in case of sugar-coated tablets, mechanised chattoo (for mixing guggulu) where required.
3.	Lavana Bhasma	150 sq. feet	Bhatti, karahi/stainless steel vessels/patila, flask, multani matti/plaster of Paris, copper rod, earthen container, Gaj put bhatti, Mufflefurnace (electrically operated), end/edge runner, exhaust fan, wooden/ SS Spatula.
4.	Capsules	100 sq. feet	Air conditioner, de-humidifier, hygrometer, thermometer, capsule filling machine and balance.
5.	Ointment	100 sq. feet	Tube filling machine, crimping machine, ointment mixer, end runner/mill (where required), SS storage container.
6.	Asava / Arishta	200 sq. ft	Fermentation tanks, containers and distillation plant where necessary, filter press
7.	Avaleh	100 sq.	feet Bhatti section fitted with exhaust fan and should be fly proof Iron Kadahi/S.S. Patila and S.S. Storage container
8.	Tail	100 sq. ft	Bhatti, kadahi/SS Patila, SS storage containers, filtration equipment, filling tank with tap/liquid filling machine

Table 13.2: List of machinery, equipment and minimum manufacturing premises required for the manufacture of various categories of Unani system of medicines

S.No.	Category of Medicine	Minimum manufacturing space required	Machinery/equipment recommended
		1200 square feet covered area with separate cabins, partitions for each activity. If Ayurveda/Siddha medicines are also manufactured in same premises, an additional area of 400 square feet will be required.	
1.	Arq.	100 sq. feet	Distillation plant (garembic), SS storage tank, boiling vessel, gravity filter, bottle filling machine, bottle washing machine, bottle drier.
2.	Habb (Pills) and tablets.	100 sq. feet	Ball mill, mass mixer/powder mixer, granulator drier, tablet compressing machine, pill/vati cutting machine, stainless steel trays/ container for storage and sugar coating, polishing
3.	Sufoof (Powder)	200 sq. feet	Grinder/pulveriser, sieves, trays, scoops, powder mixer
4.	Raughan (oils) (crushing and boiling)	100 sq. feet	Oil expeller, SS patilas, oil filter bottle, filling machine, bottle drier, bhatti.
5.	Marham, Zimad (ointment)	100 sq. feet	Kharal, bhatti, end runner, grinder, pulveriser, triple roller mill (if required).
6.	Capsule	100 sq. feet	Pulveriser, powder mixer (where needed), capsule filling machine, air conditioner, de-humidifier, balance with weights, storage containers, glass.
7.	Qutoor-e-Chashm and Marham (Eye drops, eye ointment)	100 sq. feet	Hot air oven electrically heated with thermo-static control, kettle.
8.	Each manufacturing unit will have a separate area for Bhatti, furnace boilers, puta, etc. This will have proper ventilation, removal of smoke, prevention of flies, insets, dust etc.		

MAJOR AYURVEDIC MEDICINE MANUFACTURING UNITS

A brief discussion on the major manufacturing units of India is as follows:

1. **Dabur India Limited,** Founded in 1884, has manufacturing units in the States of Uttar Pradesh, West Bengal, Bihar, Himachal Pradesh, Rajasthan and Madhya Pradesh, besides units in Nepal and Egypt. The total sales turnover of Dabur exceeds ₹ 1,000 Crores. The company is well-known for its product, **Dabur Chwanprash** and products include hair oil (Dabur Amla Kesh Thail, Vatika Hair Oil), Dabur Lal Dant Manjan and Dabur Honey. The Pharmaceutical products of the company include LivJit, Honitus, Ulgel, etc.

2. **Himalaya Drug Company** Located at Bangalore, is one of the few companies in India which undertakes extensive research programmes for the development of P and P medicines in ayurveda. This manufacturer has over forty qualified scientists and doctors who are constantly engaged in the

research work of new P and P medicines. Himalaya Drug Company manufactures around 25 products and 13 related products.

3. **Shree Baidyanath Ayurved Bhawan** Limited Located at Calcutta, popularly known as Baidyanath. The company manufactures around 700 products at 10 manufacturing units. The products are marketed through 3500 exclusive showrooms managed by qualified medical practitioners and 1000 distributors. Baidyanath has a market share of 20 per cent of the Chwanprash market. It manages Ayurvedic hospitals and two schools and publishes a monthly magazine Sachitra Ayurved.

4. Indian Medical Practitioners Co-Operative Pharmacy and Stores Limited (IMCOPS) IMCOPS was established in 1944 at Chennai. It is engaged in the manufacturing of Ayurvedic, Siddha and Unani medicines.

CONCLUSION

Government of India has made the GMP mandatory to manufacture quality formulations for Ayurvedic, Siddha and Unani drugs manufacturing units. Implementation of good manufacturing practices in ayurvedic pharmaceutical units will lead to manufacture of safe and efficacious medicines. GMP also validates the processes involved in ayurvedic pharmaceutics. It also facilitates the functioning of regularity authority and enforcement personnel and ultimately ensures the safety of Ayurvedic, Siddha and Unani medicines. GMP provides a strong base for ensuring preparation of quality medicines. These are the minimum requirements that need to be followed by ayurvedic drug manufacturers. Compliance of good manufacturing practices will increase the credibility of ayurvedic medicines in general public and it will help in global acceptance and marketing of these medicines.

Bibliography

Altemimi A, Lakhssassi N, Baharlouei A, Watson DG and David A, Lightfoot, Phytochemicals: Extraction, Isolation, and Identification of Bioactive Compounds from Plant Extracts, Plants 6, 42, 2017.

Article by Richa Shah, Regulatory Requirements for Herbal Medicines in India.

Arun N, Kadibagil Vinay R, Gazala Hussain, Saokar Reshma M, Apte Manik, Insight of Good Manufacturing Practices in Ayurveda, UJAHM, 2014, 02 (06), 51–5.

Barel OA, Paye M, Maibach IH, Handbook of Cosmetic Science and Technology, CRC Press, 2010.

Basic Tests for Drugs Pharmaceutical Substances, Medicinal Plant Materials and Dosage Forms, 1998.

Bracketing and Matrixing designs for Stability Testing of Drug Substances and Drug Products, ICH Topic Q 1 D, February 2002.

Brian Scarbrough, Dietary Supplements: A Review Of United States Regulation With Emphasis On The Dietary Supplement Health And Education Act Of 1994 And Subsequent Activity, LEDA at Harvard Law School, 2004.

Carrera JO, Junior S, Processing and Quality Control of Herbal Drugs and Their Derivatives, Quality Control of Herbal Medicines and Related Areas, 2011, 196–222.

Chandan Das, Goutam Ghosh, Debajyoti Das, Ayurvedic Liquid Dosage form Asava and Arista: An Overview, Indian Journal of Pharmaceutical Education and Research, Vol 51(2), Apr-Jun, 2017.

Chandra Nath Saha and Sanjib Bhattacharya, Intellectual property rights: An overview and implications in pharmaceutical industry, J Adv Pharm Technol Res. 2011 Apr-Jun; 2(2): 88–93.

Chintale AG, Kadam VS, Sakhare RS, Birajdar GO and Nalwad DN, Role Of Nutraceuticals In Various Diseases: A Comprehensive Review, IJRPC 2013, 3(2), 290–9.

Connor JG, Herb-Drug Interactions and How to Avoid Them, 2011 (https://www.compassion-ateacupuncture.com/author/johnbarb/).

Dhan Prakash and K. R. Gupta, The Antioxidant Phytochemicals of Nutraceutical Importance, The Open Nutraceuticals Journal, 2009, 2, 20–35.

Dharmendra S, Surendra JK, Sujata M, Shweta S, Natural Excipients—A Review, International Journal of Pharmaceutical and Biological Archives 2012; 3(5):1028–34.

Dhiraj AV, Vatsala M, Functional Foods, Nutraceuticals and Natural Products Concepts and Applications, Destech Publications, 2016.

Drugs and Cosmetics Act 1940 (URL: cdsco.nic.in/html/Drugs&CosmeticAct.pdf)

Dureja H, Kaushik D, Gupta M, Kumar V, Lather V, Cosmeceuticals: An emerging concept, Indian J Pharmacol, June 2005, Vol 37(3), 155–9.

Farrukh A, Radha M, Jeyaprakash J, and Manicka VV, Bioavailability of phytochemicals and its enhancement by drug delivery systems, Cancer Lett. 2013; 334(1): 133–41.

General Guidelines for Methodologies on Research and Evaluation of Traditional Medicine, 2000.

Gooswami A, Barroah PK, Sandhu JS, Prospects of Herbal drugs in the age of globalization-Indian Scenario, Journal of Scientific and Industrial Research, 2002, 61, 423–31.

Gopinath H, Shanmugasundaram S, Pragati KB, Brief Review on Disintegrants, Journal of Chemical and Pharmaceutical sciences, 2012, 5(3), 105–12.

Guidelines for Inspection of GMP Compliance by Ayurveda, Siddha and Unani Drug Industry, Department of Ayush, Ministry of Health and Family Welfare, Government of India, 2014.

Gupta A, Malviya R, Singh TP, Sharma PK, Indian Medicinal Plants Used in Hair Care Cosmetics: A Short Review, Phcog.Net, 2010, Vol 2(10), 361–4.

Joy PP, Medicinal Plants, Kerala Agricultural University, 1998, 1–210.

Jyothi M. Joy, G. Avinash Kumar, Naveen Kumari, A Review on Herbal Drug Interactions, International Journal of Pharmacy, 1(1), 2011, 18–31.

Kapoor VP, Herbal Cosmetic for Skin and Health Care, Natural Product Radiance, Vol 4(4), 2005, 306–14.

Krishna VA, Kumar PG, Colorants The Cosmetics For The Pharmaceutical Dosage Forms, International Journal of Pharmacy and Pharmaceutical Sciences, Vol. 3, Suppl 3, 2011.

Kunle, OF, Omoregie H Standardization of herbal medicines–A review, International Journal of Biodiversity and Conservation 2012, Vol. 4(3), pp. 101–12.

Laxmi SJ and Harshal AP, Herbal Cosmetics and Cosmeceuticals: An Overview, Nat Prod Chem Res 2015, 3:2.

Legal Status of Ayurvedic, Siddha and Unani Medicines, Govt. of India, Department of AYUSH Ministry of Health and Family Welfare Pharmacopoeial Laboratory for Indian Medicines, Ghaziabad,

Manisha P, Rohit KV, Shubhini AS, Nutraceuticals: New era of medicine and health, Asian Journal of Pharmaceutical and Clinical Research January-March 2010, Vol. 3(1), 11–5.

María LS, Elena F and Herminia D, Relevance of Natural Phenolics from Grape and Derivative Products in the Formulation of Cosmetics, Cosmetics 2015, 2(3), 259–76.

Mecocci P, Tinarelli C, Schulz RJ, and Polidori MC, Nutraceuticals in cognitive impairment and Alzheimer's disease, Front Pharmacol. 2014; 5: 147.

Minal PS, Shailesh BP, Kailaspati PC, Umesh PJ. Complementary alternative medicinal systems: An overview. SPER J Anal Drug Regul Aff 2016; 1(1):1–5.

Mohammad Y, Mohammad I, Herb-Drug Interactions And Patient Counselling, International Journal of Pharmacy and Pharmaceutical Sciences, Vol. 1, Supply 1, Nov.-Dec. 2009.

Mukherjee PK, Venkatesh M, Kumar V., An Overview on the Development in Regulation and Control of Medicinal and Aromatic Plants in the Indian System of Medicine, Bol. Latinoam. Caribe Plant. Med. Aromaticas, 2007, Vol. 6(4), 137.

Nandre BN, Bakliwal SR, Rane BR, Pawar SP, Traditional Fermented Formulations—Asava and Arishta, International Journal of Pharmaceutical and Biological Archives 2012; 3(6):1313–9.

Narayanaswamy V, Origin and Development Of Ayurveda (A Brief History), Ancient Science of Life, July 1981, Vol. I(1), pg 1–7.

Neacsu NA, Bulletin of the Transilvania University of Brasov Series V: Economic Sciences, Artificial Sweeteners versus Natural Sweeteners, 2014, Vol. 7 (56) No. 1.

Pandey MM, Rastogi S, and Rawat AKS, Indian Traditional Ayurvedic System of Medicine and Nutritional Supplementation, Evidence-Based Complementary and Alternative Medicine, Volume 2013.

Photostability Testing of New Active Substances and Medicinal Products, ICH Topic Q1B, January 1998.

Prachi SS, Amruta NA, Natural Excipients Research Journal of Pharmaceutical, Biological and Chemical Sciences, 2013, 4(2), 1346–54.

Prerna KR, Nutraceuticals-Its Current Scenario and Challenges In Dietary Supplements, World Journal Of Pharmacy And Pharmaceutical Sciences, Volume 4(7), 460–74.

Priya SP, Natural Excipients: Uses of Pharmaceutical Formulations, International Journal of PharmTech Research, 2014; Vol. 6(1), 21–8.

Purnendu P, Banamali D, Bhuyan GC, Meher SK, Rao MM, Ayurvedic Pharmaceutical Dosage Forms-A Review, International Journal of Applied Ayurved Research ISSN: 2347- 6362.

Quality control methods for herbal materials, World Health Organization, ISBN 978 92 4 150073 9, 2011, 1–173.

Quality Control Methods for medicinal plant materials, World Health Organization, 1998.

Ravi Kant Upadhyay, Nutritional, therapeutic, and pharmaceutical potential of plant gums: A review, International Journal of Green Pharmacy, Jan-Mar 2017 (Suppl), 11(1) I S30.

Ravi, Vivek Prakash, Ram Singh, A Study of Cardiovascular Diseases: Types and Risk Factor, Journal of Scientific and Innovative Research Review Article, March-April, 2013, Vol 2(2), 433–57.

Research Guidelines for Evaluating the Safety and Efficacy of Herbal Medicines. 1993.

Rina H. Gokani and Kinjal N. Desai, Stability Study: Regulatory Requirement, International Journal of Advances in Pharmaceutical Analysis IJAPA, 2012, Vol. 2(4), 73–8.

Rubaya Sultan, Manzoor Ahmad Wani and Irshad A. Nawchoo, Herbal drugs - Current status and future prospects, International Journal of Medicinal Plant and Alternative Medicine, Vol. 1(2), 2013, 20–29.

Saha CN, et al., Intellectual property rights: An overview and implications in pharmaceutical industry,J Adv Pharm Technol Res. 2011.

Sanchari C, Raychaudhuri U, and Chakraborty R, Artificial sweeteners—a review, J Food Sci Technol. 2014 Apr; 51(4): 611–21.

Sarfaraj Hussain, Patient Counseling about Herbal-Drug Interactions, Afr J Tradit Complement Altern Med. 2011; 8(5 Suppl): 152–63.

Sebastian Pole, Ayurvedic Medicine: The Principles of Traditional Practice 1st Edition, 3–363.

Shailendra P, Shikha A, Natural Binding Agents in Tablet Formulation, International Journal of Pharmaceutical and Biological Archives, 2012, 3(3):466–73.

Shalini S, Advantages And Applications of Nature Excipients—A Review, Asian Journal of Pharmaceutical Research, 2012, Vol 2(1), 30–9.

Sharma A, Shanker C, Tyagi LT, Singh M and Rao CV, Herbal Medicine for Market Potential in India: An Overview, Academic Journal of Plant Sciences, 2008, 1(2):26–36.

Sheetal Verma and S.P. Singh, Current and future status of herbal medicines, Veterinary World, 2008, Vol. 1(11): 347–50.

Shilpa P Chaudhari and Pradeep S Patil, Pharmaceutical Excipients: A review, IJAPBC, Jan-Mar 2012, Vol. 1(1):21–34.

Singh P, Mahmood T, Shameem A, Bagga P, Ahmad N, A review on Herbal Excipients and their pharmaceutical applications, Sch. Acad. J. Pharm., 2016; 5(3): 53–7.

Singh, P., Yadav, R.J. and Pandey, A. (2005). Utilization of indigenous systems of medicine and homoeopathy in India. Indian J.Med Res 122, Aug 2005, pp137–42.

Stability testing of new Drug Substances and Products, ICH Topic Q 1 A (R2), August 2003

Stability Testing: Requirements for New Dosage Forms, ICH Topic Q1C, January 1998.

Standardization of herbal medicines—A review, International Journal of Biodiversity and Conservation 2012, Vol. 4(3):101–12.

Sujata Saxena and A. S. M. Raja, Natural Dyes: Sources, Chemistry, Application and Sustainability Issues, Central Institute for Research on Cotton Technology, Mumbai, India, Springer Science+Business Media Singapore, 2014, 37–80.

Sukhdev Swami Handa Suman Preet Singh Khanuja Gennaro Longo Dev Dutt Rakesh, Extraction Technologies for Medicinal and Aromatic Plants, International Centre For Science And High Technology, Trieste, 2008.

Sumit K, Vivek S, Sujata S, Ashish B, Herbal Cosmetics: Used For Skin And Hair, Inventi Rapid: Cosmeceuticals Vol. 2012, Issue 4, 1–7.

Swaroopa G. and Srinath D., Nutraceuticals and their Health Benefits, Int. J. Pure App. Biosci., 2017, 5(4):1151–5.

Talal Aburjai and Feda M. Natsheh, Plants Used in Cosmetics, Phytother. Res. 17, 987–1000 (2003).

The Drugs and Cosmetics Act, 1940 (India), Government of India Ministry of Health And Family Welfare, As amended up to the 31st December, 2016.

Ujjwal KS, Swati ND, MIT International Journal of Pharmaceutical Sciences, Vol. 2, No. 1, January 2016, pp. 43–52 ISSN 2394-5338; 2394-5346.

Ved DK, Goraya, GS (2008). Demand and Supply of Medicinal plants in India, NMPB, New Delhi and FRLHT, Bangalore, India

Voluntary Certification Scheme for Ayush Products, GMP Requirements Based On WHO Guidelines for Ayush Premium Mark, Section III, Annex A, GMP Requirements, Version 1,1–20.

WHO guidelines for assessing quality of herbal medicines with reference to contaminants and residues, World Health Organization, 2007, ISBN 978 92 4 159444 8, 1–105.

WHO Guidelines on Good Agricultural and Collection Practices (GACP) for Medicinal Plants, World Health Organization Geneva, 2003; 80.

WHO guidelines on good manufacturing practices (GMP) for herbal medicines, World Health Organization, 2005.

WHO guidelines on safety monitoring of herbal medicines in Pharmacovigilance systems, World Health Organization Geneva, 2004, 1–50.

WHO Monographs on Selected Medicinal Plants, Vol. 1 (1999); Vol. 2 (2004); Vol. 3 (2007); Vol. 4(2009)

WHO Traditional Medicines Strategy, World Health Organization, 2002–5.

World Intellectual Property Organization, (Website: www.wipo.int/)

Yadav AK, Organic Agriculture (Concept, Scenario, Principals and Practices), National Centre of Organic Farming, Ghaziabad, 1–60.

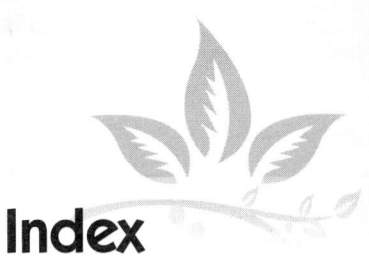

Index